P9-DNQ-816

PHARMACY

AN ILLUSTRATED HISTORY

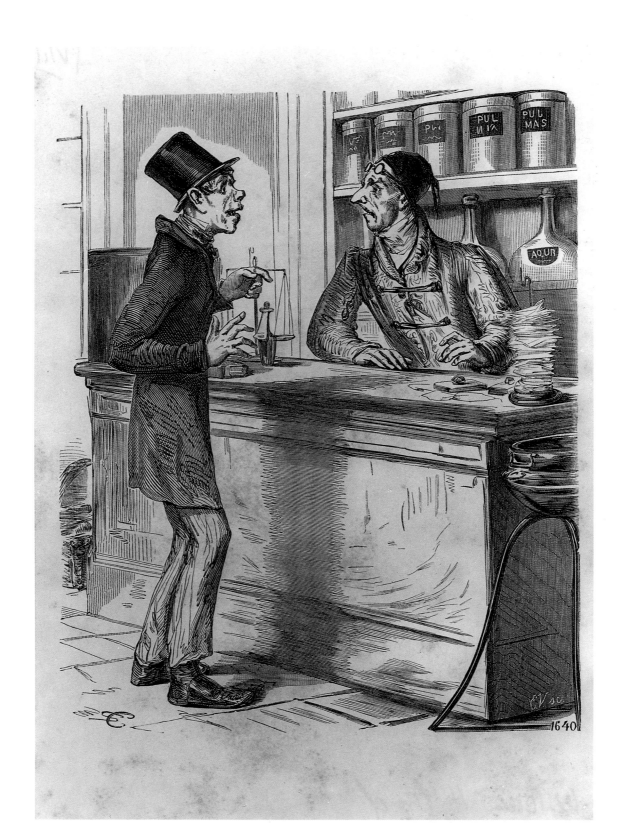

PHARMACY

AN ILLUSTRATED HISTORY

BY

DAVID L. COWEN

AND

WILLIAM H. HELFAND

HARRY N. ABRAMS, INC., PUBLISHERS, NEW YORK

To Audrey
and
To the memory of Florence

Editor: Ruth Eisenstein

Designer: Carol Robson

Photo Editor: John Crowley

NOTE ON THE ILLUSTRATIONS

Unless otherwise indicated in the captions or in the photograph credits, the illustrative material shown in these pages is from the collection of William H. Helfand, New York

Library of Congress Cataloging–in–Publication Data

Cowen, David L.
    Pharmacy: an illustrated history / David L. Cowen, William H. Helfand.
        p.   cm.
    Includes bibliographies and index.
    ISBN 0–8109–1498–0
    1. Pharmacy—History.   I. Helfand, William H.   II. Title.
    [DNLM: 1. Pharmacy—history.   QV 711.1 C874p]
    RS61.C69   1988
    362.1′782′09—dc19
    DNLM/DLC
    for Library of Congress   88–6273
                                   CIP

Illustrations copyright © 1990 Harry N. Abrams, Inc.
Text copyright © 1990 David L. Cowen

Published in 1990 by Harry N. Abrams, Incorporated, New York
All rights reserved. No part of the contents of this book may be reproduced without the written permission of the publisher
A Times Mirror Company

Printed and bound in Japan

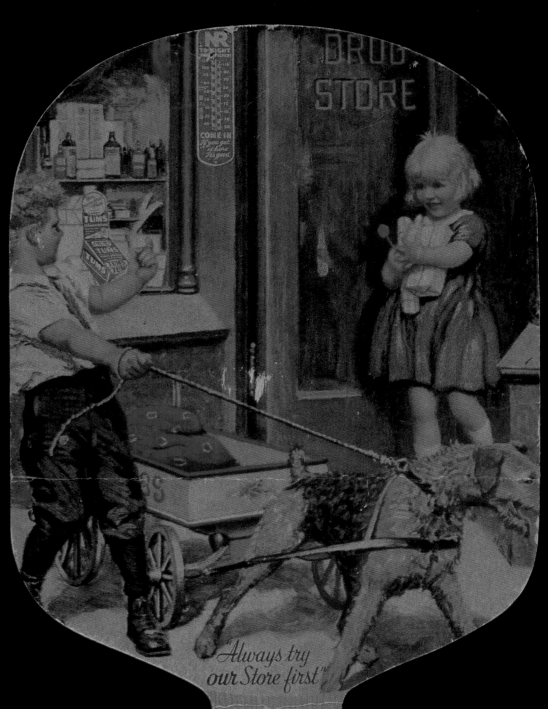

CONTENTS

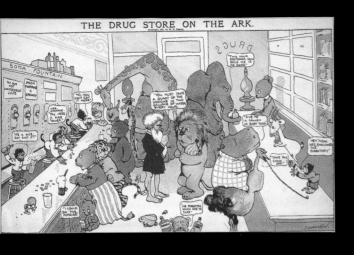

THE DRUG STORE ON THE ARK.

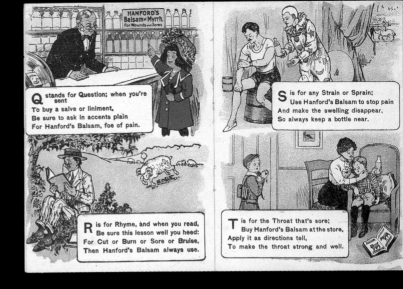

Q stands for Question; when you're sent
To buy a salve or liniment,
Be sure to ask in accents plain
For Hanford's Balsam, foe of pain.

S is for any Strain or Sprain;
Use Hanford's Balsam to stop pain
And make the swelling disappear,
So always keep a bottle near.

R is for Rhyme, and when you read,
Be sure this lesson well you heed:
For Cut or Burn or Sore or Bruise,
Then Hanford's Balsam always use.

T is for the Throat that's sore;
Buy Hanford's Balsam at the store,
Apply it as directions tell,
To make the throat strong and well.

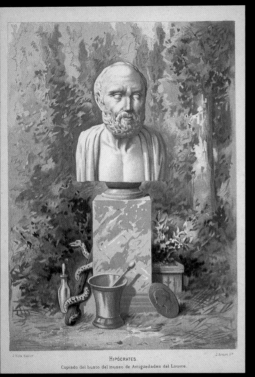

HIPÓCRATES.
Copiado del busto del museo de Antigüedades del Louvre.

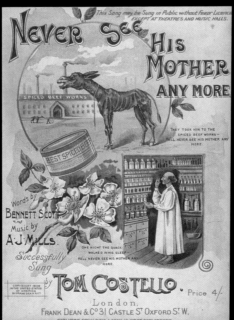

NEVER SEE HIS MOTHER ANY MORE

Words by BENNETT SCOTT
Music by A.J. MILLS.

Successfully Sung

TOM COSTELLO · Price 4/-

London.
FRANK DEAN & Co. 31 CASTLE St. OXFORD St. W.
NEW YORK. SPAULDING & GRAY. 16. WEST 27TH. STREET.

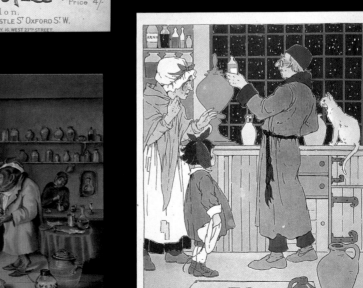

DOCTOR COMPUS MENTIS.

ADVICE GRATIS FROM 6 TILL 9

"With Doctor Compus Mentis,
I was bound apprentice,
And sweeter to me than a raspberry drop,
Was the girl I loved at the Doctor's shop."

SUNG BY

HARRY RICKARDS,
WRITTEN & COMPOSED BY TOM HAINES.

LONDON,
HENRI DALCORN & Co. 351, OXFORD STREET, W.

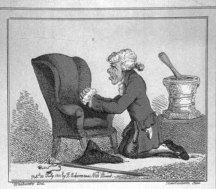

THE APOTHECARY'S PRAYER!!

O mighty Esculapius! hear a poor little man overwhelm'd with misfortunes, grant I beseech thee to send a few smart Fevers and some obstinate Catarrhs amongst us, or thy humble supplicant must shut up shop—and if it should please thee to throw in a few Cramps and Agues it would greatly help thy miserable servant, for on the word of an Apothecary I have scarcely heard the music of Mortar these two months.

Take notice also, I beseech thee, of the mournful situation of my neighbour, Crape the Undertaker, who suffers considerably by my want of practice, and loses many a job of my cutting out; enable him to bear his misfortunes with philosophy, and to look forward with new hope for the tolling of the bell.

Please those, I beseech thee, that will not encourage our profession, and Blister their evil intentions, viz. such as their cursed new-invented waterproof; and may all the coats be eaten by the rats that are so made: But pour down the Balm of Gilead on the Overseers of the village, and all the Friends of Gales.

May it please thee to look over my book of bad debts with an eye of compassion, and increase my neighbours' infirmities; give additional twinges to the Rector's Gout, and our worthy Curate's Rheumatism; but above all, I beseech thee to take under thy especial care the Lady of 'Squire Handy, for should the child prove an heir, and thy humble servant so fortunate as to bring the young gentleman handsomely into the world, it may be the means of raising me to the highest pinnacle of fortune.

SPRAGG, PRINTER, 10, BOW-STREET, COVENT-GARDEN.

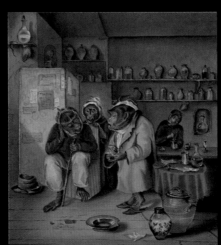

DOCTOR McSWATTLE FILLED UP A BOTTLE

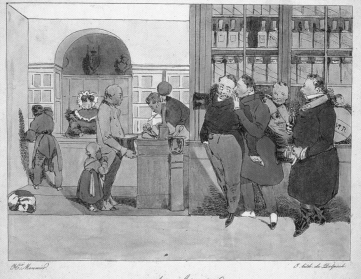

Apothicaire.

3.

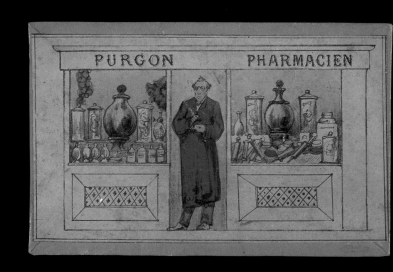

PURGON   PHARMACIEN

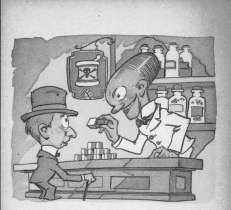

DRUGGIST

The skull and cross bones represent
Your so-called "occupation"—
You're "poison" to the universe,
A pill's in your head's location.

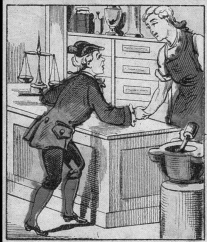

Calino asked his chemist to sell
him some strap-oil and scamper-
powder.

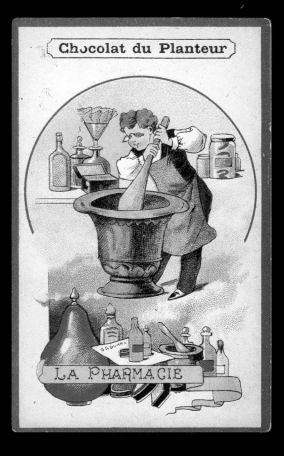

Chocolat du Planteur

LA PHARMACIE

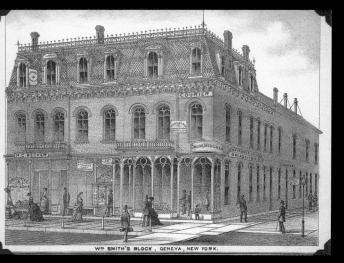

Wm SMITH'S BLOCK, GENEVA, NEW YORK.

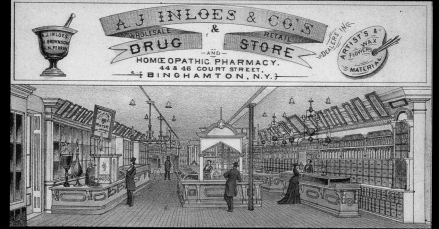

A. J. INLOES & CO'S
WHOLESALE & RETAIL
DRUG — AND — STORE
HOMŒOPATHIC PHARMACY.
44 & 46 COURT STREET,
BINGHAMTON, N.Y.
DEALERS IN ARTISTS' & WAX FLOWERS MATERIAL

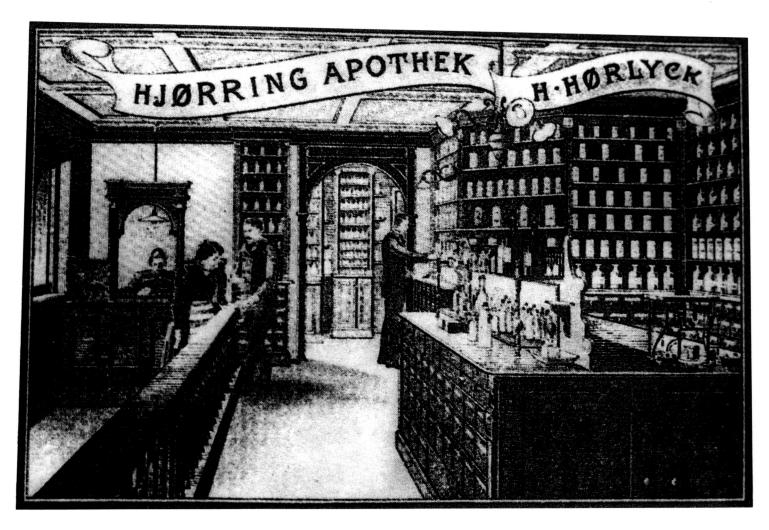

On the preceding pages, from left to right:

Page 8. TOP ROW, *The Drug Store on the Ark.* Color lithograph by James A. Swinnerton. This one-panel cartoon appeared on a comics page in the Sunday supplement of a Hearst newspaper in 1901. · Advertisement for Hanford's Balsam of Myrrh. Color lithograph from a children's booklet, *ABC Jingles.* American, 1911. MIDDLE ROW, *Hipocrates.* Lithographs by J. Armet of a sculpture in the Louvre. French, c. 1900. Armet has appropriately placed a caduceus and a mortar and pestle at the sculpture's base. · *Never See His Mother Any More.* Color lithograph. English, 1896. Cover of a song sheet; one verse tells of a quack who "walked in his sleep and went towards a shelf / Got one of his own pills and swallowed it himself! / He'll never see his mother any more . . . ." · *Doctor Compus Mentis.* Color lithograph by H. S. Maguire. English, 1873. This cover of a song sheet is one of the many comic commentaries on the health professions that delighted Victorian audiences. BOTTOM ROW, *The Apothecary's Prayer!!* Color engraving by Thomas Rowlandson after George M. Woodward. English, 1801. Among the pleas addressed to "mighty Esculapius" is one requesting that he "send a few smart *fevers* and some obstinate *Catarrhs* among us." Fry Collection, Library, Yale University School of Medicine, New Haven · *The Toothache.* Color

lithograph by G. Monkland. c. 1845. Monkeys, frequently depicted in prints satirizing human foibles, are shown here in a rural pharmacy. Rare Book Collection, Library, Harvard University School of Medicine, Cambridge · *Doctor McSwattle Filled Up a Bottle.* From *The Peter Patter Book,* a children's favorite, illustrated by Blanche Fisher Wright. English, c. 1900.

Page 9. TOP ROW, *Apothicaire.* Hand-colored lithograph by Henry Monnier. French, c. 1830 · Box cover for the children's game Purgon Pharmacien. Color lithograph. French, c. 1880. MIDDLE ROW, *Druggist.* Color lithograph. American, c. 1925. Valentines like this one were invariably sent anonymously. · *Calino's Simplicity.* Color lithograph published by Imagerie d'Epinal for the Humoristic Publishing Co., Kansas City, Missouri, c. 1910. This pharmacy scene is one of twelve depicting the stupidity of a certain Calino. In a mistranslation of two French idioms, he is really asking for a beating (strap-oil) and to run away (scamper-powder). · *La Pharmacie.* Chromolithograph advertising card. French, c. 1890. BOTTOM ROW, Views of drugstores from American county atlases. Hand-colored lithographs. c. 1876.

Prescription envelope, H. Hørlyck's pharmacy in Hjørring, Denmark. c. 1910. In Scandinavia the pharmacist does not retain the physician's prescription but returns it to the client in an envelope that serves to identify and advertise the pharmacy.
Above

Alpenkruidermaagbitter. Engraving from Elchanon Verveer, *Humoristisch Salon-Album,* Rotterdam, c. 1875. A pharmacist and his client are both confused over the name of the product in question (Alpine herb stomach bitters). The spiked prescription file (on the counter) was long used in pharmacies as a convenient way to store records.
Page 2

Cardboard fan distributed to pharmacists as a promotion piece. American, c. 1935
Page 5

PREFACE AND ACKNOWLEDGMENTS

Pharmacy is a profession with ancient antecedents, and its development in a particular society, like that of any other human institution, reflects the extent to which that society has been able to adjust to its environment through its religion, its science, its technology, and its social organization. Pharmacy did not develop in vacuo: its status and its progress in a given society depended upon the time, the people, and the cultural level of that people. The primitive concept of animism, the rationality of the classical Greeks, the spirituality of the medieval monastery, the beauty of Renaissance art, the excitement of discovery and exploration, the wondrous burgeoning of science and technology in the nineteenth century, the mind-boggling advances in high technology and genetic engineering of our own time, all—and more—have a place in the history of pharmacy and in the shaping of its character.

Pharmacy evolved into a specialized health profession, which, shorn of the commercial aspects sometimes visible in the pharmacy shop, has as its raison d'être the provision of medications. Pharmacy can be defined on three levels. First, pharmacy performs the functions of procurement, preservation, preparation, compounding, and dispensing of drugs in appropriate dosage forms. Historically, it will be seen, these activities were performed by a variety of functionaries; not until all were performed by a single practitioner in a separate establishment can there be said to have been a "pharmacist" and a "pharmacy shop." Except for the preparation and compounding of medicines, which are now almost entirely in the hands of the pharmaceutical industry, these activities are still the responsibility of the pharmacist. Pharmacy, on this level, is not only the sum of these activities and functions; it also includes the institutional, legal, and ethical bases on which these functions are carried out in the service of society.

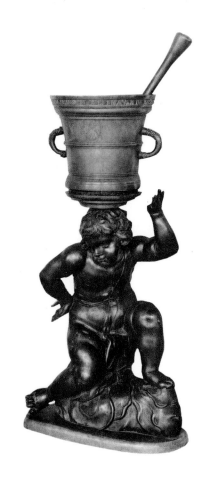

Bronze mortar and pestle on a carved wooden pedestal, a decoration from a Swiss-German pharmacy. 1686. National Museum of American History, Smithsonian Institution, Washington, D.C.

The second level on which pharmacy is to be defined is that of materia medica, or, perhaps better here, materia pharmaceutica. Pharmacy in this sense is the body of knowledge of drugs and medicines—their identification, their properties, their actions. Based historically on botany and chemistry, this scientific concept of pharmacy now also embraces the sciences of pharmacology and pharmacognosy and is concerned with such relatively new subsciences as pharmacokinetics and pharmacodynamics.

On the third level, pharmacy applies a body of experimental science to improve and develop medications. Whereas pharmacy as a profession depends on science to assure safe and effective medications and to make it possible to understand how they work, pharmacy as experimental science proceeds from that point toward a creative role. On this level, pharmacy contributes to sciences and technologies that have become to a great extent the responsibility of the large enterprise: the university laboratory, the government agency, the pharmaceutical industry.

The history that unfolds in the following pages deals with pharmacy on each of these levels. In the process, it casts light on the importance of pharmacy to the public weal, on how contemporary pharmaceutical institutions became what they are, and on the future prospects of pharmacy. For centuries, pharmacy was a relatively static profession, but it has become a changing and dynamic force in the delivery of health care.

We must first of all acknowledge an immeasurable debt to Dr. Glenn Sonnedecker, Dr. Edward Kremers (1865–1941), and Dr. George Urdang (1882–1960). Without the seminal and comprehensive fourth edition of *Kremers and Urdang's History of Pharmacy,* which Dr. Sonnedecker edited and augmented, this work would have proved an endless task.

Dr. Sonnedecker has read the manuscript and given us the benefit of his knowledge and ability. Our work has profited considerably from his cogent comments and suggestions. We take his painstaking attention as a demonstration of collegiality at its best and as a mark of personal friendship. Drs. Roy A. Bowers, Rudolf Schmitz, and Melvin P. Earles have each read portions of the manuscript, and we have used their comments and corrections to advantage. We are indeed grateful to them.

We have also had the advantage of being able to consult a great number of other friends and colleagues. All the following have answered questions or have otherwise been of help, and we express our gratitude to them: Alex Berman, Jack Cargill, Bruce R. Cowen, John K. Crellin, Susan Crowley, Allen G. Debus, Véronique Denis, Roland Errisson, David E. Fairbrothers, Richard E. Faust, Hans-Rudolf Fehlmann, Kurt Ganzinger, Alvin N. Geser, Dietlinde Goltz, George B. Griffenhagen, Michael Harris, Wolfgang-Hagen Hein, Gregory J. Higby, Ramón Jordi González, Pierre Julien, Øivind Karlsson, Dan Kushner, David Lilien, Ernst Lowenstein, Albert S. Lyons, Jean-Pierre Marliac, Bernard Mattelaer, Robert G. Mrtek, John Parascandola, Bernard Pejouan, Wojciech Roeske, John Scarborough, Gottfried Schramm, Alvin B. Segelman, Ernst W. Stieb, Jeffrey L. Sturchio, Z. L. Tang, Yngve Torud, Rossana Ventura, Armin Wankmüller, L. H. Werner, Brian A. Wills, Dirk A. Wittop Koning, and James Harvey Young.

In addition, the willing assistance of librarians, so essential to the success of any historical venture, is also most gratefully acknowledged. Our thanks go to Bernard Downey and Patricia Piermatti of the Rutgers University Libraries, to Dorothy T. Hanks of the National Library of Medicine, to Joan P. S. Ferguson of the Royal College of Physicians of Edinburgh, to Kate Arnold-Foster of the Royal Pharmaceutical Society of Great Britain, to Heather Walkiden of the Wellcome Institute for the History of Medicine, to Barbara Irwin of the University of Medicine and Dentistry of New Jersey, to Charlotte Finnerman of the Warner-Lambert Corporate Library, and to Glen Jenkins of the Cleveland Medical Library Association.

It is a great sorrow to us that Florence L. Cowen did not live to see the fruits of her unwavering encouragement and devotion. We gratefully acknowledge Florence's support and the support and help of Audrey Helfand, whose linguistic versatility has proved especially valuable.

Finally, we thank the members of the Abrams staff who have made this book a reality: Barbara Lyons, Director of Photo Research; John Crowley, Photo Editor; Neil Ryder Hoos, Photo Researcher; Ruth Eisenstein, Senior Editor; and Carol Robson, Designer. Our editor's extraordinary competence, critical acumen, and patience have earned our special gratitude, and we are indebted to our designer for the skillful and imaginative layout that enhances our text. The Abrams staff has carried our work to what, to us at least, is a most beautiful and happy conclusion.

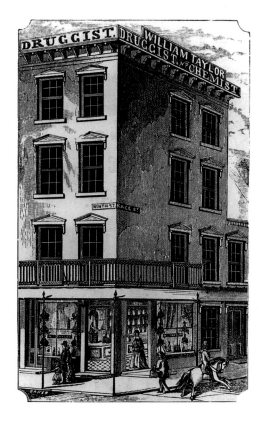

Advertisement for William Taylor, Druggist and Chemist, in Philadelphia. 1856
Above

The corner drugstore of F. Brown, Druggist, in Boston. Lithograph. c. 1850
Page 14

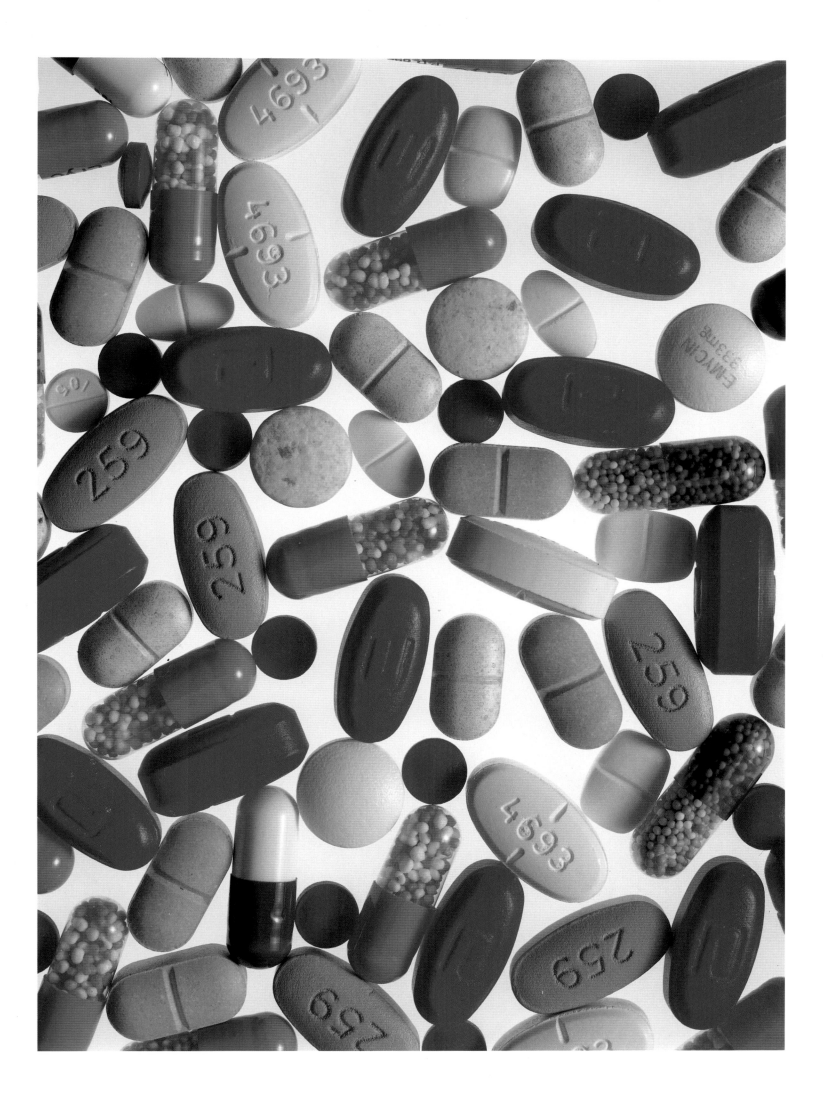

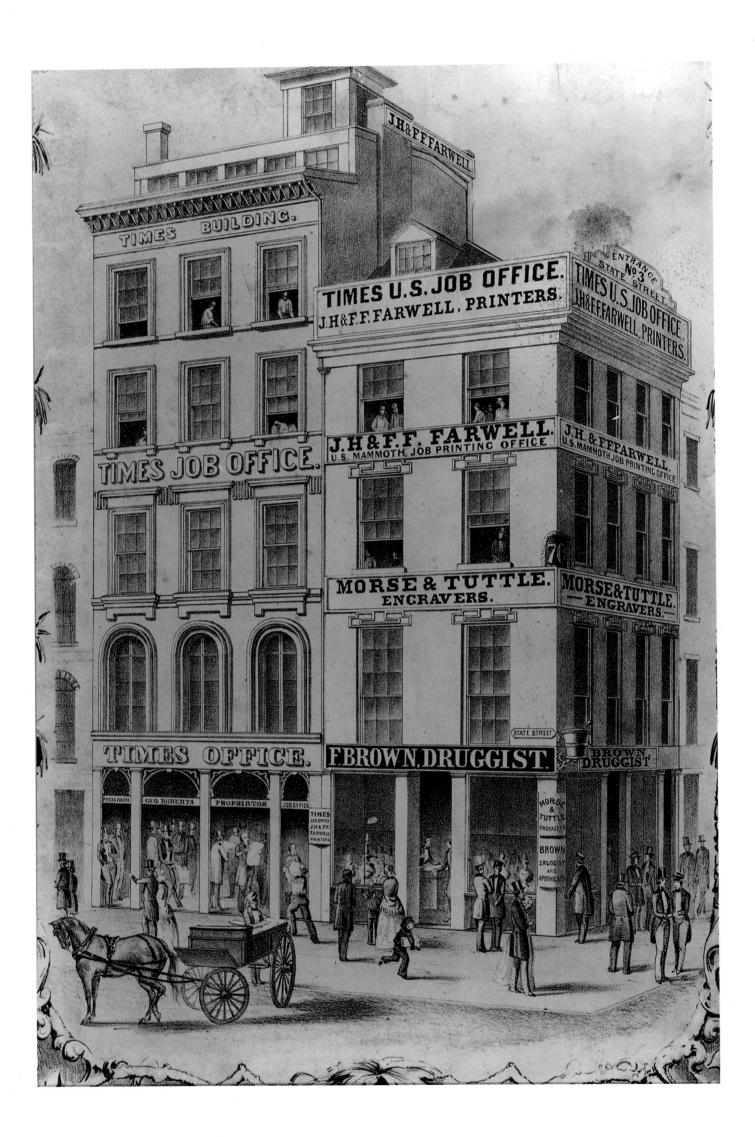

PHARMACY

AN ILLUSTRATED HISTORY

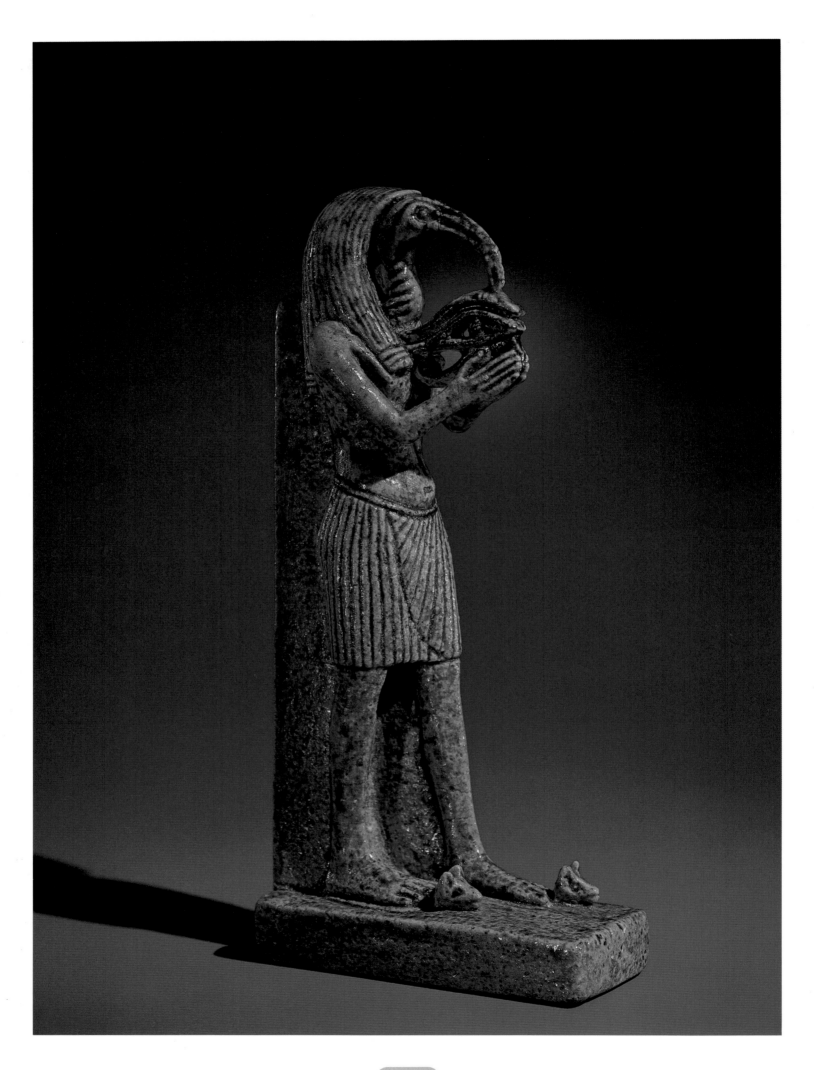

Chapter I

ANCIENT ANTECEDENTS

The origin of the word "pharmacy" is generally ascribed to the Greek *pharmakon* ("remedy"). It has been suggested that there is a connection with the Egyptian term *ph-ar-maki* ("bestower of security"), which the god Thoth, patron of physicians, conferred as approbation on a ferryman who had managed a safe crossing. The notion of an Egyptian origin has a certain romantic appeal, but in all likelihood the word "pharmacy" and its many cognates derive, like so many other scientific terms, from the Greek.

Pharmacy in a rudimentary form existed before the word. It has been said that it would be a fruitless enterprise to speculate on the origins of drug therapy and on the procedures and practices basic to that therapy. It would indeed be fruitless to attempt to determine whether some internal drive, or instinct, or some lesson learned from animal behavior, or some felicitous or hard-earned experience was the origin of human reliance on medication to cure illness and ease discomfort.

Thoth, god and physician, the inventor of science and medicine. Green faience figurine. Egyptian, 305–30 BC. The Brooklyn Museum, New York
◄

THE PRIMITIVE WORLD

Whatever the origins of drug therapy, it is certain that preliterate peoples had a considerable knowledge of medicinal plants and that, in all parts of the world, they developed therapeutic systems that combined empirical, rational, religious, and magical elements. As much as 80,000 years ago, people of the Paleolithic period were sufficiently interested in the flora around them to engrave a variety of plants and plant parts on bones and deer antlers, and 50,000 years ago a Neolithic man was buried in the Shanidar Cave in northern Iraq with clusters of flowers and herbs. The Neolithic Lake Dwellers of Switzerland cultivated or gathered two hundred different plants, not a few of which possessed medicinal qualities, and the Magdalenian artists who painted on the walls of the cave of Les Trois Frères in

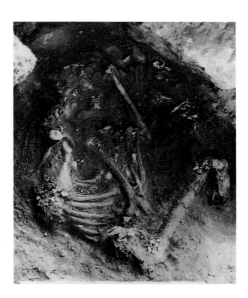

Burial of a Neolithic man found in the Shanidar Cave in the Zagros Mountains of northern Iraq. Clusters of flowers and herbs (some still valued for their medicinal properties by inhabitants of the area) were buried with the body 50,000 years ago.

Ariège, in southwest France, some 14,000 years ago added an image of a medicine man to those walls.

Disease is older than humankind, and prehistoric peoples knew their full share of illness, pain, and death. Their approach to disease and to its treatment reflected their view of the world, which was based on animism—the belief that everything has a spirit, that spiritual forces explain all phenomena, that every happening is a manifestation of spiritual forces. Because both disease and its treatment involved this world of spirits, there was a need for specialists who understood and could control the spirits—a need that led primitive societies to elevate the priest, the sorcerer, and the medicine man. The functions of these three were often combined in the same person, for it was not always easy to distinguish supernatural from natural forces. The priest-sorcerer-medicine man was trained to deal with both.

In most primitive societies disease was thought to result from the invasion of the body by evil spirits, from the intrusion of some object into the body, or from the departure of some spiritual force from the body. The medicine man, having determined which of these evil forces was at work, had next to determine why the afflicted body had been invaded or the soul enticed away. Enemies and violations of taboos, all had to be explored. Once the spirit force that was responsible had been identified, treatment was possible: the evil spirit could be banished, objects mysteriously injected into the body without injury to the skin removed, or the soul enticed back into the body.

The first step in treatment was the "oral rite": chants and noises made by a specially costumed shaman as he danced and gyrated before the patient. Then came the "manual rite." This might include performing deeds of legerdemain, attaching charms, sucking out evil from the body, giving the patient something to smell or—most important of all—something to swallow. Magic, the esoteric manipulation of nature by those initi-

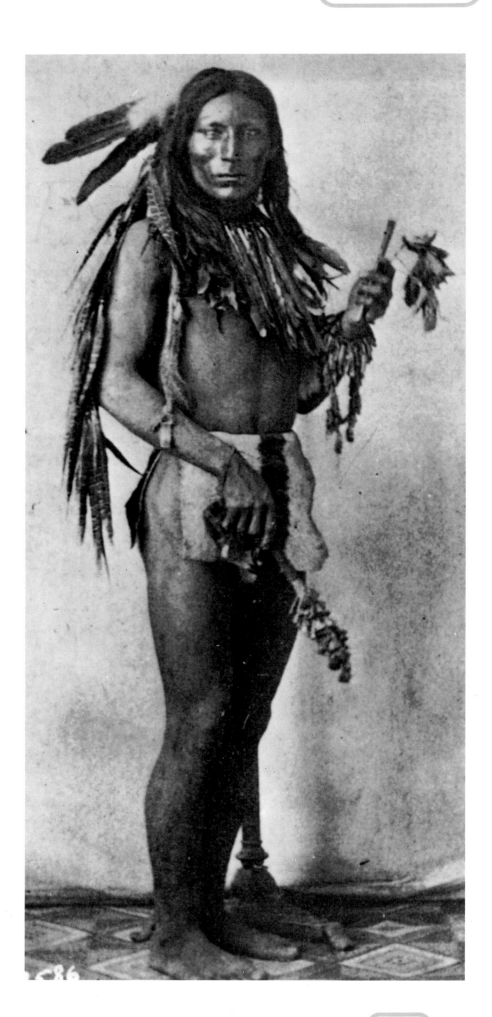

Medicine man of the Yankton Indians.
c. 1900. National Library of Medicine,
Bethesda

ated into its mysteries, was dominant, and in connection with such regimens "materia magica" is a more accurate term than "materia medica." The use among the Mano of Liberia of one word, *nye,* to connote both magic and medicine underscores this point.

In the medicine man's collection and preparation of remedies lies the beginning of pharmacy. That a medication might possess powers beyond its effect on bodily function, and that medication was needed to exorcise evil spirits, were ideas that would affect pharmacy and medicine for ages to come.

ANCIENT CIVILIZATIONS

The term "civilization" implies a more complex culture—more complex, that is, than the cultures of primitive societies. People did not arrive at a civilized state, it is generally agreed, until writing was invented, until political, social, and economic institutions developed sufficiently to provide a degree of order and efficiency, and until there was discernible progress in the arts and sciences.

Civilization developed in the major river valleys of Africa and Asia: in the Nile Valley and the Tigris-Euphrates Valley about 4000 BC, in the Indus Valley about 3250 BC, and in the Yellow River Valley about 1500 BC. Each civilization developed its own characteristics, but each grew out of previously existing cultures. This debt to precedent cultures was particularly evident in pharmacy and medicine, for although they became more organized and, to a considerable extent, more rational, the animistic-religious-magical notions of disease and its treatment did not disappear as human beings became literate, more knowledgeable, more secure, and more "civilized."

Mesopotamia

The successive civilizations of the Tigris-Euphrates region—Sumerian (c. 4000–2000 BC), Babylonian (2000–1350 BC), Assyrian (1350–612 BC), and Chaldean (612–539 BC)—made widely varying contributions to the development of pharmacy and medicine. During the entire epoch, however—that is, from the fourth millennium to the sixth century BC—certain common threads can be discerned.

In the Mesopotamian pantheon, three deities were especially associated with medicine. The god Ninazu was known as the Lord-Physician, and his son Ningishrida carried as his symbol a staff around which serpents were entwined. There was also Gula, the goddess of death and healing, who was the patroness of the physician and who was called the Great Lady of Physicians.

The gods of Mesopotamia were capable of both good and evil. They visited disease upon the sinful, and they also healed the sick; their deputies in the healing process were priest-physicians. Acceptance of the concept of sin, evident in the Babylonian and Assyrian periods, reached a pathological level of intensity among the Chaldeans. Mesopotamians believed that one could avoid disease by leading a righteous life and worshiping the proper gods—a somewhat more sophisticated version of the thinking of preliterate peoples. Like their preliterate forebears, the Mesopotamians made offerings to the ghosts of their ancestors, respected taboos, and sought to acquire the magical accessories necessary to ward off evil. There arose out of these beliefs a demonology that envisaged hordes of malevolent spirits who lived in the dark and flew through the air.

Three categories of medical practitioners can be identified in ancient Mesopotamia: the *bârû,* the seer-priest; the *âshipu,* the exorcist or incantation priest; and the *âsû,* the physician-priest. All were healers and all were priests, in conformity with the concept of disease as a consequence of sin or

Pazuzu, Assyrian-Babylonian goddess of sickness. Clay figurine, c. 1000–500 BC. The British Museum, London

transgression. Cures therefore involved a spiritual-religious purification and catharsis. The medicinal cathartic emerges from this source, and the dual nature of the cleansing—the purification of both soul and body—was to remain consciously or subconsciously ingrained in medical practice for centuries.

All this suggests that the differences between the medicine of preliterate societies and Mesopotamian medicine were differences in degree, not in kind. Yet advances in the Mesopotamian civilization—in literature, in art, in law, in mathematics, in astronomy—did not pass medicine by. Particular progress was seen in the areas of drug therapy and, of special significance for pharmacy, in the materia medica. Among the thousands of clay tablets unearthed in the region is the earliest known medical text (Museum of the University of Pennsylvania, Philadelphia), which was pressed into clay about 2100 BC. The language of the tablet is Sumerian, but the contents are thought to be older, perhaps by as much as a millennium.

This first medical text is in fact a pharmaceutical compendium: the portion that has been translated consists entirely of a set of formulas and directions for compounding. The practitioner of pharmacy is directed, for example, to "pulverize [the bark of] the apple tree and the 'moon' plant; infuse it with *kushumma* wine; let tree oil and hot[?] cedar oil be spread over it." In all, this text lists 30 different simples (simple drugs used unmixed or for making composite remedies) from animal, mineral, and vegetable sources, many no longer identifiable. Numerous pharmaceutical forms and processes, among them aqueous and oil extracts, infusions of wine, pulverization, boiling, filtering, and spreading, are referred to. Significantly, beer is the only vehicle named.

A study of some 800 tablets or parts of tablets containing medical material—from among the 32,000 in the library at Nineveh collected by the Assyrian king Assurbanipal in the seventh century BC—has revealed

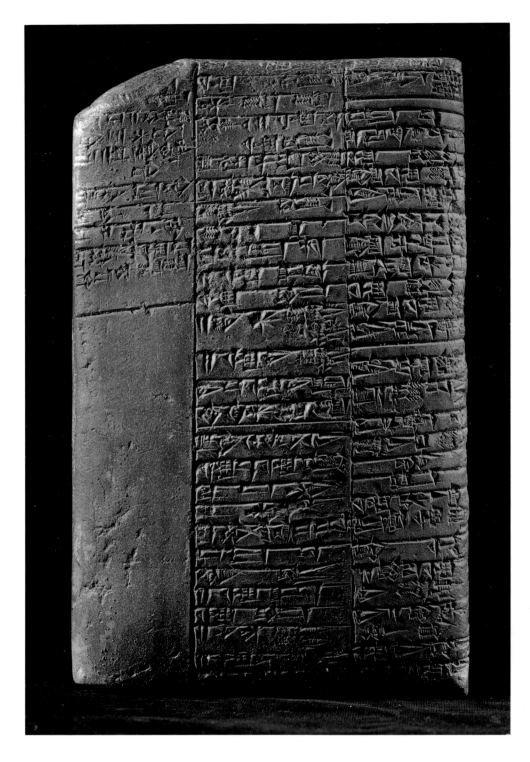

Sumerian collection of prescriptions, the earliest known medical text. Clay tablet discovered at Nippur. c. 2100 BC. University of Pennsylvania Museum, Philadelphia

Sargon II bearing a sacrificial ibex and followed by a priest holding poppies to sedate the animal. Alabaster relief. Assyrian, 8th century BC. The Louvre, Paris

►
Hammurabi receiving the code of laws from the sun-god Shamash. Bas-relief at the top of a black diorite stele. The Code of Hammurabi contained a section on ethical standards of health practitioners. Babylonian, c. 1792–1750 BC. The Louvre, Paris

roughly 250 drugs of vegetable origin, 120 of mineral origin, and 180 from other sources. Vegetable drugs, arranged by an Assyrian botanist in what has been called "an intelligent and methodical manner," made up over three-fourths of the ingredients in the recipes in the tablets. Oils, alcohols, wines, fats, honey, milk, and wax (in the order of frequency) were used as vehicles.

This suggests that it was not just natural materials but also their manipulation by various processes that was deemed of value from early times. Moreover, it is clear that there were functionaries in ancient Mesopotamia who had a knowledge of pharmaceuticals and who performed pharmaceutical tasks. At least during the Babylonian period there was apparently a special street in Sippur where retailers of drugs plied their trade.

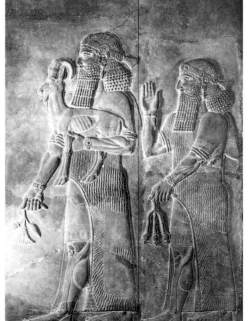

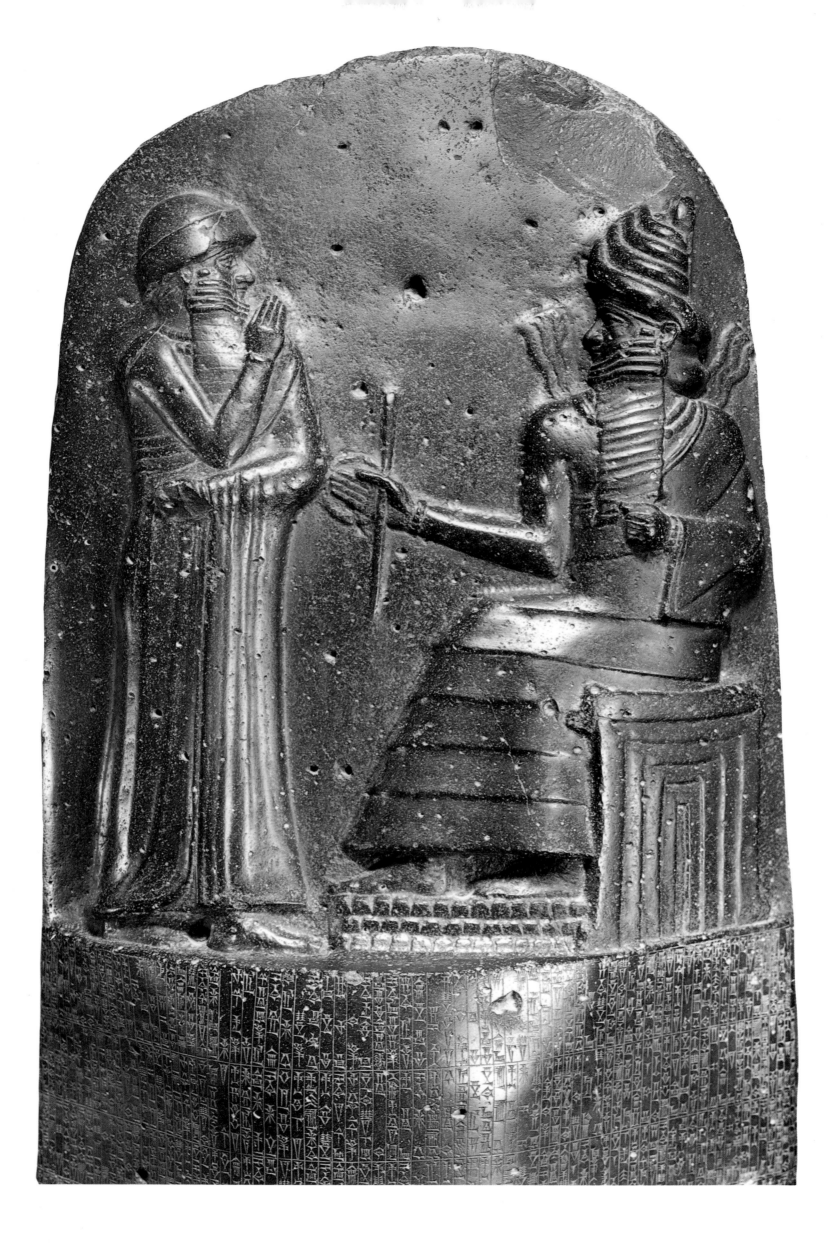

Egypt

The ancient civilization of the valley of the Nile is roughly contemporaneous with that of the Tigris-Euphrates. Egypt was protected on all sides by natural barriers to invasion, and its culture remained largely homegrown, uninfluenced by that of other societies. Egyptian civilization arose about 4300 BC and it collapsed with the fall of the New Kingdom in 1087 BC. Egypt then fell under the successive control of Libyans, Nubians, Assyrians, and Persians. With the conquests of Alexander, in the fourth century BC, Egypt became the center of the Ptolemaic Empire, which was eventually absorbed into the Roman Empire.

There were great similarities between the civilizations of Mesopotamia and Egypt, similarities that extended to pharmacy and medicine. Like the Mesopotamians, the Egyptians had an array of deities, some of whom were involved in matters of health. Two stand out: Thoth, the inventor of science and medicine and patron of physicians, and Imhotep, a mortal of the third millennium BC who was deified in Egypt during Greco-Roman times and was identified by the Greeks with their own Asclepios.

The ancient Egyptian world, like the Mesopotamian, was inhabited by spirits, demons, and evil forces. A sick person was one out of harmony with the world, having irked the gods, the dead, or the spirits. The logical way to restore harmony was by religious and magical means: prayers, incantations, and rituals not unlike those practiced by the Mesopotamians—and not so unlike those practiced by preliterate peoples. But here too medicine did not rely solely on one approach, and here too there were three kinds of practitioners: the priest, the sorcerer, and the physician. The presence of the last indicated that Egypt had developed medicine to an empirical-rational stage, but this approach was generally combined with religion and magic. The religious, magical, and empirical-rational systems of medicine operated side by side and frequently overlapped, but they were different systems.

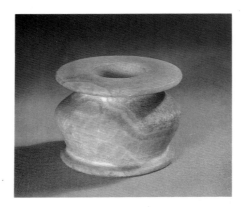

Stone unguent or cosmetic jars. Egyptian, c. 2500 BC. Museo Egizio, Turin

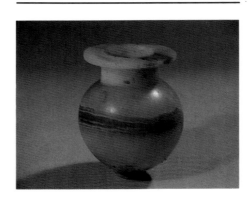

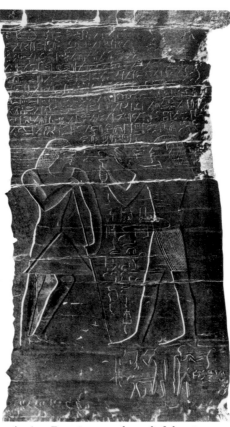

Ancient Egyptian stone bas-relief showing a priest administering medicine. Smithsonian Institution, Washington, D.C.

Our knowledge of Egyptian medicine derives largely from eleven medical papyri. Several of these have some significance for the history of pharmacy; the most significant is the Ebers Papyrus, written about 1500 BC. A collection of recipes, it contains 811 prescriptions and mentions some 700 drugs. A document over 22 yards (20.23 meters) long, it covers a variety of medical subjects. Its very size testifies to the importance of empirical-rational medicine in ancient Egypt.

This huge armamentarium of drugs comprised materials from the vegetable, animal, and mineral kingdoms. The precise interpretation of prescriptions and identification of drugs present difficulties, but Egyptologists have had considerable success in identifying many that have analogues in Western medicine. Colocynth, senna, and castor oil, for example, were used as laxatives by the ancient Egyptians. From animals came a large assortment of animal parts and excrements. Among them were pig's brain, the vulva of a bitch, fly's dirt, and crocodile's dung—all precursors of what came to be called in early modern times *Dreckapotheke*. Alum, copper, and salt are the only minerals mentioned repeatedly in the papyri.

The preparation and administration of these drugs was firmly rooted in the religious and magical practices of the time, which held that it was not the drug itself but its magical virtue, in combination with the words spoken over it, that was effective. Not surprisingly, then, the Ebers Papyrus begins with a prayer. The Papyrus Hearst, which dates from about 1600 BC, contains certain benedictions to be pronounced when preparing remedies and others to be pronounced over the measuring cup and over the ingredients, among them barley and beer. The artful physician not only selected the correct drugs but prepared them in the magically correct way and uttered appropriate words over them.

The magical effect of a drug did not always coincide with its pharmacological effect, and there came a time in ancient Egypt

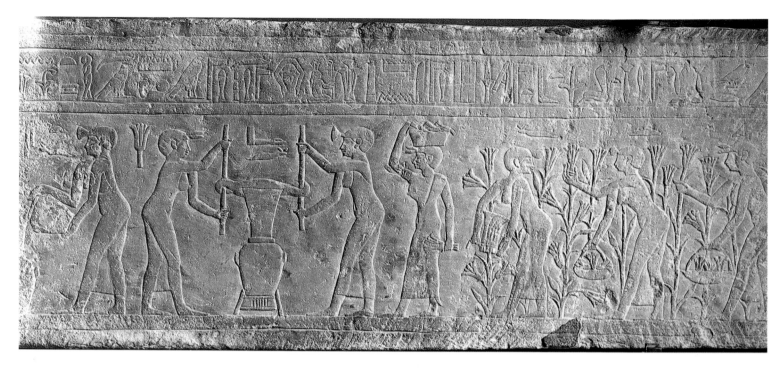

when medicine and magic separated. It is significant that the Ebers Papyrus refers to spells only twelve times, and there are even fewer references in the Papyrus Hearst. Drugs, it is clear, were increasingly administered without magic formulas, and in time drugs became the more popular form of treatment. Egypt early gained a reputation for its drugs—and its poisons. "In Egypt," wrote Homer, " . . . the fruitful soil yields drugs of every kind, some that when mixed are healing, others deadly."

For all this, there was no functionary in ancient Egypt who performed the sum total of all pharmaceutical services exclusively. There were, however, various individuals who performed specific pharmaceutical functions: collectors of drugs, preparers of drugs (this functionary was the *pastophor*), and conservers of drugs—all under the supervision of a physician. Indeed, the practitioner of medicine was largely a practitioner of pharmacy, and had the assistance of pharmaceutical functionaries.

There seems to have been a special room in the temple, the *asi-t,* for the preparation of medicines—the forerunner of the officina, the workshop of the pharmacist. More important were the royal depository and the royal laboratory, known respectively as the Royal Warehouse and the House of Life.

Bas-relief depicting servants gathering lilies and preparing perfumes and ointments. Egyptian, 650–550 BC or 450–350 BC. The Louvre, Paris

The Ebers Papyrus (detail). Discovered by Georg Ebers in Thebes in 1872, this medical compilation, completed c. 1500 BC, contains 811 prescriptions and includes some 700 different drugs. Museum of the University of Leipzig

In these establishments, drugs were collected and preserved under a Conservator of Drugs and were compounded under a Chief of the Preparers of Drugs, who was also Chief of the Royal Physicians.

The Egyptian preparer of drugs performed a variety of pharmaceutical tasks: he had to measure, to powder, to mix, to strain, and to boil. Moreover, he made his prescriptions in almost every nonparenteral dosage form: gargles, snuffs, fumigants, inhalations, poultices, enemas, suppositories,

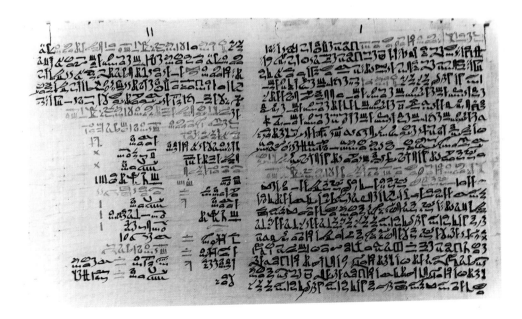

wines, ointments, decoctions, infusions, and collyria. In ancient Egypt, as in Mesopotamia, the manipulations and the artistry that were to become basic to the practice of pharmacy were thoroughly integrated into the delivery of health care.

The Ancient Hebrews

It is difficult to assess the full extent of the pharmaceutical and medical knowledge of the ancient Hebrews and of the Jews of postbiblical times, because the two main sources—the Bible and the Talmud—contain no treatises on these subjects. The Talmud does refer to a "medical book" that was "canceled" by King Hezekiah and to a scroll on pharmacology, but both had already been lost.

Situated as they were at the crossroads of the ancient Mediterranean world, between the mighty Egyptian and Mesopotamian empires, and at different times captives of both, the Hebrews were inevitably influenced by those civilizations. Like the Egyptians and Mesopotamians, the Hebrews believed in the divine force in health and disease, but with the very great difference stemming from their monotheism. God alone was the healer, and it was he who bestowed his healing gifts upon the physician.

"God hath created medicines out of the earth, and let not a discerning man reject them," said Ben Sira in Ecclesiasticus (38:4), and it is evident from the Bible and the Talmud that the Hebrews made use of a number of vegetable drugs—and especially a mineral drug, salt—that would later become familiar to Western society. One vegetable drug, the Balm of Gilead, or one by that name, remained in the pharmaceutical literature into the twentieth century.

Like the peoples of the surrounding areas, the Hebrews were influenced by prevailing superstitions and beliefs. Although at one time they did repudiate magic and attained a rational approach to medicine, during the apocryphal period (c. 200 BC–AD 100) they adopted Babylonian practices

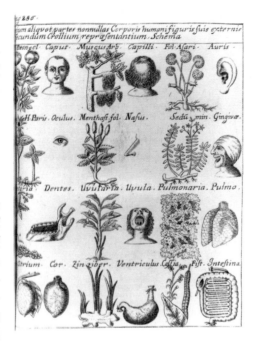

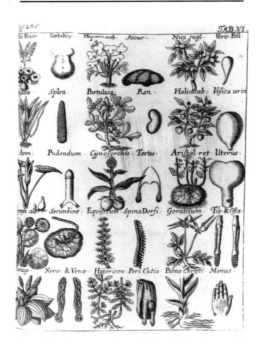

Woodcuts illustrating the "doctrine of signatures," a belief widely held, in ancient China as well as the West, that plants are divinely "signed" for the treatment of diseases of the organs of the human body that they resemble in shape, color, or general appearance. From Michael Bernhard Valentini, *Medicin Nov-Antiqua,* Frankfurt, 1713. National Library of Medicine, Bethesda

of using spells, amulets, and charms to prevent and cure disease. Jewish physicians became increasingly involved in magic and superstition, and the medications they prescribed required the support of chants and incantations. The Talmud speaks of the evil eye and of the Angel of Death that stalks in the night. Nonetheless, such notions were far less widely accepted by the Jews than by their neighbors.

It has long been assumed that pharmacy was practiced in biblical times because of references in the Bible that have been translated as "art of the apothecary" and "apothecaries." Modern translators, however, point out that the functionary involved was a *rokeakh*—a perfumer, who compounded ointments and perfumes and whose work was different from that of a pharmacist or herbalist.

China

The history of pharmacy and medicine in ancient China followed familiar patterns. The resort to magic was widespread; charms and incantations were used as well as prayers. Among the many functionaries that participated in the healing arts were the *fang shih*—a designation that has been translated as "gentlemen possessing magical recipes." The earliest known Chinese texts dealing with drugs date from the last five centuries BC. These were inscriptions on wooden or bamboo slats giving the quantities of drugs that went into prescriptions, the dosage forms, the doses, and the symptoms for which the drugs were indicated.

The early history of China is lost in legend. One of the legendary emperors, Shen-nung, who has been dated in the third millennium BC but probably lived no earlier than the fourth century BC, was credited with being the father of pharmaceutics by the scholar-ruler Liu An in the second century BC, and thereafter Shen-nung's name was applied to a good number of compilations of materia medica. For example, during the Eastern Han Dynasty (AD 25–255) the knowledge of pharmacy that had been transmitted orally since Shen-nung's time was set down in writing in compilations called *pen-ts'ao*. These often contained in their titles the phrase *Shen-nung pen-ts'ao*. The term *pen-ts'ao* has been translated variously as "materia medica," "the fundamentals of simples," and "the botanical basis of pharmacy."

These compilations continued to appear, and they culminated in the monumental *Pen-ts'ao Kang-mu* of China's great naturalist Li Shih-chen. Published in 1596, three years after Li Shih-chen's death, the work comprised fifty-two volumes and represented thirty years of work and of travel through the drug-producing provinces of the country. The compendium described well over 1,000 plants and almost 450 animal substances. It contained just under 11,100 prescriptions.

Li Shih-chen accomplished a revision and updating of the ancient materia medica, but his work was more than a mere list of drugs. With each one came a monograph giving a full description of the drug, its locale and methods of procurement, its odor and taste, the principal application, its preparation, and an "interpretation" of its value. The materia medica was classified into seventeen categories: water, fire, earth, metals and stones, herbs, grains, vegetables, fruits, woods, clothing, instruments, insects, fish, shells, birds, animals, and material from the human body. Although vegetable products predominated, animal parts and excrements were more numerous than those found in European lists—lists that the modern observer finds incredible enough. In addition, the Chinese made use of minerals to a greater extent than the people of any other ancient civilization.

In this manifold classification, and in the long list of drugs, lies the key to Chinese pharmacotherapy: the belief that there must be a remedy for every ill and that virtually everything could have a medical use. The proper drug would bring about the patient's restoration; its efficacy lay in its ability to neutralize the evil influences in the

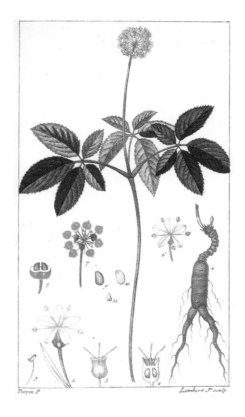

Gin-seng. Color engraving from François Pierre Chaumeton, *Flore médicale* (Paris, 1815–20), vol. 4. National Library of Medicine, Bethesda

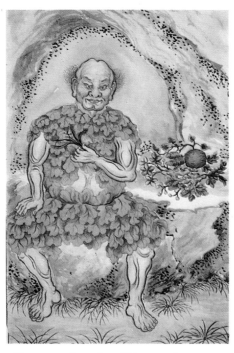

Shen-nung, legendary Chinese god-emperor credited with being the father of pharmaceutics. Watercolor (copied from an old painting in Shanghai, by a Chinese artist), 1920. Wellcome Institute Library, London

environment. In the background was the Chinese philosophical preoccupation with living forces and with their balance and imbalance. The sixth-century *Shen-nung pen-ts'ao* of T'ao Hung-ching, for example, designated drugs that corresponded to *yin* (the feminine, passive, cold, wet, and dark principle of nature) and those that corresponded to *yang* (the masculine, active, warm, dry, and light principle). Drugs were thought to be animated with helpful or harmful spirits, which affected these vital forces and their balance. Out of this developed the notion—suggestive of the Western "doctrine of signatures"—that certain drugs displayed characteristics analogous to the conditions they were to alleviate: red ingredients would be natural remedies for cardiovascular complaints, yellow ingredients for ailments involving the liver and bile.

Many pharmacies in China are still strikingly close to their counterparts of centuries ago. The contents of the shops include the materia medica of ancient days, largely herbal, as well as a good deal from animal sources. Traditional Chinese medicine still requires traditional materia medica. This materia medica has not been without influence in the West. Gingseng, ephedra, cassia bark, rhubarb, and camphor are part of the West's debt to the Chinese.

India

The civilization of India had its beginnings in the valley of the Indus about 3250 BC. Two city centers, Mohenjo-Daro and Harappa, flourished between 2800 and 2500 BC. Little can be said with any certainty about the pharmacy and medicine of these early years, for no historical records have been found. Even excavations made in this century have revealed virtually nothing definite. It can only be surmised that Indian pharmacy and medicine included religious, magical, and empirical approaches.

Harappa culture declined about 2000 BC, and after the invasion of India by Indo-

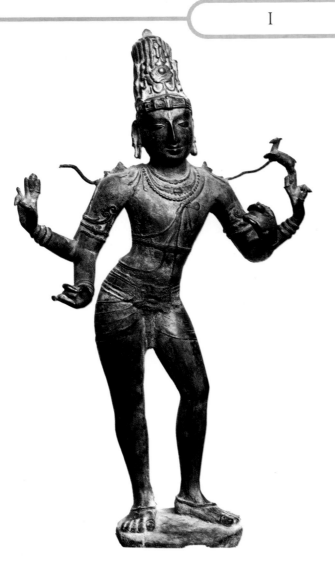

Bronze figure of Siva. Indian, 15th century. One of the two great deities of Hinduism, Siva represents both the creative and the destructive aspects of the world; he was capable of causing illness. Musée Guimet, Paris

European–speaking peoples from the northwest, about 1500 BC, the Vedic age began. Much is known of Indian civilization from then on, for Vedic culture developed a rich literature, largely religious in nature. Nevertheless, chronology is difficult to establish, especially with regard to pharmacy and medicine. Charaka, one of the two outstanding figures in the history of pharmacy in India, has been placed as early as 1000 BC by some, as late as AD 100 by others. Susruta, the other key figure, has been placed as early as 1000 BC and as late as the twelfth century AD.

The materia medica of the Vedic period is found in the *Ayurveda,* a part of the Hindu collection of religious poems and chants known as the *Atharva Veda.* The *Ayurveda* contains eight sections pertaining to medicine and health, one of which, the *Kaya cikitsa,* covers therapeutics.

The major components of the Vedic materia medica were vegetable substances. In the writings of Charaka, for example, more than 2,000 are mentioned, among them sandalwood, cinnamon, cardamom, asafoetida, ginger, pepper, aconite, and licorice—drugs and spices that were to become the basis of trade with the Romans and were later to play a consequential role in history. But the Charaka Collection was more than a list of the materia medica: it not only described the substances and their properties; it also explained their action, defined measurements and dosages, and provided for the addition of materials to make a medication pleasanter in color, taste, feel, or odor.

The development of Brahmanism and Buddhism over the centuries affected the Ayurvedic pharmacy of Charaka and Susruta. Religious writings of the period not only dealt with meditation and magic but also delved into alchemical experimentation. After AD 500, alchemy attained great significance in India, and there developed a Tantric-alchemical pharmacy whose materia medica was distinguished by an array of inorganic chemical preparations. From AD 500 to 1000 this Tantric pharmacy paved the way for a medico-chemical materia medica that was incorporated into the Ayurvedic corpus. About 1400, the compilation known as the *Rasaratnasamucchaya* appeared. In it, mercury was given special prominence, and it has been calculated that more than 5,000 preparations of mercury and other metals were known.

By the end of the fifteenth century, the Ayurvedic corpus had attained its final form. Traditional Indian pharmacy would soon be subject to foreign encroachments, however, for Vasco da Gama had landed in Calicut, on the Malabar Coast, in 1498. Significantly, native Indian pharmacy, with its long Vedic tradition, never fully succumbed to the Western invasion. In the countryside and in town bazaars and among "traditional" physicians the ancient remedies still dominate. By and large, age-old tradition, superstition, and religious beliefs have confined Western science and medicine to the large cities and Westernized universities of India.

The society of the Hellenic Greeks that flourished in the Eastern Mediterranean between 600 and 330 BC was different in outlook and organization from the societies of Mesopotamia and Egypt. The preliterate barbarians who invaded Hellas from the north around 1000 BC were surely influenced by the Minoan-Mycenaean civilization, already at its apogee on the island of Crete and on several sites on the mainland of Greece and Asia Minor.

GREEK SOCIETY: HIPPOCRATIC MEDICINE

The civilization developed by the Hellenes was individualistic, speculative, this-worldly, and concerned with concepts of liberty and aesthetics—and Greek medicine and pharmacy developed within this cultural framework. The trained practitioners of medicine and pharmacy in classical Greece sought a natural, rational, and empirical basis for their ministrations. They did this although a temple medicine did co-exist, although a "conventional piety" was to be found among medical writers, although the Hippocratic oath invoked the divine help of Apollo, Asclepios, Hygeia, and Panacea, although there were numerous magicians and charlatans who practiced medicine, and although catharsis, a common feature of Greek medical practice, had spiritual as well as medical connotations. Nature and reason were not in conflict with the divine but were manifestations of it, and at the professional level medicine was not based on religion, magic, or superstition. The momentous achievement of Greek medicine was its seeking a natural basis for disease, its causes and its treatment.

Interest in the natural causation of disease was a reflection of the concern of Greek philosopher-scientists with understanding

THE CLASSICAL WORLD

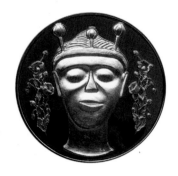

Silver medal representing opium in the series "The Medallic History of Drugs" issued in 1972 by the Medallic Heritage Society. The head on the obverse of this medal is based on that of a Minoan clay figurine of a goddess from Gazi in the Archaeological Museum in Herakleion, dated 13th century BC. The representation is linked to opium both by the three poppy capsules in the diadem and by the ecstatic facial expression. Collection David L. Cowen, Rossmoor, New Jersey

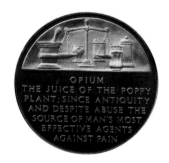

the world of nature. As early as 500 BC the Milesian school, seeking to find a single unifying principle that would explain all phenomena, came up with a variety of answers. Thales thought that the underlying principle was water; his followers added air, fire, and earth—which they defined as the primary substances from which all things derive. These four became known as the "Aristotelian elements," and for many centuries physics and chemistry as well as medicine were based on this theory of the four elements. It became the keystone of the system of humoral pathology and the pharmacotherapy that it generated.

The appellation "the father of modern medicine" is traditionally applied to Hippocrates, who was born about 460 BC on the island of Cos. There he taught medicine, and there he and his followers, collectively known as the Hippocratic school, fostered a rational and empirical approach, as opposed to a religious and magical approach, to medicine. It was through the writings of this school—the Hippocratic corpus—that the theory of humoral pathology, and its concomitant theory of drugs, became basic to the conception and treatment of disease.

Humoral pathology drew directly on the theory of the four elements: the body contained four humors, each the counterpart of one of the four elements. These four humors were phlegm, blood, yellow bile, and black bile. Not only were they the counterparts of water, air, fire, and earth, respectively; they possessed the same qualities as those elements. Thus phlegm, like water, was moist and cold; blood, like air, was moist and hot; yellow bile, like fire, was dry and hot; and black bile, like earth, was dry and cold.

Good health, like the good society, depended upon harmony, an underlying principle in Greek thinking. Good health required that the humors be in harmony; if one or another was overabundant or insufficient, illness resulted. Balance, or harmony, had been destroyed—and it was the physician's task to restore that balance. In accomplishing this task he could rely on the four qualities to indicate which humor was at fault: the qualities hot, cold, dry, and moist told the story. If the patient felt moist and cold, he had a superfluity of phlegm; if he felt moist and hot, he had a superfluity of blood; and so forth. The Greek notion of four basic temperaments reflecting the humors, derived from this system, is still evident in our use of such terms as phlegmatic, sanguine, choleric, and melancholic.

The Greek physician made use of the whole gamut of therapeutic practices and surgical techniques, physiotherapy and exercise among them. Bleeding, scarification, cupping, blistering, and the use of leeches were known. Most significant were dietary regimes and drug therapy; the salient characteristic of Greek medicine was the use of both in treating the sick.

Hot, cold, moist, and dry were more than symptoms, however; they were also the "qualities" that gave drugs their particular properties and thus were the theoretical base for pharmacotherapy. Here were the beginnings of Western pharmacology and pharmacodynamics, a system of pharmacotherapy that was to go virtually unchallenged for two thousand years.

The Greeks believed they knew both what a particular drug could accomplish in the human body and how. Drugs were directed at the particular humoral anomaly manifested by the patient's symptoms. (Here the system of curing by opposites—modern allopathy—had its rational foundation.) In a pleurisy, for example, the physician administered such drugs as aristolochia, hyssop, and cumin—drugs possessing the qualities of drying and heating and therefore capable of counteracting the moistness and coldness of the patient. As a logical outcome of the concept of humoral superfluity, cathartics, emetics, diuretics, and expectorants abounded in the armamentarium of the Greek physician.

There was no compilation of the materia medica in the Hippocratic corpus, but in the writings of the Hippocratic physicians scholars have accounted for two hundred herbal drugs, animal drugs from at least ten

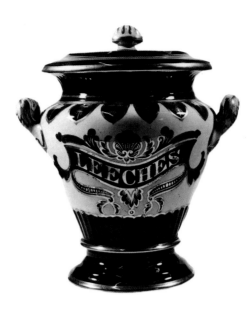

Leech jar. Porcelain, decorated in white, blue, and gold. English, c. 1850. These jars were fitted with perforated lids so that the leeches could breathe. Wellcome Institute Collection, Science Museum, London

▶

Carving of Asclepios and Hygeia on the sliding lid of a portable ivory pharmacy. The one-snake staff that Asclepios holds is—like the familiar two-snake, wing-topped staff, the caduceus— a symbol of medicine. The bowl that Hygeia holds is now a pharmaceutical symbol. 4th century. Musée Cantonal d'Archéologie du Valais, Sion, Switzerland

phyla, and about a dozen mineral drugs. The dosage forms named in these writings indicate that a high level of pharmaceutical skill and art was attained: fomentations, poultices, gargles, pessaries, pills, ointments, oils, cerates, collyria, lohochs, troches, and inhalations are all mentioned.

It is in other Greek sources—principally the works of Diocles, Theophrastus, and Dioscorides—that a systemization of the materia medica, which was largely botanical, is to be found. Diocles of Carystus, who lived in Athens in the late fourth century BC, was the most important of the *rhizotomoi*, or professional collectors of plant roots. The subjects of his writings, considerable in scope and quantity, included medical botany. His herbal, dealing with the origin, recognition, nutritive value, and medicinal uses of plants, placed far greater emphasis on pharmacy than it had received in the Hippocratic writings.

Theophrastus, who died in Athens about 287 BC, was one of Aristotle's foremost students. His botanical works, *De historia plantarum* and *De causis plantarum,* entitle him to be called the first systematic botanist. In his studies he classified plants by their leaves, roots, seeds, stems, and growing season and described and discussed some five hundred species and varieties of medicinal plants found from the Atlantic to India.

The greatest pharmaceutical guide of antiquity was that of Pedanius Dioscorides, who achieved his great work in AD 50–70. Dioscorides, who continued to be regarded as a major authority on drugs for sixteen centuries, wrote only one treatise, *De materia medica.* Altogether, Dioscorides discussed more than 600 plants, 35 animal products, and 90 minerals. Of 827 entries, only about 130 were to be found in the Hippocratic corpus; Dioscorides had added a great deal from old authorities and from what he had learned in his travels in Africa, Gaul, Persia, Armenia, and Egypt.

De materia medica set the pattern for the pharmacopoeias of later times. For each drug listed (with its synonyms), Diosco-

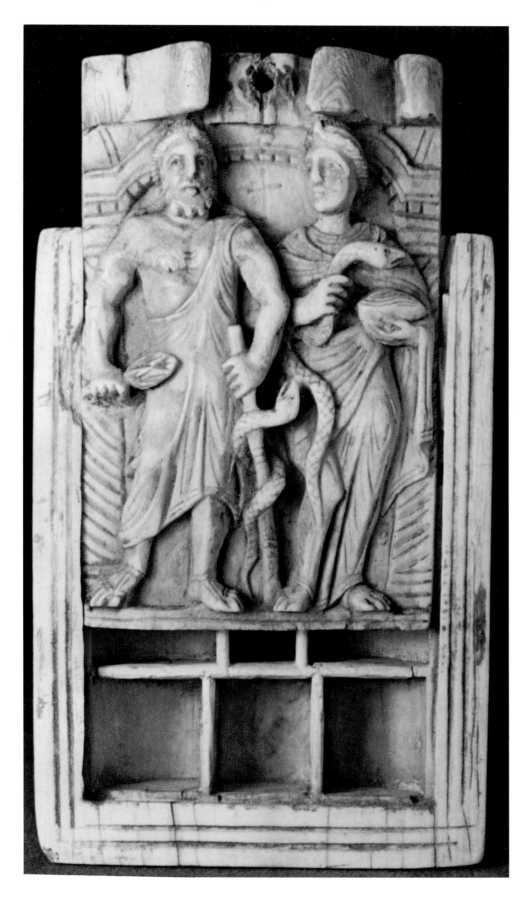

rides described its habitat; gave a botanical description; explained its properties or type of action; described its medicinal usage and side effects; gave quantities and dosages; gave instructions on harvesting, preparation, and storage; described methods of adulteration and tests for detecting adulteration; gave the veterinary, magical, and nonmedical usages; and indicated where the plant could be found. Withal, he admonished the practitioner to study each plant with attention to its habitat and seasonal differences, to prepare each medicine precisely, and to judge a medicine by its effectiveness.

Dioscorides' approach was not only rational and empirical; it was also critical, and it deserves to be recognized as the beginning of the sciences of pharmacognosy and pharmacology. His classification of drugs was based on their presumed physiological action, and he was largely responsible for determining modern plant nomenclature. More particularly pharmaceutical were such recommendations as his directions for the storage of most medicines in thick vessels of silver, glass, or horn. Liquids were to be kept in brass vessels, fats and marrows in tin vessels, and so forth. He gave directions for the compounding of simples in prescriptions; he described the making of extracts by maceration followed by evaporation; he outlined methods of expressing juices and concentrating them by exposure to the sun.

Versions of Dioscorides' work appeared, from the second century on, in Greek, Latin, and Arabic. Outstanding was a beautiful and lavishly illustrated edition, arranged alphabetically, of the *De materia medica* compiled in the year 512. With the invention of printing, a host of editions and translations of Dioscorides' work appeared, the first in 1478. By 1544, no fewer than thirty-five translations and commentaries had been issued.

Clearly, the Greeks made considerable headway in pharmacognosy, pharmacology, and pharmaco-therapeutics. However, pharmaceutical practice remained one of

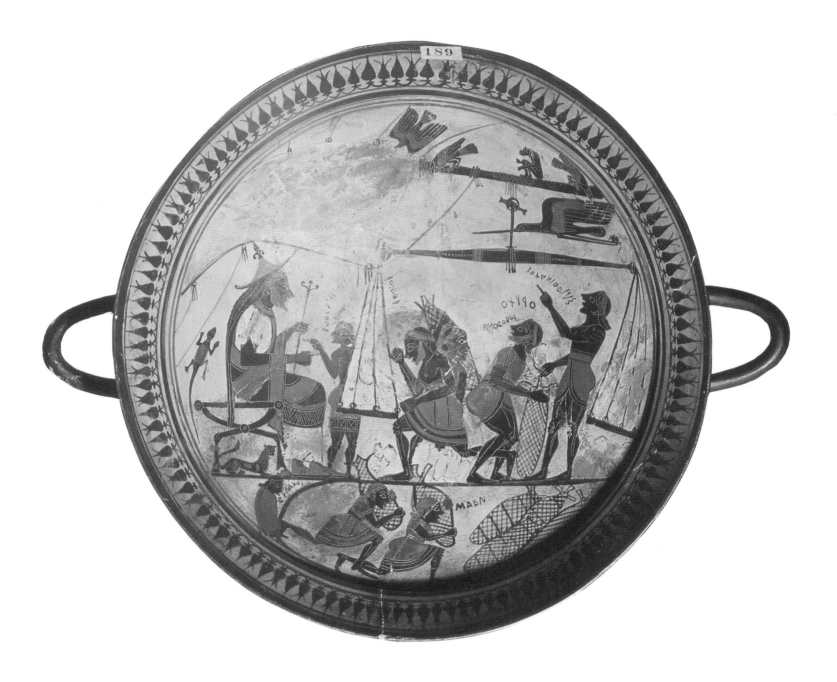

Greek bowl showing royal supervision of the weighing of the medicinal plant silphium. c. 6th century BC. Bibliothèque Nationale, Paris

the functions of the medical practitioner, although groups of collectors and sellers of drugs, and also preparers of remedies, did develop. In addition to the already mentioned *rhizotomoi,* there were the *migmatopolos,* seller of mixtures; the *pharmakopoeos,* maker of remedies; the *pharmakopolos,* itinerant drug seller who traveled from market to market; and the *myropoeos,* or *myrepsos,* maker of ointments. It is evident that as pharmaco-therapeutics became more rational, more empirical, and more scientific in its approach, the physician found it increasingly desirable to rely upon the expertise of a specialist in the preparation of remedies.

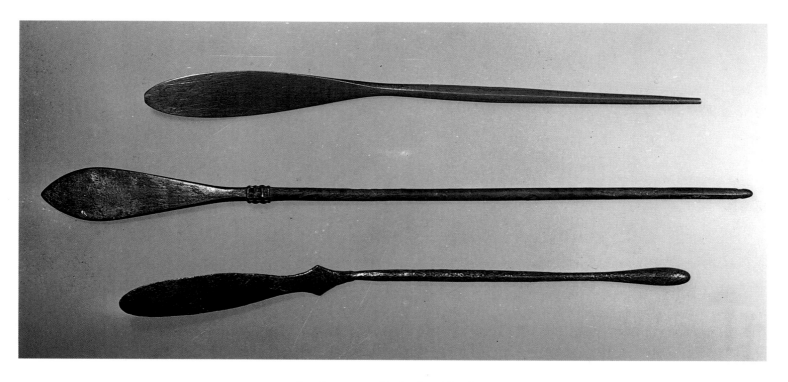

Spatulas excavated in the City of London.
Roman, 2nd century. Guildhall Museum,
London

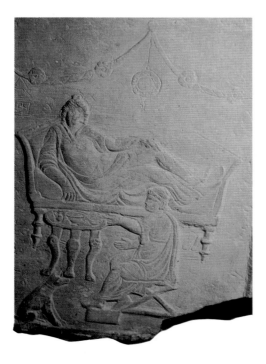

Bas-relief of Asclepios preparing medicine for a
patient. Greek, 2nd century BC

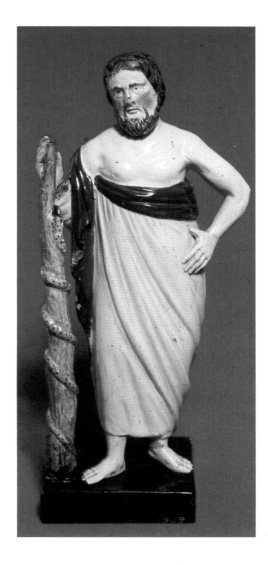

Asclepios. Ceramic Staffordshire figurine.
English, early 19th century. Wellcome Institute
Collection, Science Museum, London

THE ROMAN ORDER

Roman civilization spanned approximately a millennium: five pre-Christian centuries as the Roman Republic, five centuries as the Roman Empire. In its formative period it was in frequent direct contact with the Greek world; eventually it subjugated that world, the Eastern Mediterranean, North Africa, and Western Europe.

"Captive Greece took Rome, her captor, captive," wrote the Roman poet Horace, acknowledging that Roman society drew its major inspiration from the Greek. Nonetheless, Roman civilization, largely eclectic and imitative, and far less speculative than the Greek, succeeded in placing its imprint on every aspect of Western life.

It was certainly true of medicine that its history in Rome began with the arrival of Greek physicians. Because it is not easy to separate Greek and Roman elements, historians often resort to the term "Greco-Roman." In any case, Greco-Roman medicine was clearly an adaptation and augmentation of the Greek. In general, what the Romans added was the organization of medical and pharmaceutical knowledge and the conversion of theory into rules and dogma. Examples of the Roman contribution to medical science are such works as the *De medicina* of the encyclopedist Aulus Cornelius Celsus, the *De compositione medicamentorum liber* of Scribonius Largus, and the *Historia naturalis* of Pliny the Elder—all written in the first century AD.

This process of regularization was the work especially of Galen, who was to surpass even Dioscorides in his impact on the history of pharmacy. A Greek who was born in Pergamum in AD 129 or 130 and who died in 199 or 200, Galen was the acknowledged leader of the medical men of his time. An extremely well-trained and experienced physician, he made the city of Rome the center of his activity, and he became the friend and confidant of the emperors Marcus Aurelius, Lucius Verus, and Commodus.

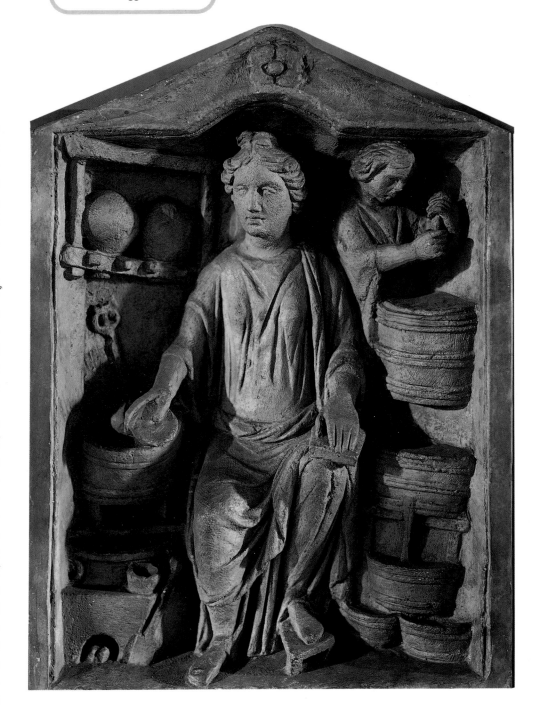

Venus saponaria. Bas-relief found at Epinal, France, showing a woman pharmacist with mortars, a furnace, and other equipment. Roman, c. 2nd century. Musée des Antiquités Nationales, Saint-Germain en Laye, France

As a physician, Galen was thoroughly Hippocratic in his outlook and he kept to the path outlined by the Hippocratic school. A prolific author, he drew on a variety of sources—only some of which he acknowledged. His knowledge of simple drugs derived mainly from Dioscorides, and he undertook the organization of Dioscorides' materia medica within the basic framework of humoral pathology.

In his great work *Methodo medendi* (*On the Art of Healing*), Galen discussed such topics as the properties and mixtures of simple medicines, compound drugs ac-

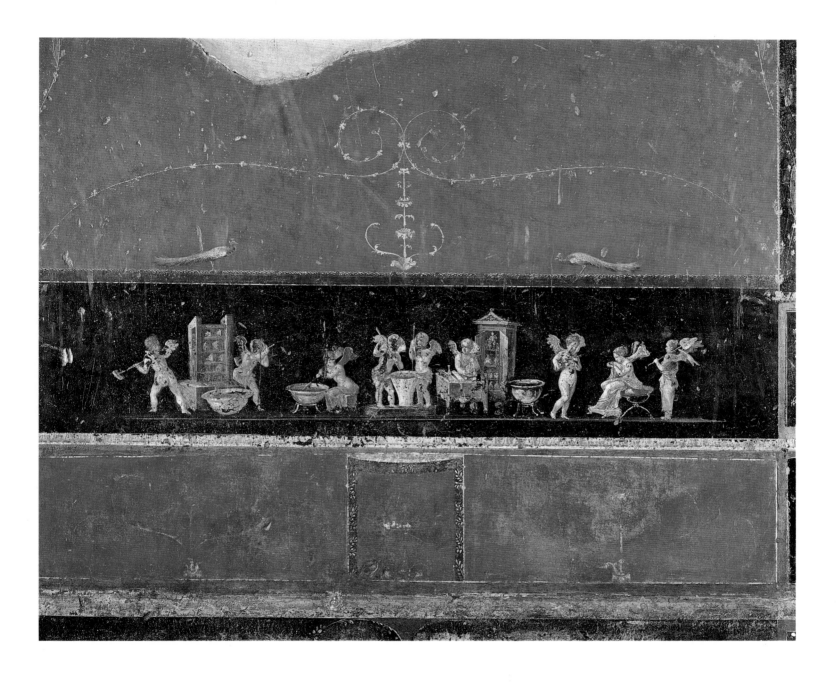

cording to the place of ailment, and compound drugs according to types. Although he assigned great value to the empirical testing of medicines, he often had to fall back on speculative conceptions. His major contribution lay in his classification of drugs by their pharmacological effects, based on their qualities in humoral pathology. In doing so, he organized the pharmacotherapy of humoral pathology into a system of rigid and dogmatic procedures and rules.

This system divided drugs into three groups. First were the simples, which Galen defined as having but one of the qualities of cold, hot, dry, moist. Each simple was fur-

Putti preparing cosmetics, using equipment similar to that for medicines. Frieze from the peristyle of the House of the Vettii, Pompeii. 1st century AD

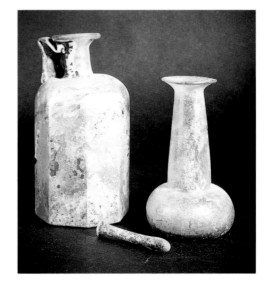

Roman glass medicine or cosmetic bottles found in Israel.

ther categorized by degree of strength, and the strengths required to treat certain diseases were indicated. Second were composites, compounded drugs that possessed more than one quality, which Galen also categorized by various degrees of strength. Third were entities, drugs that had a specific action—evacuants, emetics, and diuretics, for example.

In his medical treatises Galen described 473 drugs of vegetable, animal, or mineral origin as well as a large number of formulas for compound drugs. Three remedies that were to become universally celebrated and esteemed, although they were not original with him, were *hiera picra, terra sigillata,* and theriaca (theriac). At the beginning of the twentieth century, *hiera picra* was said to be the oldest pharmaceutical compound still in existence. Galen's formula called for aloes, to which spices and other herbs were added; with the addition of honey, the compound was made into an electuary. Its "signal Virtues" according to William Salmon, a seventeenth-century commentator, were that it was "a good thing to loosen the body, and gently evacuate Choller and other ill humors. It heats . . . drys . . . opens Obstructions, and purges thick Phlegmatick humors."

Terra sigillata, or sealed earth, was a greasy clay—containing silica, alumina, chalk, magnesia, and a little oxide of iron—found on the Greek islands of Lemnos, Melos, and Samos. Galen valued especially that from Lemnos. *Terra sigillata* was formed into large, tablet-like units upon which the seal of the place of origin was impressed. Salmon extolled these tablets as "drying, binding, sudorifick, and alexipharmick, resisting Plague, Poyson, Putrefaction and all kinds of Malignity and Venom"—and went on to list specific uses for them.

Theriaca, or treacle, was the polypharmaceutical par excellence. As used in the classical world, it contained a varying number of ingredients, sometimes more than seventy. There were periodic efforts to simplify the formula, but in the Renaissance the number of ingredients actually increased.

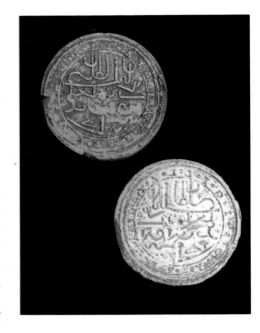

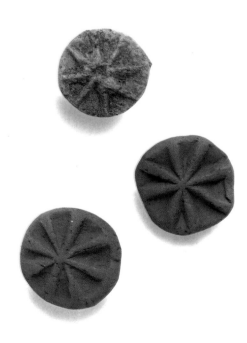

Terra sigillata (sealed earth) tablets. Lemnos, Greece, was an important source of the greasy, mineral-rich clay used throughout Europe until the 17th century as an antidote for poisons, dysenteries, fevers, and other illnesses. The tablets (here with Turkish markings) were stamped with seals indicating their place of origin. Schweizerisches Pharmazie-Historisches Museum, Basel

Originally intended as an antidote to the bites of wild creatures, theriaca eventually became a universal antidote for poisons and a remedy used in many illnesses. Its contents were largely herbal, with opium playing a prominent role, but at various times castoreum, viper flesh, and skink each found a place in the formula. The most famous of the theriacs was that called *mithridatium,* after Mithridates VI, second-century king of Pontus. Mithridates experimented with poisons and their antidotes, using condemned criminals for his subjects.

Theriaca was to become a significant article of commerce in Western Europe; Venice treacle was especially valued. The compounding of theriacs was done with pomp and ceremony by chief pharmacists under the eyes of the local Collegium medicum in the great cities of Europe into the eighteenth century. Not until 1752 did a pharmacopoeia, that of the Royal College of Physicians of Edinburgh, dare to expunge the theriacs.

Galen prepared his own remedies and was critical of physicians who relied upon others to do their compounding. He did his pharmaceutical work in a *iatreion,* as did most physicians of his time, and he stored his drugs in wooden boxes in an *apotheca,* or storeroom.

Galenic concepts dominated pharmacy and pharmaco-therapeutics until they were challenged in the sixteenth century by Paracelsus, and many of Galen's ideas held their own for a long time thereafter, despite the challenge. Galen had, after all, presented a rational approach that brought order to drug therapy. The pervasiveness of Galenic influence is indicated by the fact that various forms of vegetable drugs, those that involve no real chemical changes, are still referred to as galenicals. The preparation and testing of such medicaments has long been known as galenics.

Galen's stature as a revered figure in the history of medicine and pharmacy sometimes beclouds the fact that a sizable literature on materia medica was produced by others during the period of the Roman Empire. Aulus Cornelius Celsus, Scribonius Largus, Gaius Plinius Secundus (Pliny the Elder), and Aretaeus, in the first century, and Oribasius, in the fourth century, stand out. Although Celsus was not, in all likelihood, a physician, his *De medicina* is regarded as one of the best practical treatises on medicine in Greco-Roman antiquity. Its greatest influence was to come much later, however, for in 1478 Celsus' long-forgotten manuscript became the first medical work to appear in print.

Pliny was also an encyclopedist. His *Historia naturalis,* a vast compilation drawn from many written sources, contains interesting commentaries on the efficacy of drugs. There were, first, drugs that produced obvious physiological responses—scammony as a purge, white hellebore as an emetic. There were also drugs that in their form, color, or other characteristics exhibited a "sign" of their therapeutic value, for example, the orchidaceous plants, which, because their underground portions resembled human testicles, were used in genital complaints and as aphrodisiacs. This concept was later known as the "doctrine of signatures," and as the doctrine developed in medieval Europe the signs took on the aura of being God-given.

Pliny's commentaries on pharmacological theories went on to explain drug action on superstitious and magical grounds. The magical efficacy of his *plantae magicae* was buttressed by myths, folk tales, and legends. In addition, he described a good number of plants that served to ward off disease when worn about the body. Popular myths about the qualities of certain of these drugs have persisted into the twentieth century. In sum, Pliny is full of errors and incredibilities, but he exerted a very considerable influence on succeeding generations of scholars.

Scribonius Largus, the Roman physician whose *De compositione medicamentorum liber* was written about AD 43, presented an excellent overview of professional medical and pharmaceutical practice in imperial

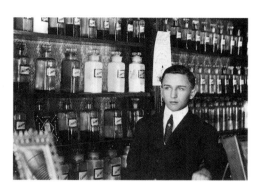

Postcard of an American pharmacist in his shop. Behind him are rows of bottles of galenicals—tinctures, solutions, syrups, powders, and other medicinals presumably derived from vegetable sources and attributed to Galen. Early 20th century

Title page of the works of Galen, published in Venice in 1556. Galen is depicted in several scenes in the border.

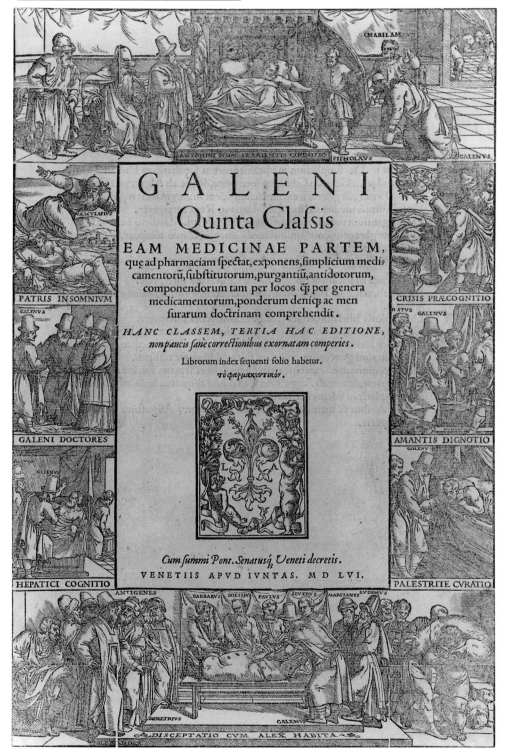

Rome. He described 242 plant, 36 mineral, and 27 animal drugs, but the main thrust of his work was the medicaments compounded from these substances. He obviously favored a polypharmaceutical approach, and his work, organized on a pharmacological basis, has been called an "early dispensatory." He is important in the history of pharmacy for the stress he placed, in the preface to his *De compositione,* on the importance and power of drugs in therapeutics.

Aretaeus, another Roman physician, probably flourished in the last half of the first century AD, but he may have lived later and been a contemporary of Galen's. Aretaeus followed conventional patterns of administering drugs that went back to Hippocrates. His rationale was different—body tone depended on the pneuma, or vital air, a spiritual element drawn in by the lungs—but the pharmacological approach was the same: the familiar purgatives, diuretics, and carminatives remained in evidence.

Oribasius, fourth-century court physician to the emperor Julian, prepared, at the emperor's request, a synopsis of Galen's works and a summary of the work of other Greek medical authorities. His *Collectorum medicinalium* included 600 drugs from Dioscorides and Galen, and it is evident that he possessed an extensive knowledge of pharmaceuticals. His major contribution, however, lay in his preservation of the essential parts of Galen's theories. He also skillfully rearranged, adapted, and simplified Galen.

Like the Greeks, Roman physicians were responsible for putting up their own prescriptions, but they too employed special preparers of remedies or owned slaves trained to do pharmaceutical tasks. Over time, ancient Rome produced a body of functionaries concerned with various aspects of pharmacy. Among those who were essentially compounders were the *pharmacopoei,* makers of remedies; the *pharmacotritae,* or *pharmacotribae,* drug grinders; the *unguentarii,* makers of ointments; and the

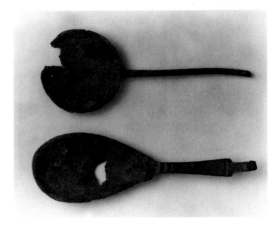

Bronze medicine spoons excavated near Augst, Switzerland. Roman, c. 2nd century. Schweizerisches Pharmazie-Historisches Museum, Basel

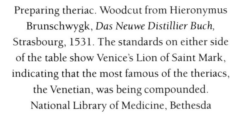

Preparing theriac. Woodcut from Hieronymus Brunschwygk, *Das Neuwe Distillier Buch,* Strasbourg, 1531. The standards on either side of the table show Venice's Lion of Saint Mark, indicating that the most famous of the theriacs, the Venetian, was being compounded. National Library of Medicine, Bethesda

pigmentarii, makers of cosmetics (who became preparers of, and dealers in, drugs). Among those who were essentially dealers in drugs were the *pharmacopolae,* sellers of drugs; the *pharmacopolae circumforaneae,* itinerant vendors of drugs; the *sellularii,* vendors of drugs who kept shops or stalls; mountebanks; and the *aromatarii,* dealers in spices. The pharmacist, as now known, had not yet evolved when the Western Roman Empire came to an end.

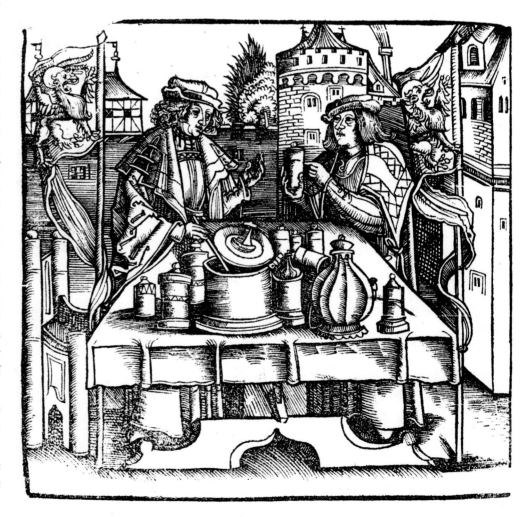

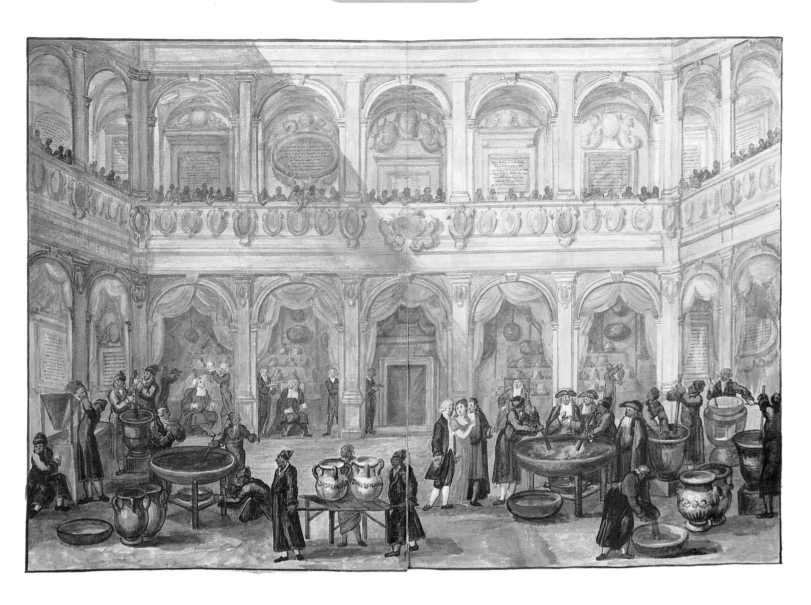

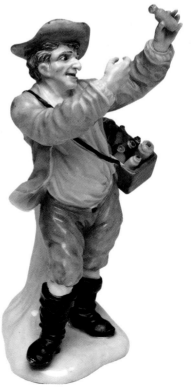

Communal and ceremonial preparation of theriac in amounts sufficient for an entire community in the late 18th century. Color engraving from Giuseppe Guidicini, *Vestiari, usi, costumi di Bologna*, 1818. Biblioteca Communale dell'Archiginnasio, Bologna

Porcelain pharmaceutical flask with mythological scene. Urbino, Italy, 1535. Museo Civico, Forlì

Porcelain figurine of an itinerant medicine seller by Simon Feilner. German (Hoechst), 1752. Collection Bahnhof Apotheke, Offenbach am Main, West Germany

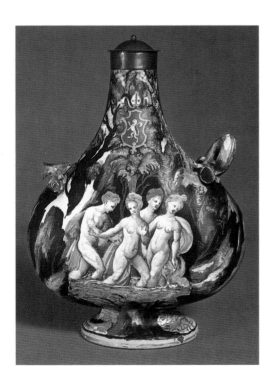

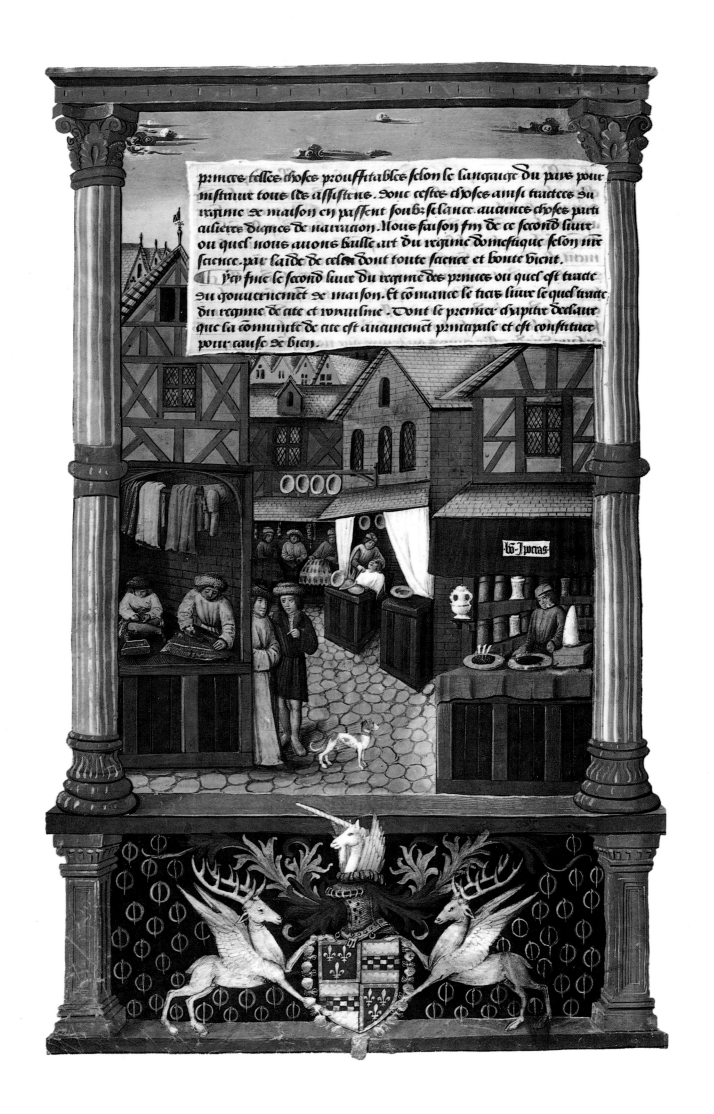

Chapter III

THE MIDDLE AGES

The collapse of the Western Roman Empire in AD 476 led to a disintegration of political authority and a concomitant cultural decline in Western Europe. The Greco-Roman heritage survived in the Eastern Empire, however, and it is to Byzantium that we must first look for the advances made in pharmacy during the Middle Ages.

BYZANTINE CIVILIZATION

While many nonrational elements of magic and folk medicine were interjected into Byzantine practices, the medicine and pharmacy of the Byzantines followed the general patterns established by the Greeks and Romans. The most important of these was the perfection and adaptation of Galen's teachings in the tradition of Oribasius. Byzantine medical writers shared a command of ancient texts and had considerable personal experience with pharmaceuticals. Chief among these writers were Aëtius of Amida, Alexander of Tralles, and Paul of Aegina.

Aëtius of Amida (on the Tigris), who lived in the sixth century, devoted the preface of his medical book to theoretical pharmacology. He edited and condensed Galen, and he brought new order to Galen's sometimes muddled classification of drugs. His contemporary Alexander of Tralles (in Asia Minor) retained Greco-Roman medical theory and the traditional materia medica, but he presented this information in new patterns based on his personal observations and experience. Paul of Aegina, who was later by half a century than Alexander of Tralles, offered a complete overview of Greco-Roman medications and made good use of Oribasius and Aëtius. Paul was active in Alexandria, and since his work was read by the Arabs he was a prime link in the

A late medieval or Renaissance street scene with an apothecary shop bearing the sign Bon Ipocras. Miniature from a 16th-century illuminated manuscript by Gillen Romain, *Le Livre du gouvernement des princes*. The sugar cone on the counter suggests that the pharmacist prepared syrups, conserves, and confections. Ms. 5062, fol. 149v. Bibliothèque Nationale, Paris

◀

transmission of Greco-Roman medicine to the Arab world.

THE ARAB WORLD: PHARMACY ATTAINS IDENTITY

In the seventh and eighth centuries, great Arab empires spread across North Africa to Spain and across the Near East and Persia to India. Arab civilization got its initial impetus from Islam, the religion founded by Muhammad, but the extraordinary culture that subsequently developed—the literature, architecture, philosophy, and science, including pharmacy and medicine—was derived from the cultures of the many nations that came under the caliphs' domination.

The achievements of Arab civilization owed much to the open-minded patronage of certain enlightened caliphs, chief among them al-Mansur, who ruled from 754 to 775 and who transferred the seat of government to Baghdad. Christians, Jews, Persians, and Moors were not only free to participate in cultural life under these caliphs; they were encouraged to do so. At its height, the Arab civilization was eclectic, cosmopolitan, and pluralistic.

Paul of Aegina was not the Arab world's only link with the Greco-Roman tradition. There were, in fact, several paths of transmission, the most significant of which was the scholarship of the Nestorian Christians. The Nestorians, whose belief concerning the Trinity differed sufficiently from orthodoxy to lead to their banishment from Constantinople in 431, established themselves in Syria, Persia, and India. They founded famous schools and translated Greek works into Syriac and Arabic.

These outstanding scholars included, in the ninth century, Jūhannā ibn-Māsawaih, who was to become well known in the West as Mesuë, Sr., and his best pupil, Hunain ibn-Ishāq. Hunain and his students translated the entire available Hippocratic corpus and works of Galen, Dioscorides, Oribasius, and Paul of Aegina. Moreover,

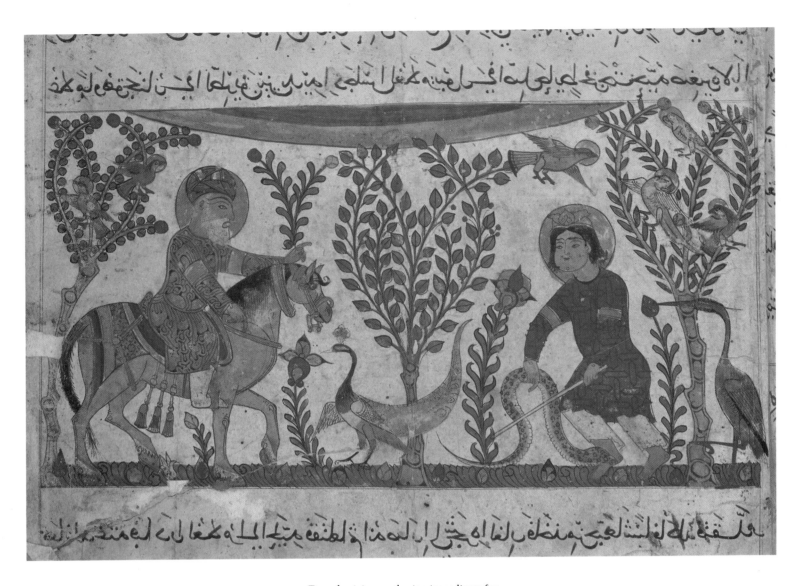

ابى لا يعفه منتمع يفت لم عملي لا لكل عمل السلح الديل ين قسا هنا ما هل ين النجمه و لو مهدمهد

قلله قفه لاله لا فلشل لع علمي لاليا الطيفف مهينا الموه المنا اننجن النافل من لظفه فعلم

Two physicians gathering ingredients for
medicines. Miniature from an illuminated
manuscript. Arabic, 13th century.
Österreichische Nationalbibliothek, Vienna

Hunain wrote over one hundred books of his own, mostly on medicine, and in his work as author and translator he epitomized the acculturation processes of the Arab world: Greco-Roman knowledge, in addition to being preserved and transmitted, was also augmented by the experience and knowledge of Arab savants.

An especially important Arab contribution was the introduction of what was essentially a new genre of professional literature: formularies intended for the use of the pharmacist and other preparers of medicines. The prototype of these formularies—compilations of formulas or recipes for medications, arranged in an orderly (usually alphabetical) fashion and including instructions for compounding and suggestions for their use—was *al-Aqrābādhīn al-Kabīr*. It was compiled by Sābūr ibn-Sahl in the Eastern Caliphate in the mid-ninth century. A product of the Western Caliphate was ibn-'Abd Rabbih's *al-Dukkan*, that

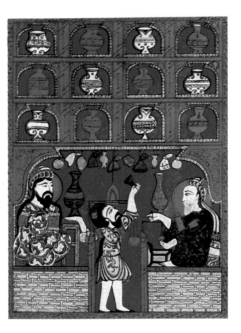

Interior of an Arab pharmacy. Miniature from
an illuminated manuscript of Dioscorides'
Materia medica. 13th century. Library,
Topkapi Museum, Istanbul

Page from a 15th-century illuminated Hebrew
manuscript of Avicenna's 11th-century *Canon
medicinae*. The center illustration shows a
pharmacy with rows of handsome drug jars on
open shelves. The insets depict bathing scenes,
bleeding, and cupping. Codex 2197. Library,
University of Bologna ▶

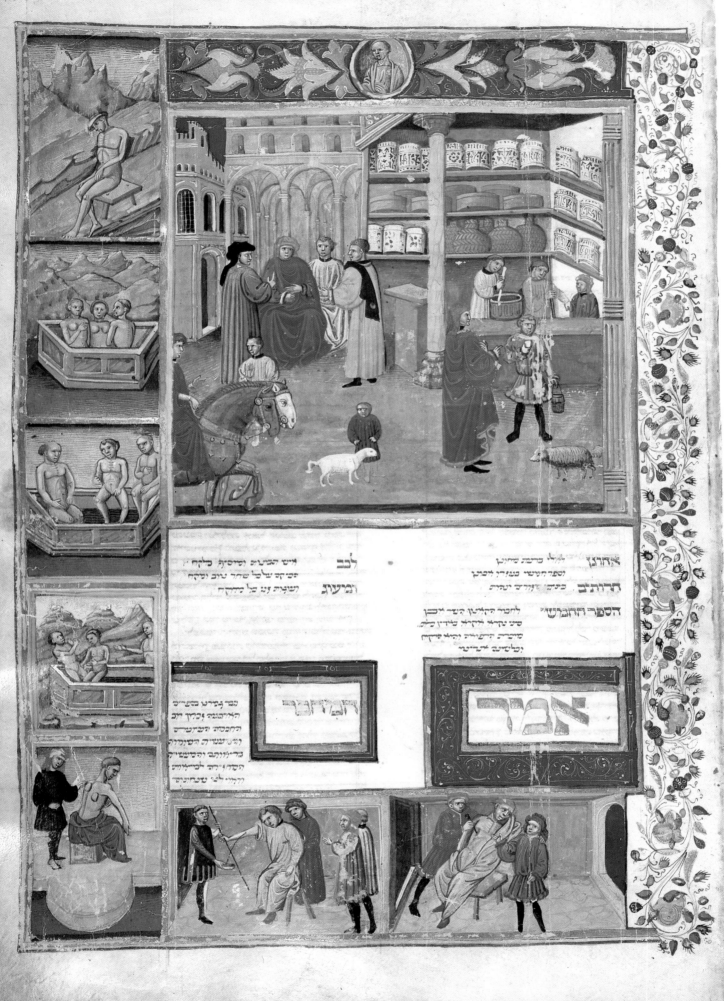

492

אהרן לב וריש המוצא וסיסת כלקח ומעוז

חרותב הספר הזומש

is, *The Apothecary Shop*. This formulary was distinguished by its description of the dosage forms to which Arabs were partial: syrups, conserves, and confections, some incorporating spices and perfumes.

Many such formularies, including some specifically intended for hospital use, were compiled during this epoch. Foremost among them was the *Dustūr bīmāristanī*, or *Hospital Formulary*, written by the Jewish physician al-Sadīd ibn Abi'l-Bajān of the Nasīrī Hospital in Cairo at the beginning of the thirteenth century. His formulary was a practical and precise work, specifying dosages and commenting on side effects and on the consequences of administering one drug in combination with another.

In the eleventh century, al-Bīrūnī was to describe more than a thousand simples in his *Kitāb al-Ṣaydanah fī al-Tibb*, or *Book of Pharmacy in the Healing Art*. His comments on the role of the pharmacist are indicative of the strides that pharmacy had made in the Arab world. Pharmacy, he wrote, is "the art of knowing . . . simples in their various species, types, and shapes. From these the pharmacist prepares compounded medications as prescribed by and ordered by the prescribing physician." Even more extensive was the thirteenth-century work of ibn-al-Bayṭār of Spain, whose *Kitāb al-Jami* named 800 botanical drugs, 145 mineral drugs, and 130 animal drugs. Ibn al-Bayṭār's contemporary, the noted Jewish theologian, scientist, and physician Moses ben Maimon, better known as Maimonides, published a glossary of drug terms and a manual of poisons.

Much more than merely a formulary, or compilation of the materia medica, was the *Minhāj al-Dukkān wa Dustūr al-'yān*, or *Handbook for the Apothecary Shop*, written in Cairo in 1259 or 1260 by the Jewish pharmacist Abū al-Munā Kohen al-'Aṭṭār. Intended to provide instruction for his son, the handbook included recipes for syrups, remedies to aid digestion, remedies missing in other formularies (particularly fumigations, inunctions, and liniments), pharmaceutical weights, and drug synonyms; it

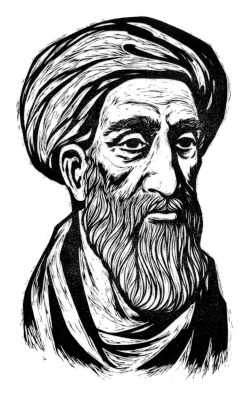

Avicenna. Woodcut by Walter Brooks, American, c. 1967

covered, as well, the acquiring and storing of drugs, the examination and testing of drugs, and the duties, social responsibilities, moral conduct, and shop practices of the pharmacist.

The pharmaco-medical literature of the Arab world included encyclopedias, commentaries, and original contributions by a number of scientists and physicians, and these had a greater impact on medicine than on pharmacy. Outstanding in this literature were the writings, in the ninth to tenth century, of al-Rāzī, known as Rhazes, a Persian physician and the first Muslim to become involved in translating and augmenting the writings of Greek and Roman authors. His major works are known by their Latin names as *Liber medicinalis* and *Continens medicinae*. In the latter, which consisted of fourteen volumes, Rhazes summarized all the available texts on therapeutics that he could assemble from the translated literature. Rhazes took particular interest in dosage forms, and he recommended pills as an agreeable means of taking medicine. He is credited, too, with being a pioneer of scientific chemistry; in his work the Arabic store of drug knowledge reached its zenith.

Another Persian, the philosopher and physician ibn-Sīnā, known as Avicenna, sought to unify all medical knowledge in his enormous eleventh-century *Canon medicinae*. Two of the five books of the *Canon* dealt with pharmaceutical matters: the second book was on simples, the fourth on compounds. These two books contained an extensive list of simples, a treatise on poisons, sections on the preparation of medicines, and a long list of medicinal recipes. Much came from Dioscorides and Galen, but Avicenna's own additions and augmentations are impressive. His materia medica included drugs used by Arabs, Persians, and Indians as well as Greeks. Avicenna is particularly noted in pharmacy for introducing the gilding and silvering of pills.

The influence of Avicenna cannot be overstated. The *Canon* was translated into Latin in the thirteenth century and later printed and reprinted throughout Europe.

Arabic editions of it are still available. After Avicenna, until well into the eighteenth century, every pharmacopoeia or work on the materia medica fell back on his work. For six centuries he was acknowledged as second only to Galen in medicine and pharmacy.

A noteworthy scholar of the tenth century was Khālaf al-Zahrāwi, known as Albucasis, who produced the thirty treatises collected in *al-Taṣrīf,* a manual for students and practitioners. A majority of these treatises were heavily pharmaceutical, none more so than the twenty-eighth, which is known by its Latin title, *Liber servitoris.* Largely devoted to medicinal chemistry, it became a handbook for pharmacists, generations of whom battened on its rich polypharmacy. This work served as an important avenue for the transmission of Arab pharmacy to Western Europe.

These scholars of the Arab world did more than translate and compile: their writings made original and significant contributions. The first was the introduction into the materia medica—and transmission to the West—of drugs from the Near East, the Orient, and Africa. Mainly vegetable, these included drugs long used in the Mediterranean area and drugs introduced through the extensive trade the Arabs had developed with the Far East. Demand for such products in the West eventually had worldwide consequences, encouraging exploration and trade at levels never previously contemplated.

The high value placed on these drugs, the extensive trade that developed in them, and the wide dissemination of knowledge of them are all evident in the manuscript antidotaries and receptaries of early medieval Europe. In the ninth and tenth centuries, even before Arabic medical writings were translated into Latin, monks were copying prescriptions calling for drugs that could have originated only in the Near East, the Far East, or Africa. There is evidence that more than routine copying by monks was involved; the drugs mentioned were actually being used. Some of them, such as

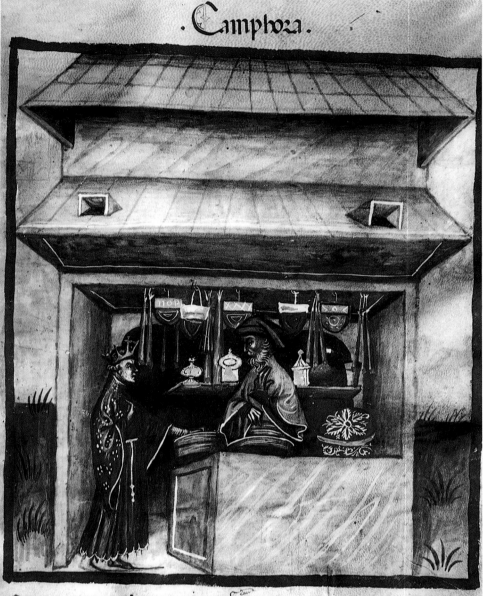

A pharmacist dispensing camphor to a patron. The containers hanging from the ceiling of the small shop probably held crude drugs. Miniature from an illuminated manuscript of the *Tacuinum sanitatis,* perhaps Veronese, c. 1400. Ms. serie Nov. no. 2644. Österreichische Nationalbibliothek, Vienna

ambergris (from the Arabic *ambar*) and camphor (from the Arabic *kāfoūr*), were unknown to the materia medica of the ancient and classical worlds.

A second original contribution of the Arab world was in pharmaceutics proper: the introduction of dosage forms new to the West, a contribution made possible by the fact that in the Arab world the art of the apothecary had progressed beyond the stage of grinding, mixing, and dissolving. New dosage forms demanded of the pharmacist new knowledge and new skills; ma-

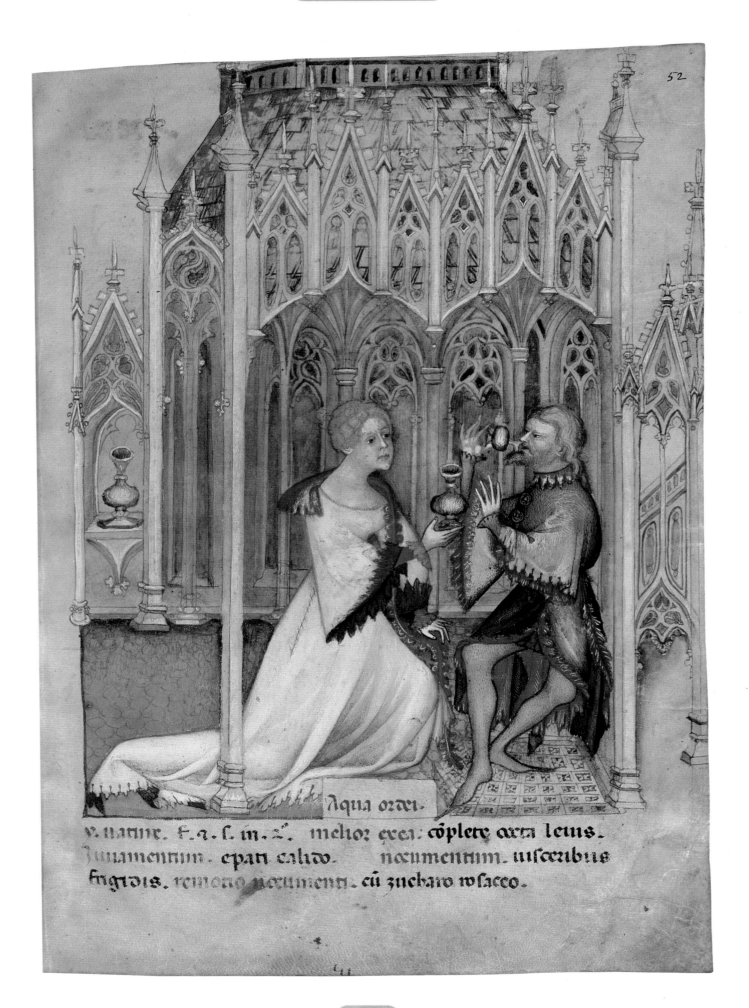

52

Aqua ordei.

v. natnre. f. q. f. m. 2. melior erea. coplete orta leuis.
Inuamentum. epati calido. nocumentum. uisceribus
frigidis. remoto nocumenti. cu zucharo rosaceo.

41

terials could no longer be collected in the vicinity or grown in a local herb garden. Among these new, or newly variegated, dosage forms were syrups, conserves, confections, juleps, and electuaries—all of which made use of sugar or honey and all of which confounded the old notion that only bitter medicines were efficacious. In addition, flavoring extracts like rosewater, orange and lemon peel, and tragacanth enhanced the pharmacist's art.

The Arab apothecary's art was further enriched by the close connections that developed between pharmacy and alchemy. These led to a wider knowledge of chemistry and to the use of chemical processes and chemical apparatus by the pharmacist. Alchemy's origins antedated those of Arab civilization itself, going back to Egypt, Syria, and Persia. Over time, alchemy developed its own set of philosophical concepts, drawn in part from Gnostic teachings in the first and second centuries and religious notions of the fourth and fifth centuries. The alchemists sought to discover the substance—the so-called philosopher's stone—that could both transmute base metals into gold and provide an elixir of life, endowing human beings with immortality.

The beginnings of Arab alchemy have traditionally been attributed to a shadowy eighth-century physician and alchemist, Jābir ibn-Hayyān, also known as Geber. There is reason to doubt the authenticity of the works purportedly by him; they may have been written by later Arab alchemists. From these works we learn that in making their potions Arab alchemists used pots, retorts, stills, crucibles, stoves, bellows, and tongs, as well as the usual mortars and pestles. In addition to distillation, they knew the processes of sublimation and calcination, of melting and compressing, and of

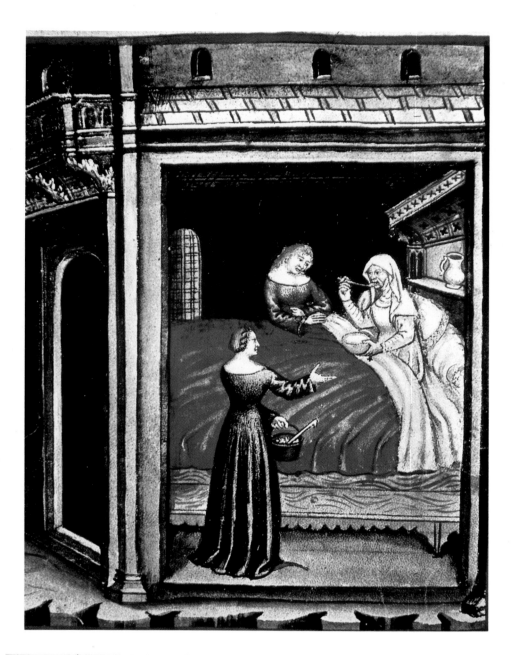

A patient taking barley water, a medicine that remained in the pharmacopoeias until early modern times. Miniature from an illuminated *Theatrum sanitatis.* 15th century. Ms. 4182, fol. 183, Biblioteca Casanatense, Rome

A patient about to drink a preparation of barley water, or *orgeat (Aqua ordei).* Miniature from a late-14th-century illuminated manuscript of the *Tacuinum sanitatis,* a Latin translation of an Arabic treatise. Ms. Lat. 1673, fol. 52. Bibliothèque Nationale, Paris

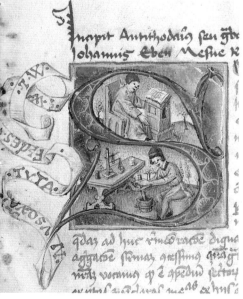

Page from an illuminated manuscript of the *Antidotarium* of the pseudo-Mesuë. 15th century. The curves of the letter S frame a physician at his desk and a pharmacist preparing a medication in a mortar. Ms. K.B.Msc. 20. Zentralbibliothek, Lucerne

the purification and cleansing of minerals. The reputation of Arab alchemy was so great in medieval Europe that alchemical writings as late as the thirteenth century were ascribed to Jābir.

While all these advances were significant, they cannot match Arab civilization's greatest contributions to pharmacy—the attainment of professional identity and independence by the pharmacist and the introduction of the pharmacy shop. Exotic drugs, expanded drug trade, increasing dependence on chemistry and chemical processes, complex formulas, elegant dosage forms, and pleasing flavoring agents, all meant that the practice of pharmacy was changing—indeed, that it had to change. A new specialist was arising, the pharmacist, who knew drugs and where to get them, who was able to recognize their quality and genuineness, who could compound them, and who could put them up in attractive and easy-to-take forms, *secundum artem.*

Medicine also made great strides in the Arab world: surgery, ophthalmology, and other specialties developed; centers of medical education arose in Baghdad, Cairo, and Damascus; great hospitals were established throughout Islam to provide health care as well as education and training for physicians. In such a milieu the physician necessarily came to rely on others to perform pharmaceutical tasks, and the pharmacist filled this need.

The pharmacy shop—operated by a pharmacist performing the totality of services associated with his profession—apparently first appeared in Baghdad, which Caliph al-Mansūr had founded in 762 and made the capital of his empire and a great center of scientific and intellectual activity. The decade 775–785 is the earliest period for which there is documentation of the existence and operation of *dakākīn al-ṣayādilah,* privately owned pharmacy shops.

The original Arab pharmacists, or *ṣayādilah,* had no formal medical or pharmaceutical education. It was not until the ninth century that a class of educated pharmacists developed and pharmacy attained recogni-

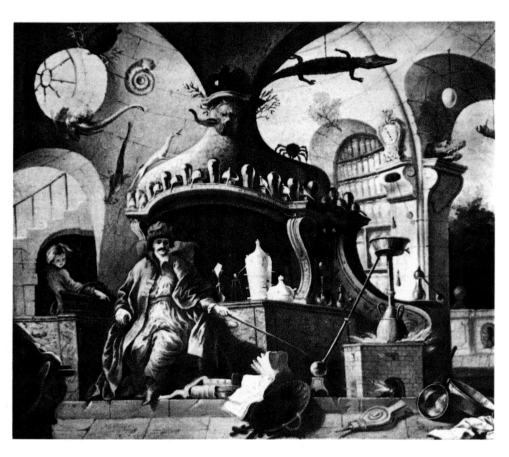

La Pharmacie. Engraving by Louis Cochon after Jacques de Lajoue. French, c. 1750. This allegorical representation of pharmacy strongly suggests its close relation to alchemy. Collection Bouvet, Paris

Distillatio. Engraving by Philipp Galle after Stradanus (Jan van der Straet). Dutch, c. 1580. Distillation is the central operation, but other activities are going on in this alchemist's laboratory. National Library of Medicine, Bethesda ▶

Trade card of Richard Siddall, Chymist. Engraving by R. Clee. English (London), 1781. Siddall's trade card incorporates a version of Louis Cochon's engraving *La Pharmacie.* Banks Collection, The British Library, London

Distillation laboratory. Engraving illustrating the many varieties of retort designs. English, 18th century ▶

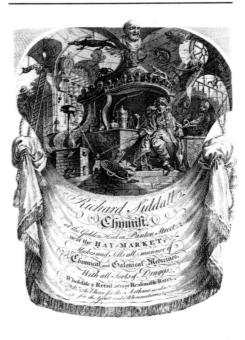

tion as a profession. Qualified pharmacists were given licenses to set up shop near army camps—and the unqualified were excluded. But drug dealers and spice and perfume sellers far outnumbered educated pharmacists, and the line of demarcation between spicers and perfumers, the *aṭṭārīn,* and the *ṣayādilah,* was not easily drawn. Physicians, fearful that their prescriptions would not be handled properly by untrained *aṭṭārīn,* continued to put up their own compounds or have them prepared under their direct supervision.

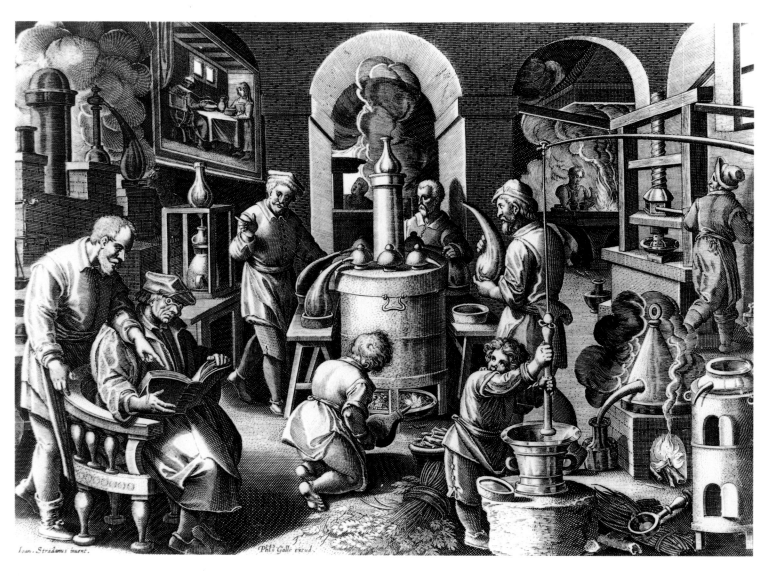

Ioan. Stradanus invent.

Phls Galle excud.

PLATE XXXIX

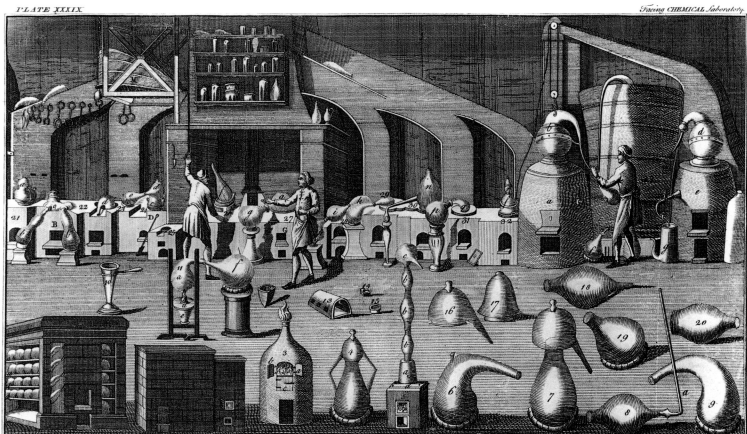

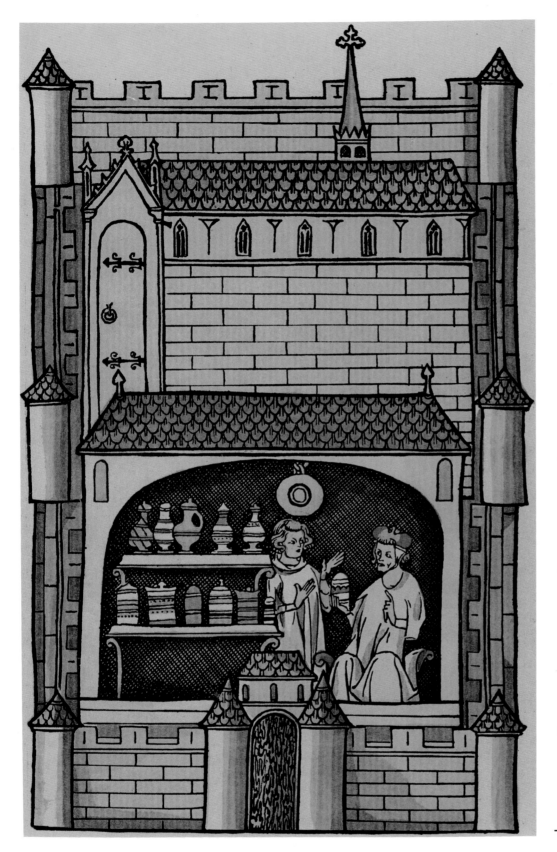

Miniature from an illuminated manuscript of a surgical treatise by Rogier of Salerno. As was typical of medieval pharmacies, the shop depicted opens directly on the street. French, 13th century. Sloan ms. 1977. The British Library, London

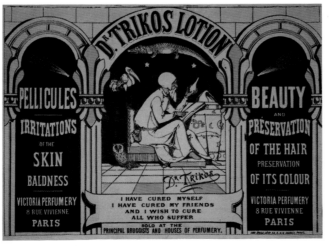

Poster advertising a French product, Dr. Trikos Lotion for skin and hair, to the British market and featuring an alchemist in his laboratory. Color lithograph. French, c. 1885

Nevertheless, pharmacy was practiced on a professional level in the ninth century in cities of the Arab world. At the Nūrī Hospital in Damascus, where there was a well-equipped pharmacy, doctors wrote out prescriptions that were then dispensed by pharmacists. Early in the tenth century, in Tunisia, the physician Ishāq ibn-'Imran wrote prescriptions to be filled at privately owned pharmacy shops. In Seville, in the second half of the twelfth century, the physician Abū Bakr al-Zuhrī similarly relied on professional pharmacists to fill his orders. The development of hospitals played an important role in the separation of pharmacy from medicine. By 1190, the great hospital in Marrakesh had a special section designed as a pharmacy. Trained pharmacists, who held staff appointments at the hospital, manufactured, compounded, and dispensed drugs, many of them made from herbs grown in the hospital's own garden.

To the long list of contributions made by the Arab world to pharmacy can be added the fundamental delineation of the duties, character, and responsibilities of the pharmacist. No calling can truly regard itself as a profession until it has formulated and accepted a code of ethics. The *Minhāj,* or *Handbook,* of al-'Attar presented, in thirteenth-century Cairo, just such a code. With pride and compassion al-'Attar offered a pharmaceutical deontology as well as instructions on the management of the pharmacy shop. In managing the pharmacy itself, cleanliness was paramount. The pharmacist must be certain to clean the balances and pans daily and keep all weights, measures, and vessels clean. The shop was to be kept well stocked and the display attractive; the inventory was to be watched carefully, and deteriorated materials were to be replaced. Finally, the pharmacist was admonished to keep his profits moderate.

As to moral obligation, al-'Attar declared that pharmacy had a decisive role to play in helping the sick, relieving pain, and restoring health. The pharmacist "ought to have deep religious convictions, consideration for others, especially the poor and needy, a

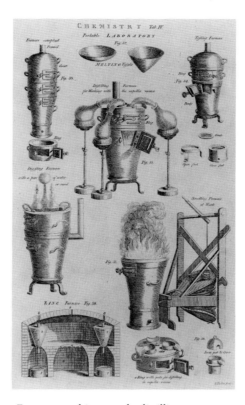

Furnaces, melting vessels, distilling apparatus, and other equipment used in a pharmacy laboratory. Engraving by I. Taylor. English, c. 1840

sense of responsibility and be careful and God-fearing." He must be friendly, honest, thoughtful, slow to anger, modest, and patient. The ideals set down by Abū al-Munā Kohen al-'Attar gained greater respect with each passing century. Numerous manuscript copies of the *Minhāj* exist, and it was printed twice in the nineteenth century and twice in this century, the last time in 1932.

CLASSICAL AND ARAB PHARMACY MOVE TO THE WEST

The Germanic tribes that dominated Western Europe after the collapse of the Roman Empire in the West added little to the medicine and pharmacy that the classical and the Arab world had developed. Christianized Europe fell back on the healing power of faith and religious relics and on traditional folk medicine.

The learning of Rome and Byzantium was not completely lost, however; the age was not entirely "dark." In an era dominated by unquestioning faith there was little to encourage the development of science, but there was one group of literate institutions—the monasteries. In these repositories of learning the monks worked to acquire and preserve ancient knowledge. Foremost among the religious scholars was Cassiodorus, sixth-century chancellor of Theodoric, king of the Ostrogoths; in one of the monasteries he founded in southern Italy the monks were set to studying and copying manuscripts. In his *Institutiones,* Cassiodorus directed the monks to acquaint themselves with the works of Dioscorides and to read the works of Hippocrates, Galen, and others. He advised them to "learn the characteristics of the herbs and the compounding of medicines," and admonished them to "place all your hopes on the Lord."

The precedents Cassiodorus established in southern Italy were adopted by most Benedictine monasteries. Benedictine monks, who knew Latin but not Greek, copied what was available of the writings of Roman and Byzantine authorities. Several important herbals and treatises came out of this monastic tradition, among them the didactic poem entitled *Hortulus,* written by Walafrid Strabo, abbot of Reichenau in the ninth century; *De viribus herbarum (Macer floridus),* most often attributed to Odo of Meung, abbot of Beauprai at the end of the eleventh century; and the *Physica* and *Causae et curae* of Hildegard, twelfth-century abbess of Bingen.

A recipe literature also developed in the vernacular. Old English, Irish, French, and German works appeared, with Roman, Celtic, and Teutonic folk medicine much in evidence. Anglo-Saxon leech books are outstanding examples of this genre of herbal literature. ("Leech" in Old English meant physician.) In addition to making these literary contributions, monasteries gave a specific and important impetus to the development of pharmacy by establishing their own herb gardens and pharmacies.

A great change in Western attitudes toward pharmacy and drug therapy took place with the transmission of Arabic and Greek compilations, in their entirety, to Western Europe. Two centers of learning arose: one at Salerno, in southern Italy, where a medical center attracted both patients and students in the tenth century; the second at Toledo, in Spain, where a school of translators was founded by Archibishop Raymond in the eleventh century.

At Salerno, Constantine the African (said to be a merchant turned monk), who was fluent in Arabic, Persian, and Greek, encouraged his students to translate into Latin everything that came into their hands. For the first time, complete works, rather than fragments copied in the monastic scriptoria, became available in Western Europe. At Toledo, the scholar Gerard of Cremona was responsible for the translation of Hippocratic works and the works of Galen, Avicenna, Rhazes, and many others. He introduced Avicenna and Rhazes to the West, and he made the work of Dioscorides available.

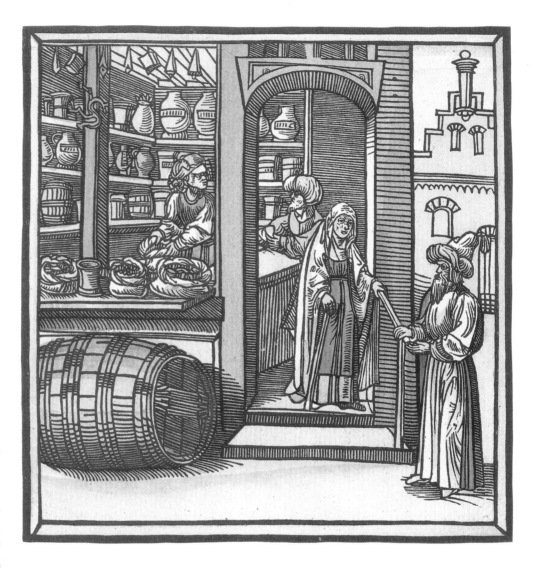

Woman leaving an apothecary shop. Color woodcut from Quiricus de Augustis, *Dlicht d'Apotekers,* Brussels, 1515. National Library of Medicine, Bethesda

The school of Salerno, which can be called Europe's first university, was responsible for major contributions to medicine and pharmacy, not just for the translation of medical texts. Even before Constantine came to Salerno, the *Passionarius Galeni* was compiled, probably by the Italian physician Gariopontus. Other treatises of considerable influence date from this period. In the tenth century a Jewish physician named Donnolo produced an antidotary based on Arabic sources, and in the middle of the twelfth century the Italian physician Mattheus Platearius issued a book on the materia medica known by its incipit as the *Circa instans;* this may have been a revision and enlargement of a work by Constantine. Sometime before 1100, the anonymous *Antidotarium magnum,* or *Great Antidotary,* appeared, with a listing of 485 drug formulas.

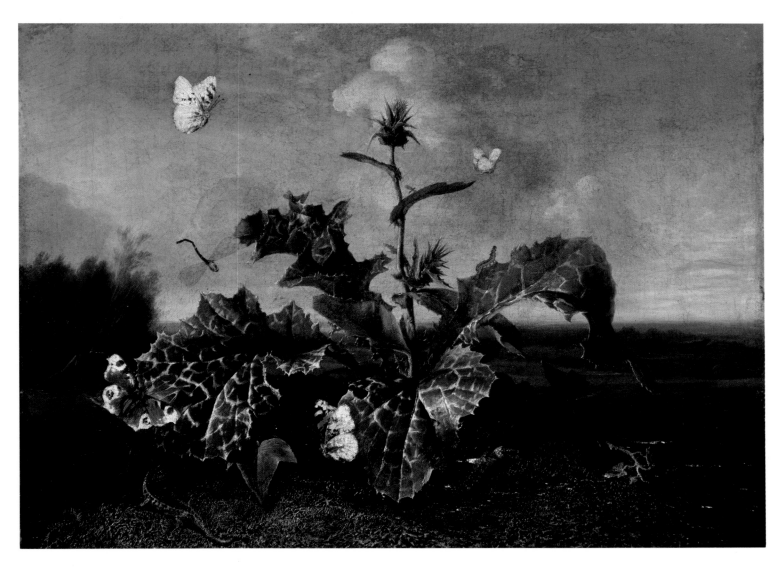

Burdock plant. Painting by Otto Marseus Van Schrieck. Dutch, 17th century. Saratov State Art Museum, U.S.S.R.

Of these, it is interesting to note, some 200 were uncomplicated remedies apparently intended as a *pharmacopoeia pauperum,* that is, recipes for the poor.

The *Antidotarium Nicolai,* which was compiled a century or so later at Salerno, was a trimmed-down version of the *Great Antidotary.* Written perhaps as early as 1169 and certainly no later than 1244, the *Antidotarium Nicolai* was intended for students of medicine—and indeed it became a required text in Paris in 1270.

In its early versions the *Antidotarium Nicolai* contained 115 drug formulas; in later versions there were up to 175. Its major thrust was possibly to provide recipes for medicaments that could be made up in quantity once or twice a year by a *stationarius* or a *confectionarius* under the supervision of a physician. These concoctions had

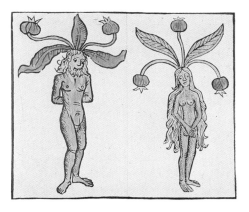

Mandragora (mandrake) plants represented as human figures. Color woodcut from the Mainz, 1491, printing of the *Hortus sanitatis.* National Library of Medicine, Bethesda

a sugar or honey base, which meant that they would keep for long periods and could be dispensed as required. The *stationarius* and the *confectionarius* were dealers in drugs and precursors of the pharmacist; the *statio,* the place where they compounded their medicines, was a forerunner of the pharmacy shop.

Another influential product of Salerno was a manual on health, the *Regimen sanitatis,* which was revised and augmented about 1300 by the physician Arnald of Villanova. It is of interest in connection with the history of pharmacy because it contains pharmaceutical as well as dietary rules. Less well known, but containing several illustrations of pharmaceutical interest, is the *Tacuinum sanitatis,* another manual of health. The known manuscripts of this work are of Italian origin, written in the late fourteenth

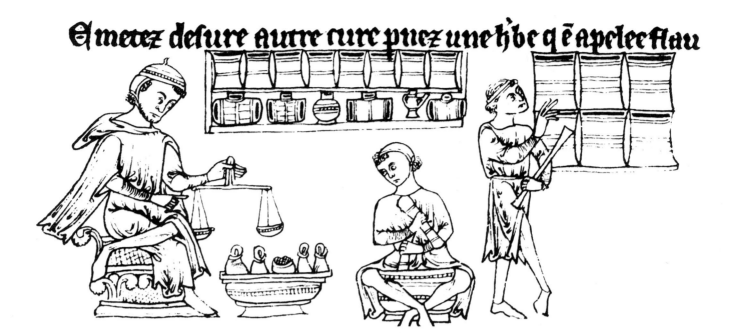

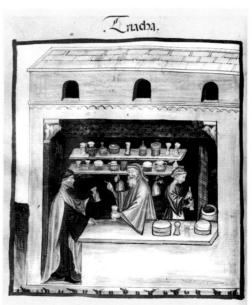

century and based on an Arab source dating from the eleventh century.

The later Middle Ages saw a plethora of writers producing works relating to medicine and pharmacy. Some of this increased activity was connected with the rise of universities—at Salerno, Padua, Paris, Bologna, Oxford, Cambridge, and Montpellier before the fourteenth century and at Prague in 1347. University-associated giants such as Arnald of Villanova, Roger Bacon, Albertus Magnus, and Ramon Lullius, all contributed to the literature of medicine and pharmacy.

Two other works of the later Middle Ages are particularly worthy of attention. In the thirteenth century there appeared a text attributed to Geber (Jābir) and an *Antidotarium*, or *Grabadin*, attributed to Mesuë. The work attributed to this Geber (usually called pseudo-Geber) reflected not only Arab knowledge but also the European chemistry of the late thirteenth century. The *Grabadin* of this Mesuë (usually called pseudo-Mesuë or Mesuë, Jr.), probably written in northern Italy, was for centuries the authoritative work on the composition of medicaments and was used in virtually every European pharmacy. The attribution of these texts to long-dead Arab scientists indicates the profound and enduring influence of Arab medicine and pharmacy and

Pharmacy scenes depicting the selecting, weighing, and grinding of drugs and their preparation at a brick oven. From a 13th-century French manuscript. Signature 0.1.20. Trinity College Library, Cambridge, England

An apothecary selling theriac to a client. Miniature from an illuminated manuscript— perhaps Veronese, c. 1400—of the *Tacuinum sanitatis*, a translation into Latin of an Arabic manual of health. The affluent appearance of the purchaser is in keeping with the costliness of the medication. Ms. serie Nov. no. 2644. Österreichische Nationalbibliothek, Vienna

the high esteem in which the Arab contributions were held.

THE EMERGENCE OF THE PHARMACIST AND THE PHARMACY SHOP

It is impossible to pinpoint the exact time and place in which the term "apothecary" and its various cognates first appeared in Western Europe. We do know that there was an oath required of *éspeciadors* (or *apothecayres*) in the city of Montpellier, France, in 1180. Ordinances and oaths pertaining to pharmacy were in effect in Marseilles between 1231 and 1253, in Avignon in 1242, and in Arles in 1245. In Melfi and Venice, ordinances were passed in 1231 and 1258, respectively. These ordinances and oaths arose in response to the perceived need to include the activities of the pharmacist in the regulation of medicine, thus bringing the pharmacist under the control of the medical police. It is no coincidence that the earliest attempts at regulation occurred in southern Italy, in the neighborhood of the medical school at Salerno, and at Montpellier in France, where there was also a medical school.

Guilds of pharmacists came into existence in this period. Pharmacists and physicians shared a guild in Florence by the end of the twelfth century; a guild of pharmacists existed in Verona in 1221; and guilds of pharmacists joined with spicers were to be found in thirteenth-century Paris, Avignon, and Dijon. Like all guilds, these sought to maintain a monopoly within the town, to protect the quality and integrity of their products, to establish and maintain prices, to control the training and length of service of apprentices, to establish rules for clerk and journeyman, and to control admission to the status of master in the guild. The last entailed an examination and usually the demonstration of a "masterpiece" (the compounding of a complex prescription). Such examinations were required by Marseilles in the thirteenth century and by a Parisian ordinance of 1484.

In mid-fourteenth-century Italy, guilds of pharmacists were granted monopolies on some two hundred different articles, from books to wax candles. Pharmacists also served as undertakers in fourteenth-century Italy—a testament to the difficulty the pharmacist had in earning a living from pharmaceutical work alone. The guild of pharmacists in Rome, founded as the Universitas Aromatariorum in the Middle Ages, designated as the Corporazione degli Speziali di Roma by papal decree in 1429, renamed the Nobile Collegio degli Speziali dell'Alma Città di Roma in 1602, is still in existence as Il Nobile Collegio Chimico Farmaceutico Romano.

Thus pharmacists in medieval Europe found a place of their own within the organization and purview of the town economy. Where there was not a sufficient number of pharmacists to form a guild, the pharmacist, in order to be able to operate within the town, joined a guild of another calling. In England, for instance, apothecaries and spicers (the terms were almost synonymous in the late thirteenth century) joined with the pepperers—dealers in pepper and spices—in what became known as the Company of Grocers. From the fourteenth

Regulations governing pharmacies promulgated by the burgomaster, council, and guild masters of Basel. Included were a provision that the apothecary—"man or woman"—take an oath before two witnesses when selling poison, to guarantee that no harm would result from the sale, and a provision prohibiting physicians from owning pharmacies. Early 14th century. Staatsarchiv, Basel

Veduta del Tempio di Antonino e Faustina in Campo Vaccino (View of the Temple of Antonino and Faustina in the Campo Vaccino). Engraving by Giovanni Battista Piranesi. Italian, 18th century. Now a church in the Forum in Rome, this former temple serves as the headquarters of Il Nobile Collegio Chimico Farmaceutico Romano, the guild of Roman pharmacists founded in 1429. ▼

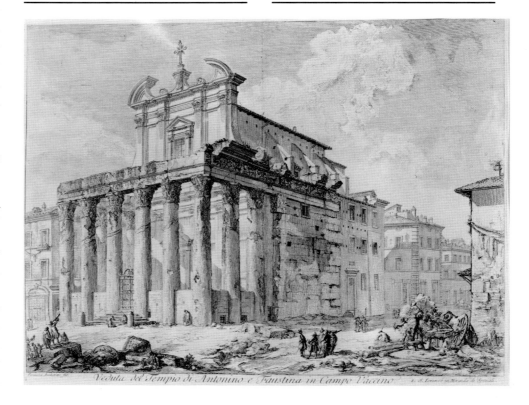

Veduta del Tempio di Antonino e Faustina in Campo Vaccino.

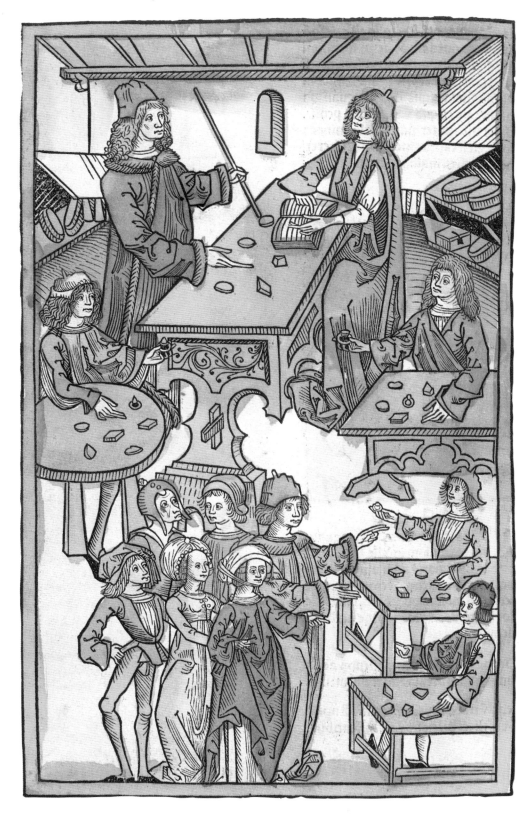

Precious stones being purchased from the master and his apprentices in a lapidary shop. Woodcut from the *Hortus sanitatis,* Mainz, 1491. National Library of Medicine, Bethesda

Facade of a 14th-century German pharmacy in Bad Frankenhausen am Kyffhäuser, home office of the Kyffhäuser Laboratorium, whose product the analgesic Doloresum is advertised on the reverse of the card

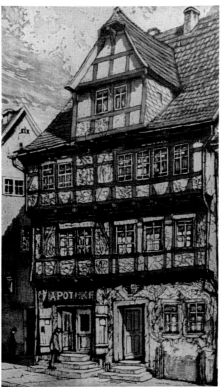

century on, apothecaries were recognized as a special section of the company; it was not until 1617 that they were chartered independently.

A crucial point in the history of pharmacy in the Middle Ages came between 1231 and 1240, with the issuing of a series of edicts—the *Constitutiones*—regulating the medical profession. These edicts, promulgated by the Holy Roman Emperor Frederick II, included what has been called the Magna Charta of pharmacy, for they separated pharmacy from medicine and legally recognized pharmacy as a separate profession for the first time in Western European history. The *Constitutiones* also set down certain requirements that were to become general throughout Western Europe: for the protection of the public, the pharmacy shop and practice were to be subject to official inspection, usually by the local or regional Collegium medicum, and the pharmacist was obliged, under oath, to prepare drugs of uniformly good quality.

The *Constitutiones* established two principles that were to be commonly accepted in parts of Western Europe (but did not, for example, influence Anglo-Saxon countries): first, a limiting (often on the basis of population) of the number of pharmacies that could operate in a given area and, second, the fixing of prices by the government. These two regulations were to be especially important, for they promoted the economic well-being of pharmacists and raised their social status. The edicts of Frederick II and the oaths and ordinances already mentioned defined the functions of pharmacists, their relation to the medical profession and to public health, and their moral responsibilities.

The shop of the European pharmacist of this period reflected Arab influence. (It is noteworthy that while at the time the term

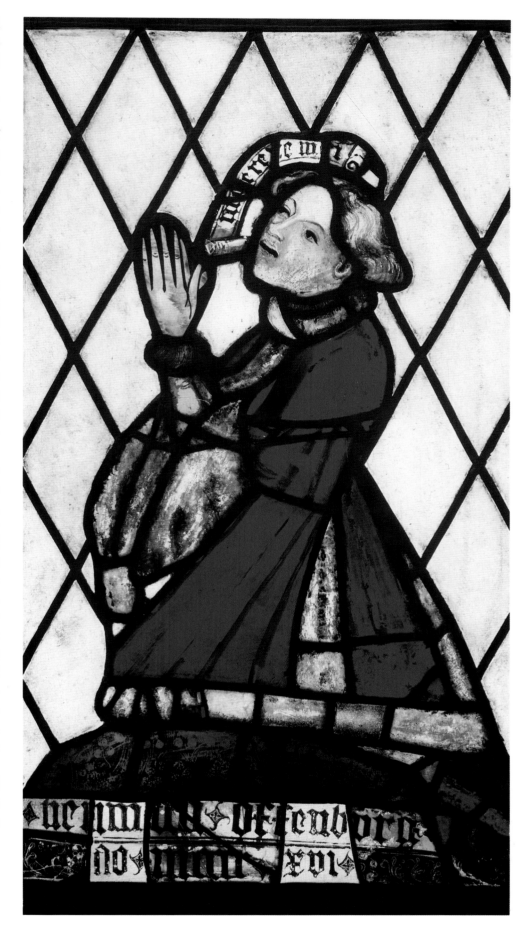

Portrait of the pharmacist Herman Offenburg. Stained-glass window formerly in the Kartauserkirche, Basel. 1416. Schweizerisches Pharmazie-Historisches Museum, Basel

apothecarius was being used in Marseilles, elsewhere terms like *éspeciador, espicier, speziale,* and spicer were in use, demonstrating the early association of the pharmacist and the spicer.) The shop in question was usually small, stall-like, and open to the marketplace. The counter folded up and helped to shutter the shop at night. Mortars and pestles and balances might be on display on the counter; behind it were shelves containing simples and prepared compounds. Drugs were in boxes, bottles, ceramic containers, or bags made of leather. The containers, which often bore distinguishing marks or names, were displayed on the shelves; bags might be suspended from the shelves or walls. Contemporary manuscript illustrations and miniatures show these shops as not unattractive, but the pharmacy shop did not attain spaciousness and true elegance until the Renaissance.

Medieval physicians prescribed about a thousand natural substances, mainly of plant origin. The materia medica of the Middle Ages was essentially that learned from the Greeks and Romans, as augmented by the Arabs. Herbalism was practiced at both the professional and the folk level. Although the theory of humoral pathology continued to be the basis on which drugs were prescribed, other explanations for the efficacy of certain drugs—some typical of the medieval mind—were in evidence. For example, the doctrine of signatures, now emphasizing the notion that God had marked—that is, "signed"—certain things in ways that indicated their therapeutic values, was generally accepted. Derived from ancient concepts of sympathetic magic, the doctrine also encompassed belief in the magical powers of names. Thus the plant stonebreak was deemed useful as a lithontriptic. A related concept attributed *virtu* (power) and *vis occulta* (hidden power) to certain drugs. Moreover, the idea that compound drugs gained power through the act of composition, a power greater than the properties of the constituents—a concept expounded by Galen and Avicenna—

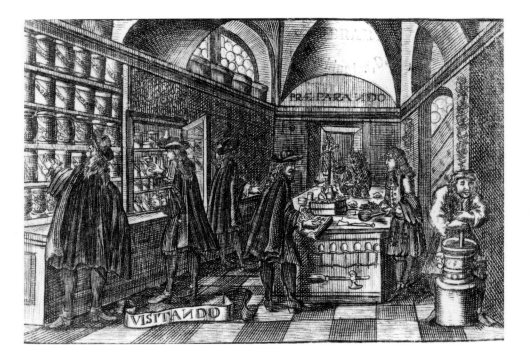

Salutis emporium. This engraving, the lower half of the frontispiece of Johann Michaelis, *Opera medica chirurgica* (Nuremberg, 1688), depicts the annual inspection of a pharmacy's stock to assure the quality and availability of the required drugs. National Library of Medicine, Bethesda

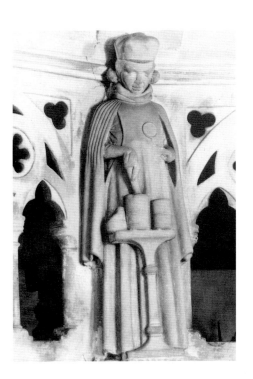

Stone statue of an apothecary in the Münster of Constance, West Germany. 13th century

gained such credence at Montpellier and elsewhere that it attained the status of empirical fact in the late thirteenth century.

The discussion of pharmacy in the Middle Ages cannot be concluded without some reference to a few special and exotic remedies that gained particular fame, among them unicorn's horn, mandrake, and precious gems. The unicorn was a ferocious mythical beast that could be captured only with the help of a young virgin of noble birth. Water or wine drunk from a cup that had been fashioned from its horn would protect the drinker from disease, injury, fire, and poison. Taken internally, powdered horn was prescribed for epilepsy, impotence, barrenness, the plague, smallpox, worms, and many other ills. It remained in favor until the eighteenth century. The pharmacist, no less gullible than others, substituted horn of rhinoceros, stag, oryx, and, especially, the tusk of the narwhal for unicorn horn. The last, a tusk several feet long, was often displayed in shops and became a symbol of pharmacy. The words Einhorn Apotheke still appear on shops in Germany.

The mandrake root sometimes bears an uncanny resemblance to the human form. Mandrake root was said to possess occult powers, and since it could resemble both the male and the female physique, it found use as an aphrodisiac and as a remedy for barrenness. Its main uses, however, were as an anaesthetic and anodyne. Fancies surrounding mandrake reached their height in the late Middle Ages—especially in Germany, where *Alraune,* mannequins carved out of the root, became symbols of divine favor. *Alraune* could confer invisibility, make the poor rich, bring their owners good fortune in love, and heal any disease. Mandrake remained in fashion until the seventeenth century.

The use of precious stones in medicine can be traced back to ancient civilizations. The brilliance, color, and rarity of gemstones caused special virtues to be attributed to them. As amulets, gems could ward off illness; as medicine, they possessed miraculous healing powers. In his *De lapidibus,* Marbode, the eleventh-century bishop of Rennes, described the marvelous medicinal and magical properties of sixty precious stones.

Thus the Middle Ages in Western Europe saw a perpetuation of the classical materia medica, augmented by that of the Arabs. Added were myth, magic, and faith, all of which had roles in medieval medicine and pharmacy. Nonetheless, for all this involvement with the occult, pharmacy in the Middle Ages made fundamental strides. These included the separation of pharmacy from medicine and the concomitant rise of the pharmacist as a functionary providing the whole range of pharmaceutical services; the establishment of the pharmacy shop; the rise of pharmaceutical organizations interested in promoting the economic wellbeing and professional competence and integrity of the practitioner; the recognition of the role of the pharmacist in providing health care and of society's need for the pharmacist; and the introduction of pharmacopoeial literature, which helped establish drug standards and defined the scope and ethics of the profession.

Page from a manuscript of *De Herba vettonica* by Antonius Musa, with miniature depicting the gathering of mandrake. 13th century. The mandrake root, which sometimes resembled the human figure, was said to emit so horrendous a shriek when pulled that the hearer might die of fright—hence the dog. Ms. 573, fol. 15v. Wellcome Institute Library, London

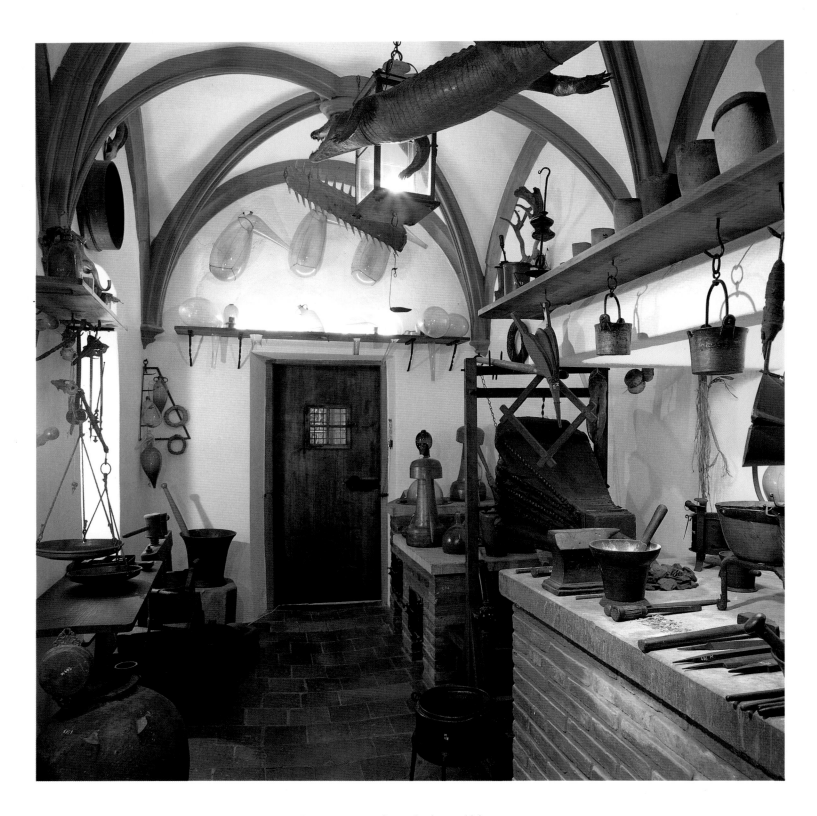

Reconstruction of an early chemical laboratory
with objects from the 17th through the 19th
century. Schweizerisches Pharmazie-
Historisches Museum, Basel

There is no sharp demarcation between the Middle Ages and the Renaissance. The late Middle Ages gave way to a changing society in the fourteenth century, but the changes were not without medieval antecedents. The notion equating the Renaissance with a rebirth of interest in the classical world hardly does justice to the impressive achievements of the period from 1350 to 1650. Although the advances that occurred in art, literature, philosophy, education, religion, and science during the Renaissance did have some classical foundation, they went far beyond Greek and Roman influence. Moreover, the Renaissance involved an outlook on life that was diametrically different from that of the Middle Ages: religion and otherworldliness dominated medieval times; secularism, individualism, and humanism characterized the Renaissance.

A PHARMACEUTICAL REVOLUTION

This new spirit and cultural ferment affected medicine and pharmacy in many ways; indeed the Renaissance was to see a challenge to the classical-Arab-medieval pharmacy that, when met, was to bring about change drastic enough both in kind and in degree to be called a revolution. The prime mover behind this revolution was Theophrastus Bombastus von Hohenheim, a sixteenth-century Swiss-born physician, philosopher, social theorist, alchemist, astrologer, rabble-rouser, and self-styled friend of necromancers and witches. In the spirit of the age, von Hohenheim blithely assumed the name of Paracelsus, by which he is known in history. He did this to point up his claim to superiority over the great Celsus, whose *De medicina,* first printed in 1478, was very popular.

Paracelsus roundly condemned the medical practice and medicine of his day,

THE RENAISSANCE

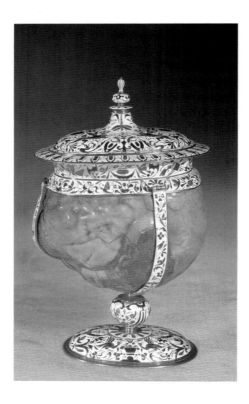

Goblet made from a bezoar, with enameled gold base, cover, and mounting. Austrian, c. 1600. Bezoars are concretions found in the stomachs and other organs of a variety of animals; those from Persian and Indian goats were valued most highly. The size of the bezoar forming the bowl of this goblet suggests that it came from a much larger creature. Genuine bezoars were costly and found places in the curiosity cabinets of the wealthy. In the Middle Ages the stone was purported to be a universal antidote and to possess remarkable detoxifying powers.
Kunsthistorisches Museum, Vienna

and he questioned everything—even the four Aristotelian elements. In their place Paracelsus named three nonmaterial principles of the human body: combustibility, the "sulfur" principle; liquidity and volatility, the "mercury" principle; and stability and solidity, the "salt" principle. Galenic humoral pathology was thus rejected; it was replaced by a new theory of disease and pharmacotherapy, one developed by the Paracelsians. This theory reflected the religious and mystical convictions of the master, whose "chemical philosophy" held that disease was a localized abnormality, not an imbalance of humors. The abnormality was a natural—that is, chemical—manifestation, and it was to be treated chemically. The body was a chemical laboratory, its chemical processes dependent upon a vital force, the *archaeus*. Disease was a morbid state of the *archaeus* that occurred when the chemistry of the body was disturbed; it could be righted by chemical remedies.

Consequently, tinctures, extracts, and essences played an important role in Paracelsian drug therapy. They were "chemicals" in that they were substances that had been transformed by the art of mixing and separating, often with the aid of fire, but with little chemical reaction as now understood. The separation of the pure from the impure was sought, as were chemical processes that would bring out the essential qualities of the drug, its spiritual as well as its chemical "quintessence."

In addition, a large number of metallic compounds were used by the Paracelsians, who proposed them on a fundamentally different basis and presented a new approach to pharmacotherapy. This new approach involved not only a reliance on chemical remedies but the suppositions that there was a specific remedy for each illness and that like cured like (as opposed to the Galenic concept of contraries). The theory that like cured like—related to the doctrine of signatures, to which Paracelsus was partial—was responsible for the use of such remedies as Oil of Man's Skull for epilepsy.

Basic to the preparation of medicines during this period was the art of the alchemist. Paracelsus gave impetus to a trend, in evidence since the time of the Arabs, that saw the art of pharmacy become increasingly associated with alchemy and hence with chemistry. The Paracelsians developed distillation techniques that were suitable for volatile substances, and thereafter the use of alcohols, spirits, essences, and oils increased significantly. Strong mineral acids were also discovered, among them oil of vitriol and aquafortis. Finally, metallurgical advances provided supplies of mercury, antimony, and lead, and lesser amounts of arsenic, iron, gold, copper, cobalt, bismuth, and zinc. From these were produced new compounds like corrosive mercuric sublimate and calomel.

These advances in pharmaceutical chemistry had to be taught to the physicians who were to use the new drugs and, especially, to the pharmacists who were to prepare them. Several works provided the needed instruction. One was the *Basilica chymica* of Oswald Croll, published in Frankfurt in 1608 or 1609 and issued many times thereafter in Germany and in Switzerland, France, and England. This influential volume, which contained a strong defense of Paracelsus, included an essay on the doctrine of signatures. It also listed drugs and gave directions for their preparation.

Another influential work was the *Tyrocinium chymicum* of Jean Beguin, printed in Paris in 1608. Even more popular than Croll's opus, it went through some fifty editions and was translated into both French and English. The growing rapport between chemistry and pharmacy is evident in Beguin's statement, in the *Tyrocinium,* that "Chymistry is the art of dissolving natural mixed bodies, and of coagulating them when dissolved, and of reducing them into salubrious, safe and grateful medicaments."

Two other important publications of the seventeenth century were the *Pharmacopoea medico-physica* by Johann Schroeder, first issued in Ulm in 1641, and the *Ortus medicinae* of Jean Baptist van Helmont. The

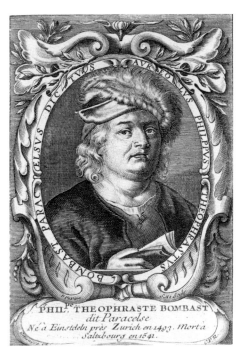

Portrait of Theophrastus Bombastus von Hohenheim (1493–1541), known as Paracelsus, father of the pharmaceutical revolution that questioned Galenic ideas and emphasized chemical remedies. Engraving by Michel Odieuvre. German, c. 1750

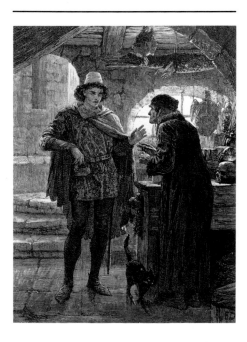

Romeo and the Apothecary. Engraving by Quesnel after a painting by Frank Dicksee. British, c. 1875. In Act V, Scene 1, of Shakespeare's *Romeo and Juliet,* Romeo offers an apothecary the exorbitant sum of forty ducats for a dram of poison. The apothecary accepts: "My poverty, but not my will, consents."

Ortus medicinae, published in Amsterdam in 1648, contained a section on the dispensing of "modern" remedies directed to the pharmacist. The seventeenth-century pharmacist thus became something of a chemist (as well as botanist), and the pharmacist's workplace became a chemical laboratory where the processes of distillation, evaporation, incineration, sublimation, and lixivation were put into practice.

PARACELSIANS VS. GALENISTS

The fame that Paracelsus enjoyed during his lifetime rested on accounts of near miraculous cures that he had accomplished. Following his death, in 1541, his fame grew, and within a century hundreds of Paracelsian texts, almost all of which referred to chemical remedies, had been published. By the end of the sixteenth century there was a whole new body of literature on the materia medica.

Most Paracelsian physicians and authors were Germans, but events in France and in England had a significant impact on the history of pharmacy. Because the Paracelsian approach to medical knowledge differed so fundamentally from what had become accepted, a major confrontation developed between Paracelsians and the entrenched medical establishment. The confrontation was sharpened by the impact of the humanists, who disdained the works of Dioscorides and Pliny, both highly popular in the late Middle Ages, and exalted works that were less generally known, particularly the physiological and anatomical treatises of Galen.

In France, the confrontation, aggravated by the fact that many Paracelsian physicians were Huguenots, was particularly acrimonious. The late sixteenth and the early seventeenth century saw the battle fought in the courts and in the press. Polemical exchanges between the antagonists were translated from Latin into French and later into German and English. And as this dueling continued, tension grew between the medical faculty of the University of Montpellier, which was Paracelsian, and that of the University of Paris, which had remained staunchly Galenist. The chemical physicians persisted and continued to gain adherents throughout the country.

Title page of the *Pharmacopoeia Londinensis* (a hand-dated 1639 reissue of the first edition, of 1618). Portraits of Hippocrates, Galen, Mesuë, and Avicenna emphasize the traditional and authoritarian nature of the materia medica.

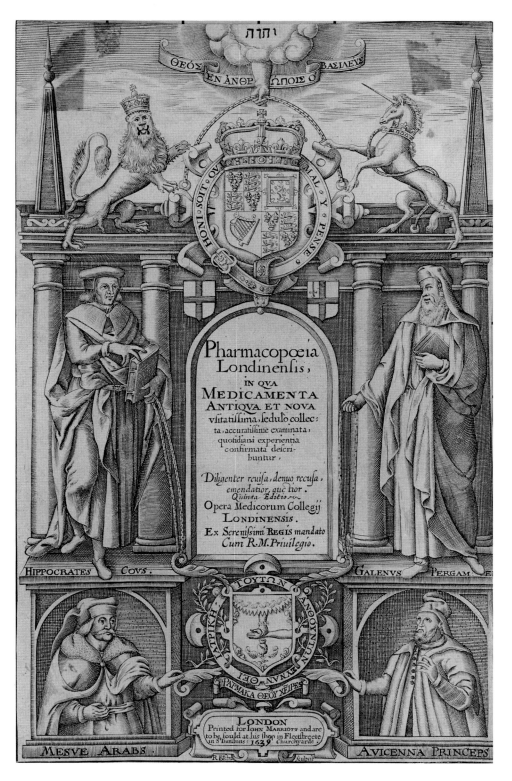

In England, the confrontation was less tempestuous. Polemics and debate there were, but the medical establishment—the Royal College of Physicians of London—was more willing than its Parisian counterpart to accept chemical remedies. The Royal College, however, insisted that it would decide which chemical remedies were acceptable and how they were to be prepared. To assure compliance by the pharmacists, the Royal College developed its own pharmacopoeia, the *Pharmacopoeia Londinensis*.

Planned as early as 1589, the *Pharmacopoeia Londinensis* did not appear until 1618, and then was largely the work of a French Huguenot physician, Theodore Turquet de Mayerne, who had been educated at Montpellier and who had had his difficulties with the Parisian traditionalists. The Royal College's pharmacopoeia accepted the "more recent" chemical remedies that "might be a servant to the dogmatic medicine" and that "might act as auxiliaries." Included were metals and minerals that had been in the materia medica at least since the time of Dioscorides, although only for external use. Included also were such Paracelsian remedies as *crocus metallorum* (crocus of antimony), *vitrum antimonii* (vitrified antimony), *mercurius vitae* ("mercury of life"—butter of antimony), *turbith minerale* (mercuric sulfate), and, probably the most recent of all, *mercurius dolcis* (calomel). This willingness to make a place for chemical remedies and use them as well as the traditional galenical armamentarium was a typical Elizabethan compromise.

IATROCHEMISTRY

The disputatious literature of the Paracelsians and their antagonists of the early seventeenth century was widely read by the foremost European scholars. The issue had shifted from the anti-Galenism of the Paracelsians to their new philosophical concepts, which sought to replace ancient knowledge with "true" religion and with chemically based observations of nature.

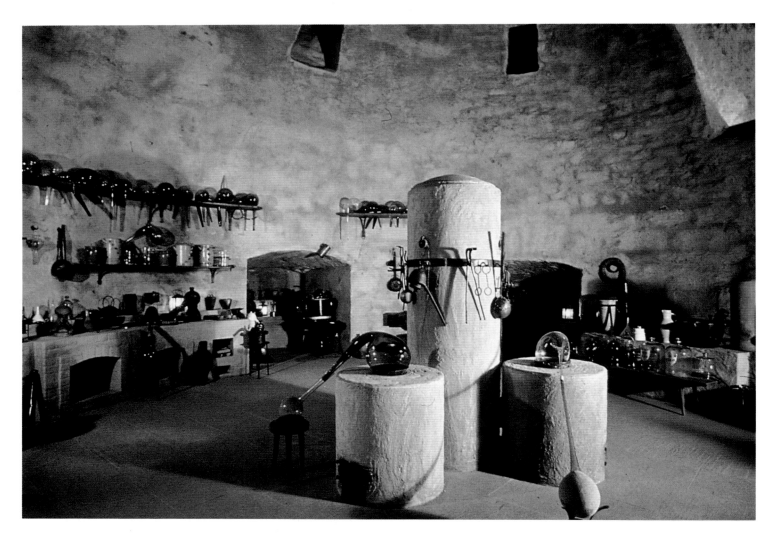

Reconstruction of an early chemical laboratory with objects from the 17th through the 19th century. Deutsches Apotheken-Museum, Heidelberg

Chemically prepared medicines had come to stay. Van Helmont—who is regarded as the founder of the iatrochemical school—propounded a medical system that, encompassing the idea of the vital force, the *archaeus,* reflected the notion that illness indicated chemical changes in the body. These notions led to the medical theory of François de Boë, known as Sylvius, in the seventeenth century. Sylvius postulated a series of fermentations that took place in the body with the ingestion of food. These, influenced by the temperature of the body and by its vital spirit, determined the acid/alkaline balance of the body. Good health obtained when alkalinity and acidity were in the proper proportions, in quantity and quality. Illness was an "acrimony," an excess of one or the other, and balance could be restored by drugs—chemical drugs—of a contrasting nature. This was the essence of iatrochemistry, and iatrochemical physi-

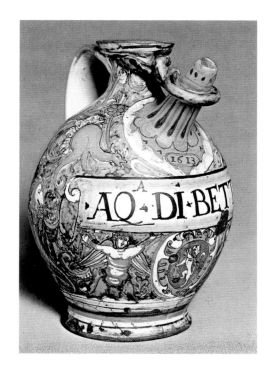

Ceramic syrup jar labeled *Aqua di Bettonica* (Wood Betony Water). Faenza, 1613. Museo Civico, Castello Sforzesco, Milan

cians not only prescribed many new agents but found a rationale for prescribing many older ones.

NEW AND OLD WORLDS AND NEW DRUGS

The Renaissance has already been described as an age of excitement—excitement arising from new scientific advances, new artistic and architectural developments, changing political and economic forms, and new religious ferment. There

Woodcut showing plants being gathered, dried, chopped, and distilled for medicines, while physicians are in consultation and a patient is being attended. From Adam Lonitzer, *Kreuterbuch,* Frankfurt, 1593. National Library of Medicine, Bethesda

was adventure and excitement beyond Europe, too—and wealth to be gained—in the exploration of the New World and in the discovery of new paths to older worlds. Western Europeans were eager to circumvent the Venetians' monopoly on trade with the Near East, a trade in which drugs and spices were of prime importance. This eagerness, combined with thirst for power in the nation-states of the West, dynamic new national economies, and the sheer vigor of the emerging mercantilist system, drove the Spanish, Portuguese, English, French, and Dutch into competition for new worlds, new trade, and new colonies.

Drugs and spices played an important role in all this, for the Venetian monopoly

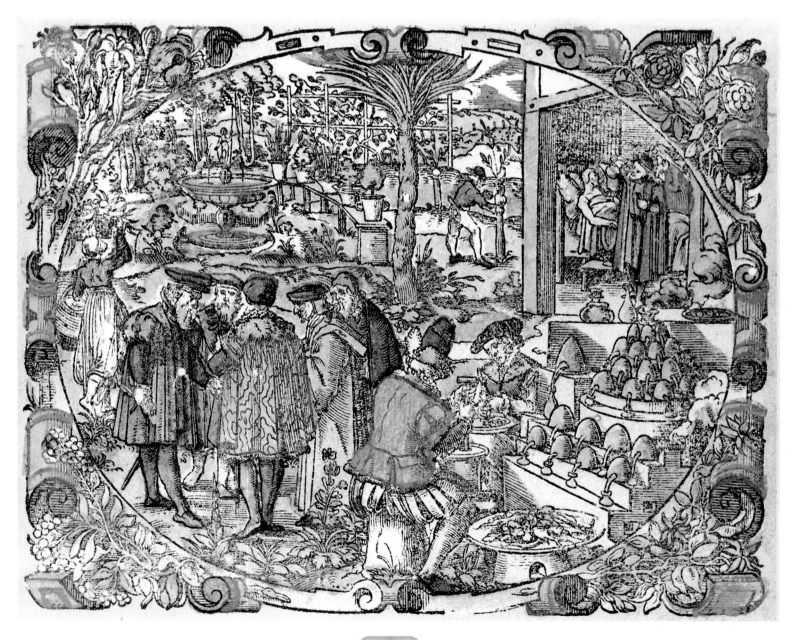

made drugs from the Near and Far East extremely costly. More than mere gain was involved here: new worlds could potentially mean new drugs, and returning adventurers often regaled European courts with stories about the exotic plants they had encountered, many of which were said to possess miraculous curative powers. Ship captains and "sea hawks" were well aware of the potential value of finding new sources for old drugs and of discovering new drugs. In January 1570, for instance, Philip II of Spain directed the physician Francisco Hernández, bound for America, to gather all the information he could "from all physicians, surgeons, Spanish and native herbalists ... and ... obtain an account of all medical herbs, trees, plants, and seeds." Similarly, in 1585 the British captain Richard Hakluyt ranked "men skilful in all kinds of drugs" second only to "men skilful in all mineral causes" on his list of the thirty-one kinds of men he needed for a forthcoming expedition.

Even before Hernández sailed for Mexico, an Aztec physician, Martin de la Cruz, compiled an herbal in his native language, and in 1552 another Aztec, Juannes Badianus (described only as "an Indian from Sochimilco"), translated it into Latin. The Badianus Manuscript, which is in the Vatican Library, did not appear in print until 1935, when an English translation was issued. A work that did find its way into print was a book by Garcia da Orta, who was forced out of his native Portugal by the Inquisition, traveled extensively in the Middle East, and published *Coloquios dos simples, e drogos he cousas medicinais da India* in Goa in 1563. In its pages the botany and materia medica of India found their way to the West for the first time. Da Orta's work was soon followed by the two books of Nicolás Monardes, *El uno que traicté de todas las cosas que traen de nuestras Indias Occidentales* and *Segunda parte del libro de las cosas,* published in Seville in 1565 and 1571, respectively. A 1574 publication combining both books was soon translated into Latin, Italian, French, and English. Some fifty issues of it

The Guaiac Seller. Woodcut from the title page of Ulrich von Hutten, *Von der wunderlichen Arzney des Holtz Guaiacum.* Strasbourg, 1519. National Library of Medicine, Bethesda

have been recorded. The welcome that Monardes' descriptions of the medicinal plants of Spanish America received is indicated by the title of the English version, published in London in 1577: *Joyful Newes out of the Newe Founde Worlde.*

The magnitude of the new challenge—there was a professional imperative to find a counterpart for each of the over 600 plants discussed in Dioscorides' *De materia medica* and also to fit each plant into the Galenic system of humoral pathology—is apparent from the fact that Hernández collected and described more than 3,000 plants in his seven years of travel through New Spain. He classified each according to its obvious physiological effect (for example, purging and sweating), and he sought to assign Galenic classifications to each (hot, hot and moist, cold, cold and dry, etc.). Hernández may even have tried out some of these drugs clinically in the Royal Hospital for Indians in Mexico City.

These new drugs were to give pause to the conservative medical faculty of the Uni-

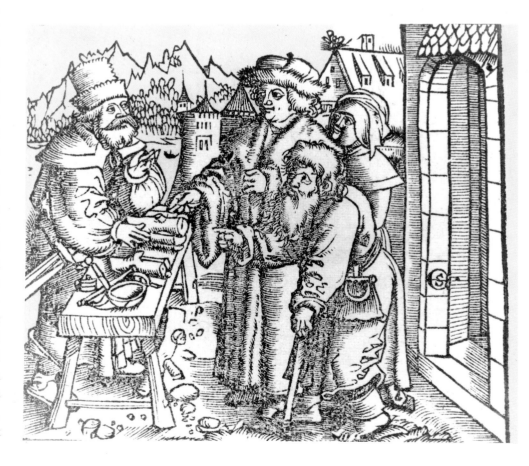

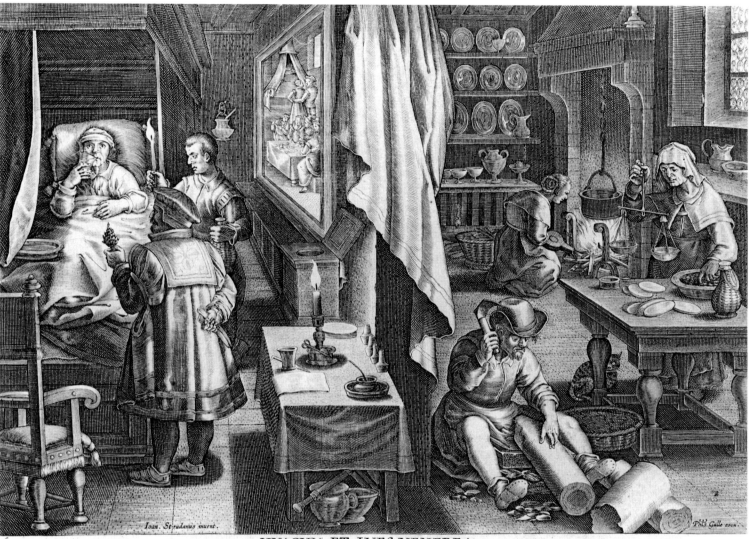

IoaN. Stradanus inuent.

6.

HYACVM, ET LVES VENEREA.

Grauata morbo ab hocce membra mollia   Leuabit ista sorpta coctio arboris.

versity of Paris. Already troubled by the inroads of iatrochemistry, they were further disturbed when drugs that were not part of the traditional materia medica began arriving from distant parts of the world. Thus cinchona, the Peruvian bark, was to be characterized in the seventeenth century as "an impertinent innovation" by Guy Patin, a leader of the faculty opposition to Paracelsianism and the new drugs.

During the Age of Discovery the armamentarium of European physicians was enriched both by more plentiful supplies of exotic drugs, such as camphor, ginger, and rhubarb, and by drugs previously unknown to them. Outstanding among the new resources acquired in the sixteenth century were guaiacum, introduced by the Span-

Hyacum et lues venerea (Guaiac and the Plague of Venus). Engraving by Philipp Galle after Stradanus (Jan van der Straet). Dutch, 1570. The preparation of guaiacum for the treatment of syphilis is shown at the right: the resinous raw material is chopped, weighed, and boiled. At the left, the patient is taking the medicine.

iards from the West Indies; jalap and mechoacan, introduced by the Spaniards from Mexico and sent to Europe in large quantities; capivi, introduced by the Portuguese from Brazil; balsam of Tolu and balsam of Peru, introduced by Monardes; winterian, introduced by the British from the Strait of Magellan; sassafras, whose discovery in southeastern North America has been attributed to the Spanish and to the French; and sarsaparilla, which Monardes said was imported into Seville from New Spain. Sassafras is of special interest, both for the "sassafras rush" that ensued and for the great profits that Sir Walter Raleigh was to gain from the bark and wood—until prices fell sharply because of the ubiquity of the tree. Coca leaves, another American drug, were not to find medicinal use until the nineteenth century, but the perversion of cocaine (extracted from the leaves in the nineteenth century) into an agent of personal and social destruction in our own time was presaged by the denunciation of the chewing of the leaves in 1563 by the Audiencia, the ruling body of Lima, as "un delusio del demonio," since it diverted the natives from the true God.

The greatest of the discoveries was cinchona. It was the Jesuits in Peru in the seventeenth century who were responsible for recognizing its antimalarial properties. It is not likely that the natives knew the value of the bark, and the myth that the Countess of Cinchona introduced it into Spain after it cured her of malaria has long since been discredited.

The same period also marked the introduction of the European materia medica to the Orient. Starting in the seventeenth century, the Dutch brought Western medicine and Western drugs to Japan. Theriac, oculi cancri, and nux vomica, among others, found a place in the Japanese materia medica by the end of the eighteenth century—a debt the Japanese were to repay in 1887 with the isolation of ephedrine from *Ephedra sinica.*

HERBALS, PHARMACOPOEIAS, AND HANDBOOKS

One of the most notable products of the printing press, in its infancy in the fifteenth century, was the herbal. A significant feature of the herbal was the illustrations, intended to help Renaissance botanists differentiate the flora of Northern Europe from that of Southern Europe and the Mediterranean region. The earliest printed herbals probably appeared in 1477; by 1483, illustrated herbals had appeared.

Herbals in Dutch and in German, as well as Latin, soon followed. Especially note-

Woodcut by Hieronymus Brunschwygk from the *Hortus sanitatis,* Augsburg, 1496. While a pharmacist studies his book of recipes, a physician points to the ingredients he wants. National Library of Medicine, Bethesda

worthy was the *Gart der Gesundheit,* also known as the *Herbarius zu Teutsch,* issued in 1485. The woodcuts in it were handsome illustrations, well drawn from life. In 1491, a much larger version of the *Gart der Gesundheit* appeared under the title *Hortus sanitatis.* It included sections on the action of drugs and sections on animals and minerals. A French translation of the *Hortus,* called the *Arbolayre,* was published in Besançon in 1487–88. *Le grand Herbier en françois,* published in Paris about 1500, derived its figures from the *Hortus.* In England, the *Hortus* appeared as the *Grete Herbal;* it was published in London in 1526, with the stated aim of "enformynge how men may be holpen with grene herbs of the gardyn and wedys of the fildys as well as by costly receptes of the potycaryes prepared."

However, it was the *De materia medica* of Dioscorides that had the greatest impact in the early Renaissance. By the mid-sixteenth century his work was available in a great many editions and translations, some with commentaries. Of the many editions of Jean Ruel's Latin translations of Dioscorides, the first appeared in Paris in 1516. These were used by Pietro Andrea Mattioli, who issued the first of several Italian editions in 1544. Mattioli's version added marginal commentary and much-needed synonyms in Greek, Arabic, German, and French. He was in regular correspondence with a good many European botanists and absorbed into his work many new findings of Renaissance botany, thereby helping to dispel some of the confusion that had entered the materia medica of Dioscorides in the centuries of translation and retranslation. If Dioscorides provided the Renaissance with the key to the ancient materia medica, Mattioli was his prophet. It has been estimated that 32,000 copies of the early editions of Mattioli were printed in Venice alone.

Mattioli was not the only translator of and commentator on Dioscorides. Amatus Lusitanus, a Portuguese Jewish exile, published *In Dioscoridis . . . de materia medica . . . enarrationes* in Venice in 1553 and in Lyons

menſch nütze mag auch ſchwäger fro
wē zů behůtē od̉ zů beſchirmē/ vñ dari

mag d̉ gemeī mā es ſy vff ſchlöſſer od̉
vff landē ſie habē apotecken od̉ kein.

Von den ſimplicibus oder entzigē ſtückē zů
bewaren d̉ menſchē vor der peſtilentz doch zů gelaſſen medritatum vñ tiriana.

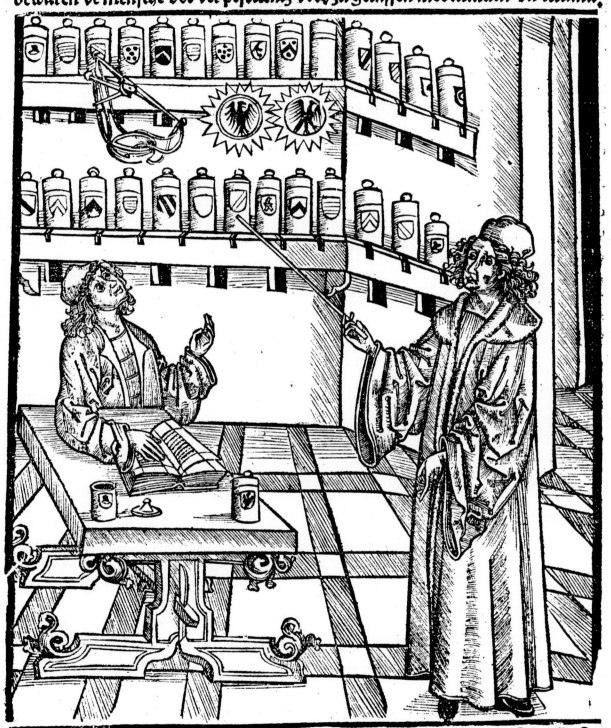

A Opfer von dem
krut mā leſen iſt d̉z ein burger
zů Baur̉ der groß vnd vil huß

geſinds hett der floch nie kein ſterben
der peſtilentz vnnd ſtarb auch nie kei
ner vß ſeinem huß/ d̉er ward auch
gefraget von einem wyſen mann. wie

in 1558; his temerity in taking issue with Mattioli on certain matters subjected him to a tirade of vilification by Mattioli, a not atypical reaction, at the time, to criticism. There were also the commentaries of Valerius Cordus, called the *Annotationes* [also *Adnotationes*] *in Dioscoridis de medica materis libros,* published, usually in conjunction with other works, in Frankfurt in 1549, in Paris in 1551, and in Strasbourg in 1561.

This hardly completes the account of Renaissance herbal literature. Among the many whose books were part of the flood of herbals published in the sixteenth century were Otto Brunfels, Hieronymus Bock, Leonhart Fuchs, Rembert Dodoens, and Jacobus Theodorus Tabernaemontanus. It must be remembered that herbals were only part of the pharmaceutical literature of the time; the works on chemistry of Croll, Beguin, van Helmont, Hieronymus Brunschwygk, Conrad Gesner, and others were also part of the literature of the age.

Another genre that proliferated during the Renaissance was the pharmacopoeia (sometimes titled dispensatorium or enchiridion). There were works by individuals, collective works by several authors, and works by medical and pharmaceutical organizations and authorities. Whatever the source, official or unofficial, the early pharmacopoeia was intended to do several things: first, it was to set down the formulas that were considered standard by the issuing authority; second, it was to give directions for compounding to the pharmacist; third, and most important, it was to give the physician control over the composition and strength of the drugs he prescribed and oversight of the practice of pharmacy. Early pharmacopoeias were all produced by physicians or medical groups. Not until the late eighteenth century did pharmacists begin taking over the responsibility of putting out pharmacopoeias.

It is now customary to consider the pharmacopoeia a collection of drugs, formulas, and directions that are mandatory for physicians and pharmacists in a given jurisdiction by virtue of a decree or enactment of

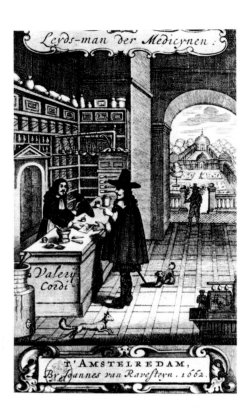

Title page of the *Leyds-man der Medicynen,* a Dutch translation of the *Dispensatorium* by Valerius Cordus, 1662, showing a Dutch pharmacy with an adjacent herb garden.

Portrait of Pierre Quthe. Painting by François Clouet. French, 1562. A Parisian apothecary and scholar, Quthe had a famous botanical garden, to which the open herbal on the table alludes. The Louvre, Paris ▶

government authorities. Without this legal sanction such a collection should be termed a receptary or formulary, regardless of its actual title. Thus the Florentine publication of 1499, a milestone in the history of pharmaceutical literature, properly called itself the *Nuovo receptario.* It emanated from the guild of physicians and pharmacists of Florence, and it was binding on the members of the guild, but it lacked government sanction, as did the *Concordie apothecariorum* of the Collegium Pharmacopolarum of Barcelona, issued in 1511.

The distinction of having the first official pharmacopoeia goes to the city of Nuremberg, where municipal authorities made the *Dispensatorium pharmacopolarum* of Valerius Cordus the official pharmacopoeia for the city in 1546. Other cities soon followed: Augsburg in 1564, Cologne in 1565, Florence in 1567, Rome in 1583.

The pharmacist's handbook is a third genre in the body of pharmaceutical literature. An example is the *Dispensarium ad aromaticus* of Nicole Prévost, printed in Lyons between 1478 and 1488; in addition to describing the simples and 575 composites, it contained a pharmaceutical vocabulary. The major work in this area—and the one which demonstrated that the art of pharmacy had achieved independent status—came from Italy. There, in the middle of the fifteenth century, the physician Saladin di Asculi wrote his *Compendium aromatariorum,* published in Bologna in 1488. The work covered all the scientific, practical, and institutional aspects of pharmacy, as distinct from medicine, and earned the reputation of being an indispensable vade mecum. It became a model for later textbooks. Jean Renou's *Institutionum pharmaceuticarum,* which appeared in Paris in 1608 and at least six times thereafter in France, Germany, and Switzerland, was clearly based on Saladin.

Saladin's work was followed in Italy by the *Lumen apothecariorum* (*Light of the Apothecaries*) of Quiricus de Augustis, published in Turin in 1492. This work was enlarged and called the *Luminare majus*

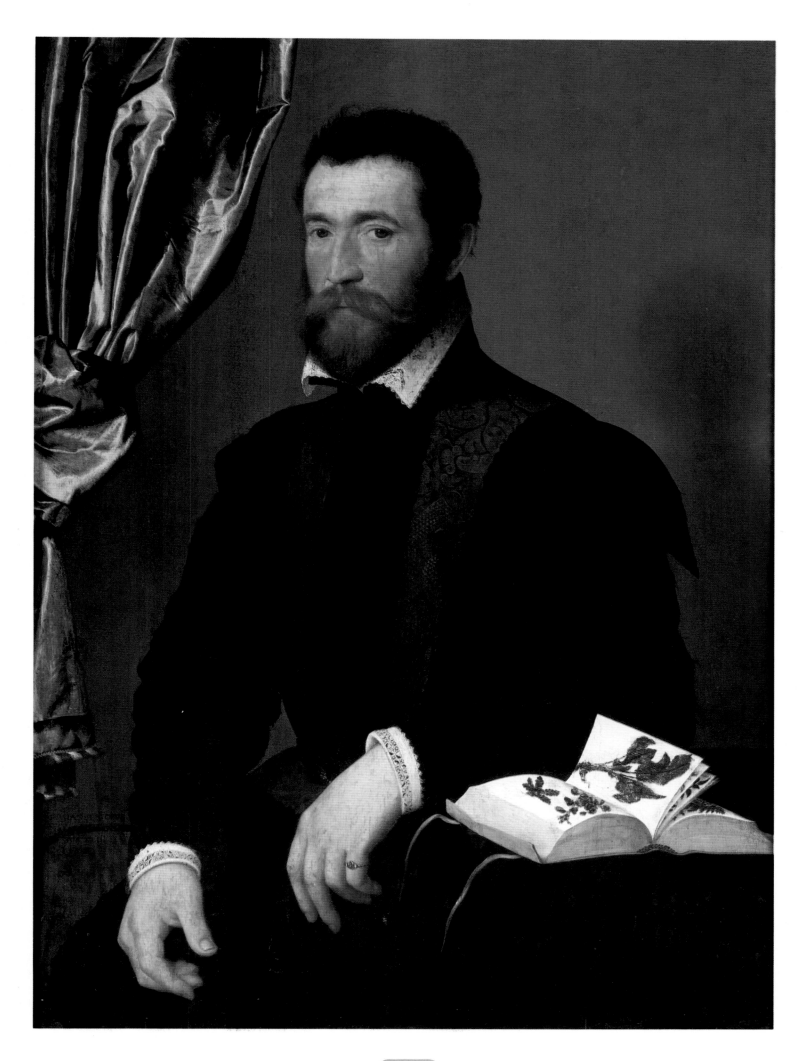

(*The Greater Luminary*) by the pharmacist Jacobus Manliis de Bosco. Published in Venice, it became recognized in several European cities as the authoritative guide to the practice of pharmacy. It was followed by similar works by other pharmacists: Paulus Suardus in Italy, Pedro Mateo in Spain, and Michel Dusseau in France.

UNIVERSITY EDUCATION

Materia medica was naturally a subject of study at the medical schools of medieval and Renaissance Europe. Padua and Bologna actually established separate chairs in the subject in the 1530s, and in the 1540s Padua and Pisa established the first university botanical gardens. As early as 1536, Paris required pharmacy apprentices to attend two lectures a week given by a member of the faculty of medicine, and those aspiring to the status of master pharmacist at Poitiers were required, in 1588, to attend lectures in the art and science of pharmacy for one year.

The beginnings of university education in pharmacy go back to Montpellier. In the early sixteenth century the eminence of Montpellier's pharmacists, and the availability of private courses given by prominent physicians, drew students interested in pharmacy to that city from all over France. In 1550 a regulation prohibited such private courses and required teachers to lecture publicly to students of surgery and pharmacy. By 1588, the guild of pharmacists had received permission from the university to establish and maintain a drug collection for teaching purposes, and a master pharmacist, Bernardin Duranc, was designated as "demonstrator." University education in pharmacy was further advanced with the establishment of chairs in botany and anatomy in 1593 and of surgery and pharmacy in 1601. It is not surprising that Montpellier, having favored the new chemical remedies, should have created a chair of pharmaceutical chemistry in 1675.

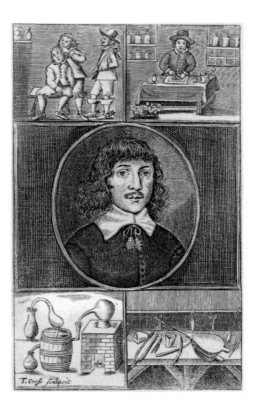

Portrait of Nicholas Culpeper by Thomas Cross. English, c. 1680. Culpeper (1616–1654), an apothecary's apprentice, became a popular London astrologer-physician and a prolific medical writer. His unauthorized English translation of a London pharmacopoeia (1649) was the first full-size medical book published in America (Boston, 1720).

And it is no more surprising that in the late sixteenth century a letter from the faculty and administration of the university attesting to the fact that its bearer had satisfactorily completed course work there was a true mark of distinction for a pharmacist.

THE PHARMACIST

The Renaissance saw the decline of the medieval city-state and the emergence of a larger political unit, the nation-state. Western European society began to reflect the ethnic, linguistic, cultural, and nationalistic particularism that was to characterize the European scene in modern times. Pharmacy was no exception to this trend.

Both the practice of pharmacy and the role of the pharmacist varied considerably from country to country. In Italy, as might be expected, traditions dating from the time of Frederick II prevailed during the Renaissance. In 1429, a papal edict reiterated the responsibility of the Corporazione degli Speziali di Roma to oversee the training of pharmacists, to regulate the location of pharmacies, and to set prices for medicines. Although a complete separation of pharmacy and medicine was technically in effect in Italy—and commercial association between the two groups was forbidden in Rome and other cities—in Florence a physician could employ a pharmacist and a pharmacist could employ a physician. Elsewhere in Italy it was likewise possible for a physician and a pharmacist to establish a joint enterprise and share profits. That such relationships continued for centuries is confirmed by a famous eighteenth-century canvas in the Accademia in Venice, Pietro Longhi's *La Bottega dello Speciale*—although there is a question as to which figure is the physician and which the pharmacist.

In Spain the guilds of pharmacists gained in strength, and their professional activities and associations received royal sanction. An intriguing regulation in Barcelona prohibited the practice of pharmacy by anyone who had not been active in the profession for two years, and in 1548 members of the Barcelona Colegio, or guild, were required by law to study botany and make a quarterly investigation of the local flora. The Spanish pharmacists' guilds assumed responsibility for policing their own members. When, in the late sixteenth century, a Barcelona pharmacist was found to be making up compositions that lacked required ingredients, stocking medications that were old, valueless, and unfit for use, and falsely labeling certain products, he was barred forever from his profession and deprived of the right to hold public office. His false medicines were burned and his share of the money in the guild treasury was confiscated. The town crier proclaimed the delinquent pharmacist's downfall through every street of the city.

In Renaissance France, the pharmacist did not enjoy the same friendly relations with physicians and officials as were usual in Italy and Spain. The French pharmacist was often called an *épicier* (the appellation *apothicaire,* which first appeared in 1270, did not come into general use until about 1400). The title *épicier* indicated the pharmacists' close association with the spicers. There were constant jurisdictional disputes between the two groups. At times the law recognized a distinction between them: pharmacy, a 1514 statute said, "requires much art, science, experience and knowledge of drugs as well as of compounding of prescriptions that enter the human body." At other times pharmacists and spicers were forced into the same guild, as they were by a law promulgated in 1560. Although it did not put an end to the differences between the two, a royal decree of 1777 finally separated the pharmacists and spicers; the Collège de Pharmacie was established and the spicers were permitted to engage in the wholesale trade in drugs and to trade in herbs.

More vituperative were the quarrels between physicians and pharmacists. Physicians contended that pharmacists were

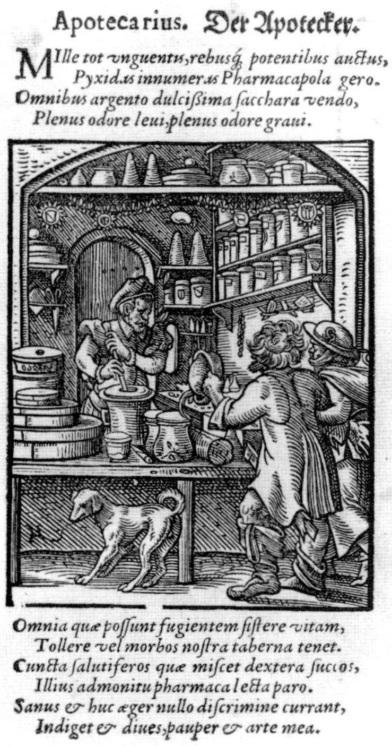
Apotecarius. Der Apotecker.

Mille tot unguentis, rebusq́ potentibus auctus,
Pyxidas innumeras Pharmacapola gero.
Omnibus argento dulcißima ſacchara vendo,
Plenus odore leui, plenus odore graui.

Omnia quæ poſſunt fugientem ſiſtere vitam,
Tollere vel morbos noſtra taberna tenet.
Cuncta ſalutiferos quæ miſcet dextera ſuccos,
Illius admonitu pharmaca lecta paro.
Sanus & huc æger nullo diſcrimine currant,
Indiget & diues, pauper & arte mea.

Page from a book of trades, *Eygentliche Beschreibung aller Stände auf Erden*, by Hans Sachs, published in Frankfurt in 1568, with woodcut illustration *Apotecarius. Der Apotecker* by Jost Amman. Ars Medica Collection, Philadelphia Museum of Art

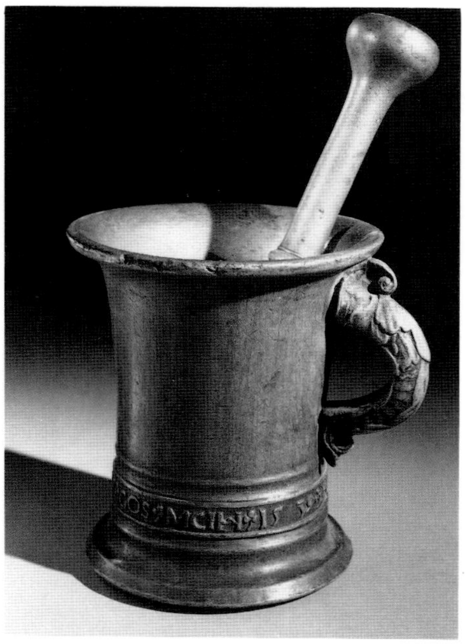

Bronze mortar and pestle. German, 1533. National Museum of American History, Smithsonian Institution, Washington, D.C.

ignorant of their calling, that they diagnosed and prescribed although not qualified to do either, and that they were constantly making errors in compounding and dispensing. The chief antagonist of the pharmacists was Symphorien Champier, a physician who favored the use of native plants and rejected Arab authorities. About 1513 he issued his *Myroel des Apothecaires,* whose subtitle reveals his position: *The mirror of the apothecaries and druggists in which is demonstrated how the apothecaries commonly make mistakes in several medicines contrary to the intention of the Greeks . . . on the basis of the wicked and faulty teachings of the Arabs.* When pharmacists responded in kind to the *Myroel,* a war of tracts began that was to spread to England and Germany.

The disputes between French pharmacists and physicians continued well into the seventeenth century. The pharmacists' chief antagonist now was the head of the Paris faculty, Guy Patin, whose disapproval of cinchona has been noted. He accused the pharmacists of fostering both chemical remedies and the new plant drugs from abroad, which the faculty opposed. Pharmacists, then as now, felt that it was their responsibility and right to fill any prescription properly proffered. The quarrel was at its height when, in 1625, there appeared a low-priced manual, *Le Médecin charitable,* written by a physician named Philibert Guibert, which gave directions for the procurement of raw materials and for compounding. This work of popular pharmacy went through numerous French editions and was translated into other languages. Its popularity led Patin to declare, in 1649, that the pharmacists of Paris had been ruined by this do-it-yourself pharmaceutical manual. The pharmacists managed to hold on, nevertheless, and the medical faculty eventually had to concede the value of the newer remedies.

In England, the pharmacist, usually called "apothecary," had been associated with the spicer since the Middle Ages. Edward I's apothecary held the title of Especer le Roy, and Queen Margaret's apothecary was known as Peter the Spicer. In fourteenth-century London, the apothecary was allied with the guilds of pepperers, grocers, and spicers. In other British cities and towns, apothecaries were to be found in a variety of guilds, including that of the mercers and merchants, as well as that of the spicers and grocers. In the provinces, the most important guilds for the development of pharmacy were those of barbers, surgeons, and apothecaries.

There was to be no significant change in these arrangements until early in the seventeenth century. In 1614, Gideon Delaune, apothecary to Anne of Denmark, queen of James I, petitioned the king for a charter that would give apothecaries independence from the Company of Grocers. The king, on the advice of Sir Francis Bacon, chief law officer, recognized that while "Grocers are but merchants, the business of an Apothecary is a Mistery." The charter was not granted, however, until the king's personal physician—who was also the president of the Royal College of Physicians—gave his approval. Physicians saw this separate charter as a way of limiting the practice of the apothecary and denying him the right to prescribe. The royal charter was granted in 1617 and at that time the Worshipful Society of Apothecaries of London came into existence. The charter gave expression to the raison d'être of pharmacy: the society was established so as to rely on the "educated and expert" rather than on "Empirics and unskilful and ignorant men [who] do make and compound many unwholesome, hurtful, deceitful, corrupt, and dangerous Medicines...to the great peril and daily hazard of the lives of our Subjects."

The new status of the apothecary in London, the merging of the apothecary and the surgeon in the provinces, Scotland, and Ireland, and the shortage of trained physicians throughout Britain led to the British apothecary's increasing involvement in the practice of medicine. This was achieved with a semblance of legality by the apothecary's charging only for the medication dispensed, not for consultation or diagnosis.

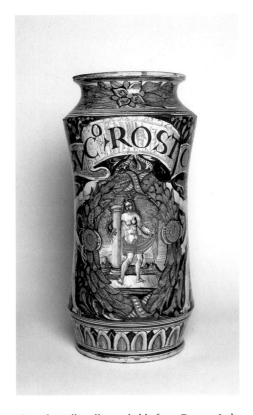

Porcelain albarello, probably from Deruta, Italy. c. 1550. In the 16th century Deruta was known for its production of pottery painted in blue and yellow luster and for the use of traditional majolica motifs. Schweizerisches Pharmazie-Historisches Museum, Basel

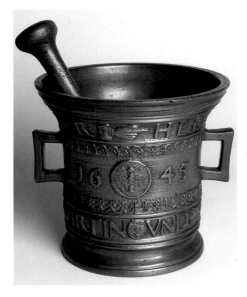

Bronze mortar and pestle. Swiss, 1645. The bands at the top and bottom give the names of the pharmacist, Rudolf Klinger, and his wife. Schweizerisches Pharmazie-Historisches Museum, Basel

Nevertheless, the development was fraught with potential conflict between physicians and apothecaries. The position of the apothecaries was greatly enhanced during the Great Plague of 1666, when most physicians fled London and most apothecaries stayed behind, but friction was to continue into the eighteenth century.

In sharp contrast to the largely self-governing guild systems prevailing in other countries, the development of pharmacy in the German states was characterized by governmental control of the profession. By 1600, some two hundred German towns had ordinances regulating pharmacy, all essentially following a pattern going back to the *Constitutiones* of Frederick II. Within a century most German states had imposed statewide controls, and thereafter state approval was required for opening an apothecary shop. In exceptional cases the owner of an *Apotheke* did not have to be a pharmacist, but the manager of the shop had to be an approved pharmacist who had taken the pharmacist's oath. The compounding of drugs had to follow recognized formulas, and *Arzneitaxen*—sometimes an integral part of the ordinances, sometimes separately issued—fixed the prices that could be charged. These official price lists, stipulating the drugs a pharmacist had to be prepared to provide and the prices he was allowed to charge for them, were known in at least ten German cities before 1500, and such lists were common thereafter in various German cities and states. Indeed, *Arzneitaxen* for all of Germany, often revised, were in effect from 1871 to 1980.

The pharmacist was granted a *privilegium* by the authorities, permitting him to operate a shop at a certain location. The privilege varied. It could be personal and end with the removal or death of the pharmacist; it could be heritable; it could be salable; it could even involve a particular building. Whichever form the privilege took, the pharmacist was granted a monopoly in compensation for the strict regulation of his performance. The system had a double purpose: to make it worthwhile for the

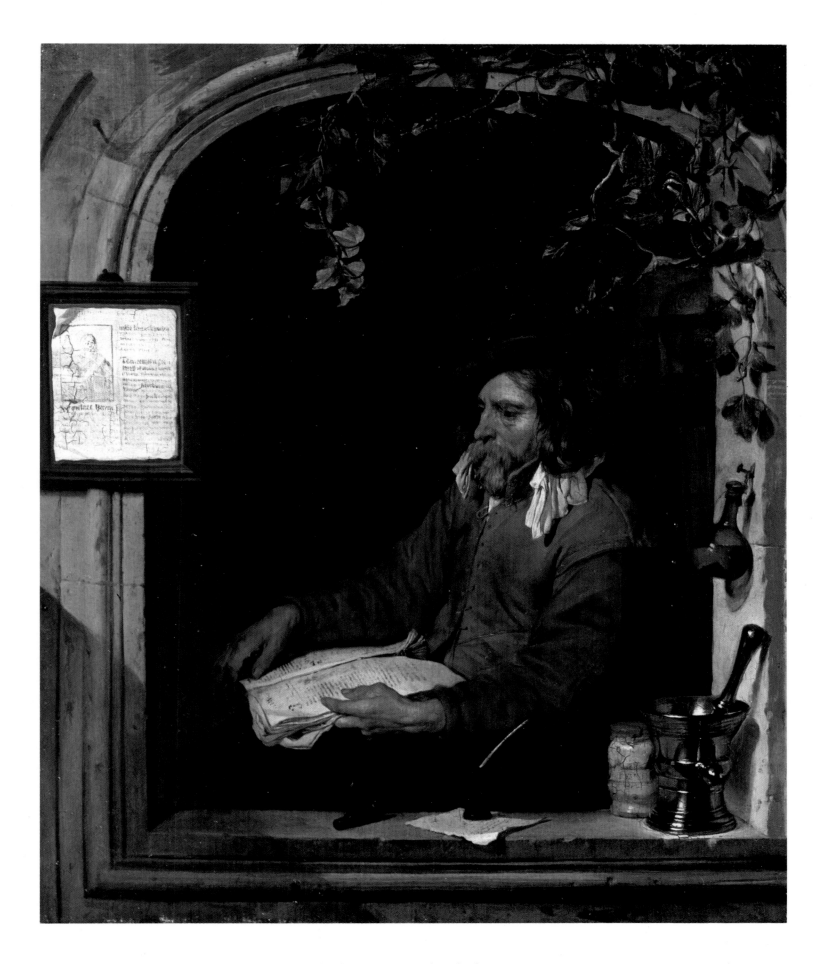

The Pharmacist. Painting by Gabriel Metsu.
Dutch, c. 1660. The Louvre, Paris

pharmacist to locate in a particular area and to attract a pharmacist to the area so that pharmaceutical services would be available to the public. This is not to say that the German pharmacist had no competition; there were peddlers, *Wunder* doctors, theriac shopkeepers, and retail grocers and hardware dealers known as *Materialisten*. The purpose of the *privilegium* was to assure the pharmacist of a reasonable, if not exceptional, income. Although the *privilegium* was supplanted by a later system of concessions, vestiges of it were to be found in Germany until after World War II. Still another kind of pharmacy was also to last into the twentieth century—the *Ratsapotheke* or *Stadtapotheke*, the municipally owned shop in which the pharmacist was an employee or lessee.

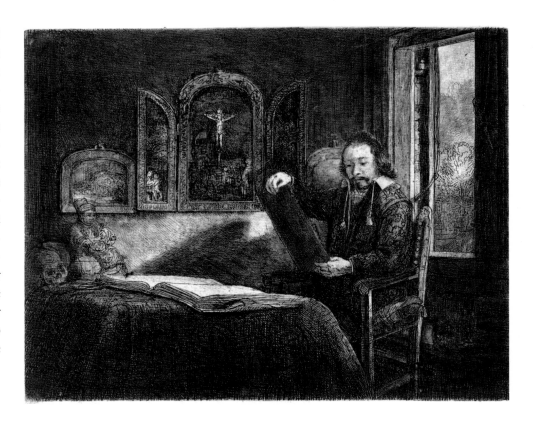

COURT PHARMACY

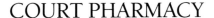

Portrait of Abraham Francen, Apothecary. Etching by Rembrandt. Dutch, 1656. A close friend of Rembrandt's, Francen was an art dealer as well as an apothecary. His name appears on many documents concerning the artist's financial troubles after 1655. Ars Medica Collection, Philadelphia Museum of Art

The appointment of personal apothecaries by kings and princes came into practice in the Middle Ages. In England the office of Royal Apothecary goes back to the time of King John, who ruled from 1199 to 1216; the position carried with it prestige and honor as well as high remuneration. In France, likewise, monarchs appointed royal apothecaries, who were charged with attendance on all the members of the royal family. The court apothecaries of the German princes had responsibilities that included not only attendance on the royal family but accompanying the sovereign on his travels and into battle. These court pharmacists bore the title of *Hof Apotheker* or *Reise Apotheker*. In Austria the practice was somewhat different: there are sixteenth- and seventeenth-century records of royal pharmacy shops, rather than pharmacists, receiving royal appointments. Royal pharmacies were often established within royal or princely palaces. The *Farmacia Real,* the royal pharmacy of Philip II of Spain, founded in 1594, has been preserved in the Palacio de Oriente in Madrid.

Royal apothecaries primarily performed pharmaceutical services. About 1306, Richard de Montpellier, apothecary, or *especer* (spicer) to Edward I, is known to have prepared, as prescribed by the king's physician, 282 pounds of electuaries, 106 pounds of white powder, plus ointments, gums, aromatics, oils, turpentines, a plaster, medicated wines, and a special electuary containing ambergris, musk, pearls, precious gems, gold, and silver. Henry VI's physicians, not to be outdone, prescribed electuaries, potions, syrups, confections, laxatives, clysters, suppositories, cataplasms, gargles, fomentations, embrocations, ointments, plasters, waxes, and rubifacients.

The royal apothecary—and the court apothecary as well—had other functions in addition to pharmaceutical ones. He sometimes served as confectioner, fruiterer, and perfumer, and he was also involved in embalming. James I of England was embalmed by an apothecary, either Lewis Le Mire or John Rumler. The life-style of the royal apothecary can be gauged from the fact that the entourage of Rumler's wife on a trip to France in 1624 included four servants.

PHARMACY AND CHRISTIANITY

Monastic Pharmacy

Monasteries remained important centers of pharmacy throughout the Renaissance. In those monasteries that survived the Reformation, their pharmacies lasted well into the nineteenth century. The monastic pharmacy, or at least the part seen by its public clients, was often very elegant. The pharmacy of S. Giovanni Evangelista in Parma, which opened to the public in 1201, was regularized as part of the church and monastery of S. Giovanni Evangelista in the seventeenth century and was operated privately into the nineteenth century. It had cases and shelves of carved walnut and decorative lunettes depicting Apollo, Mercury, Galen, Averoës, Hippocrates, Asclepios, Aëtius, Dioscorides, Avicenna, Mesuë, and twelve Parmesan physicians of the sixteenth and seventeenth centuries. Latin inscriptions on the lunettes and over the doors, and the manifold mortars, pestles, jars, jugs, and scales, attested to centuries of pharmaceutical activity.

Monastic pharmacies, which were all too frequently the only source of medical care for the poor, nonetheless stirred resentment among secular pharmacists who had opened shops nearby. However, the monastic pharmacy played an important role, as is indicated by the number of monastery-derived medicaments that attained general recognition. Best known was Jesuit powder (cinchona), but Capuchin powder (sabadilla, larkspur, and tobacco) also gained a considerable reputation as a destroyer of lice, and Carthusian powder (kermes mineral) became greatly esteemed in France for its emetic and deobstruent properties.

Another indication of the importance of monastic pharmacy is the development that has been called "the pharmaceutical industry of the monasteries." In the sixteenth century the pharmaceutical arts practiced

A portion of the facade of a pharmacy in Lemgo, West Germany, formerly a wing of the town hall. Remodeled in 1612, it is an outstanding example of High Renaissance architecture. Two of the five female figures on the whole facade and six of the ten philosophers, physicians, and scientists can be seen. The visible portion of the inscriptions reads: "Cease from sin and He will make you well. Then let the doctor come to you, for he was created by the Lord." The inscriptions continue: "Medicines come from the Lord and it is the Apothecary who prepares them."

by the brothers to supply their own needs—especially their interest in aqua vitae—and the needs of nearby communities blossomed into industrial and mercantile activities. In 1508, Florentine Dominicans began the manufacture of aromatic waters and oils. In 1534, Francis I of France enjoyed and spread the fame of the liqueur made by the Benedictines in Fécamp that bears their name, and the Carthusians of the monastery of La Grand Chartreuse originated the well-known liqueur named for that locale. The Benedictines of the area near Pernay, France, have been credited with the discovery of the process of making champagne.

Related to monastic pharmacy were pharmaceutical services rendered by the religious in hospitals and infirmaries established by various orders. The hospital was an institution developed and run by the religious, and it usually relied on the services of a pharmacist (brother or sister) who worked in a room of the hospital designated as a pharmacy. In Spain such pharmacies, controlled by religious orders, were distrib-

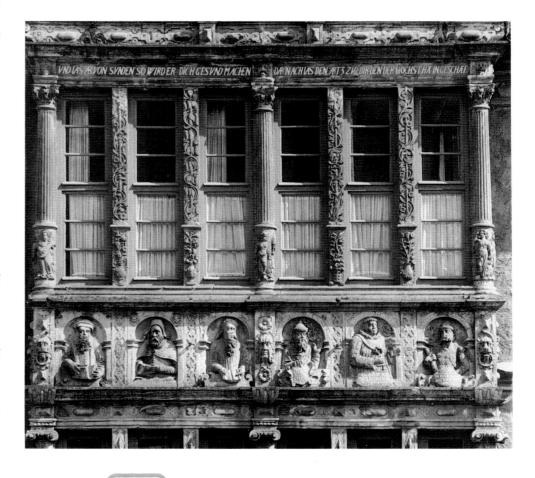

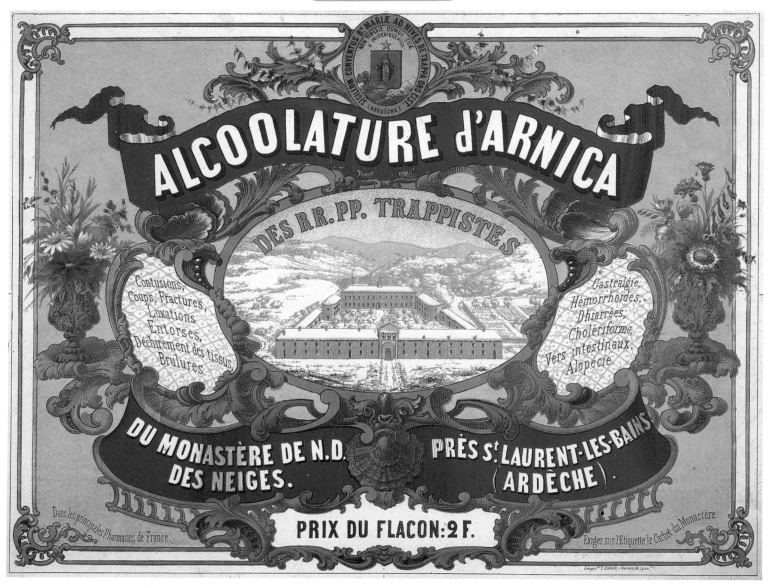

Poster for Alcoolature d'arnica. Color lithograph. French, c. 1875. At the Monastery of Notre Dame des Neiges near Saint-Laurent-les-Bains, Trappist monks prepared this product, recommended for many external and internal ailments.

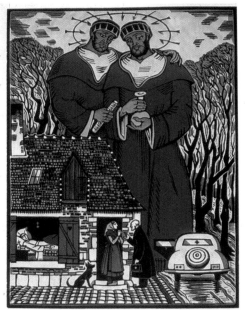

Saint Côme et Saint Damien. Color lithograph by Jean Chièze. French, c. 1935. A modern rendering of the patron saints of medicine and pharmacy.

Saints Cosmas and Damian. Painting by Adriaen Isenbrant. Bruges, c. 1525. Following the tradition, Saint Cosmas, holding a urine flask, is depicted as a physician, and Saint Damian, holding a jar, as an apothecary. Collection Van der Wielen, Hilversum, the Netherlands

Lo Speziale (The Pharmacist). Painting by Pietro Longhi. Italian, c. 1770. Galleria dell'Accademia, Venice ▶

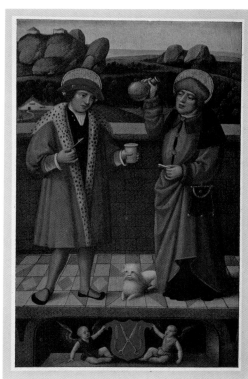

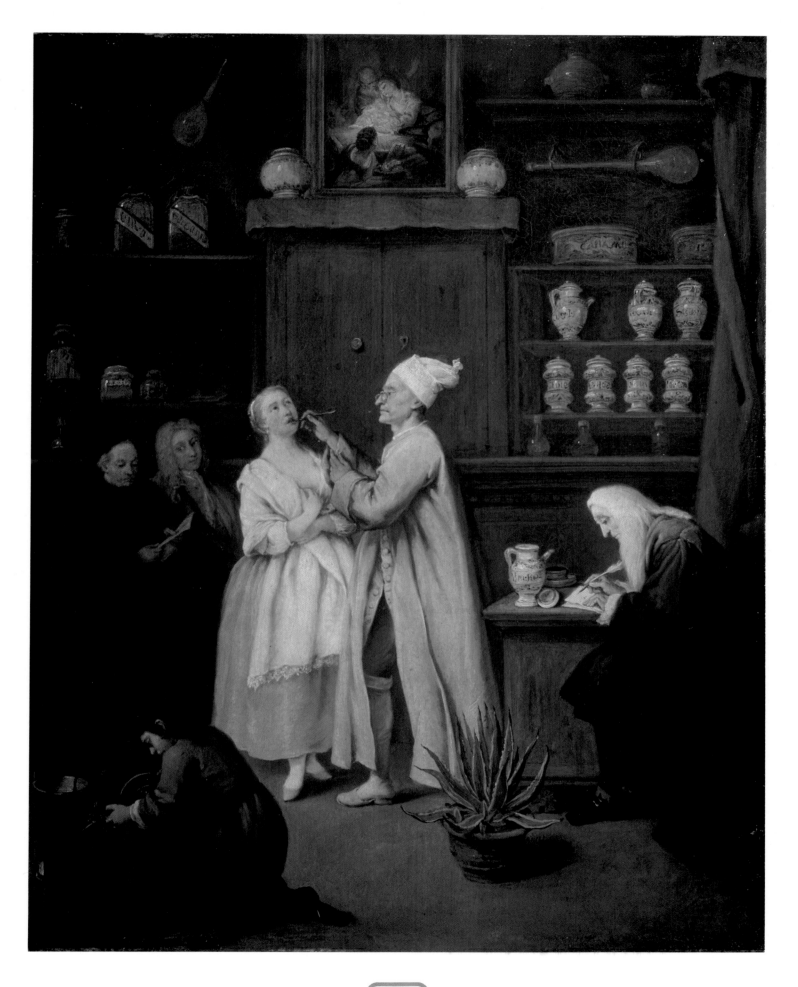

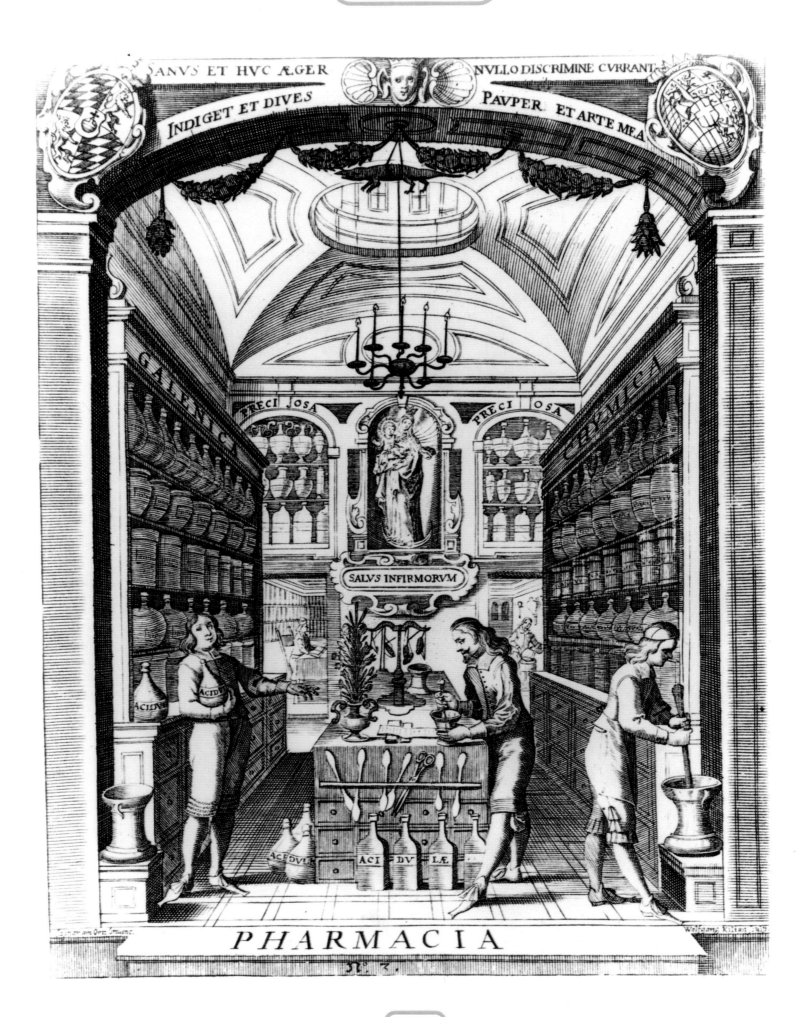

SANVS ET HVC ÆGER   NVLLO DISCRIMINE CVRRANT

INDIGET ET DIVES   PAVPER ET ARTE MEA

PRECIOSA   PRECIOSA

SALVS INFIRMORVM

ACIDVLÆ

PHARMACIA

uted throughout the land; by the middle of the sixteenth century there was a pharmacy in the Benedictine Hospital de San Juan in Burgos, and in 1587 the Hospital de San Hermenegildo in Seville was described as having "a large and curious shop with all the medicines known to Spain." In Vienna the Brothers of the Order of Good Samaritans established a *Krankenhaus* and pharmacy in 1614. Twenty years later, when three Augustinian nursing sisters arrived in Quebec to labor in the hospital there, they performed the whole gamut of pharmaceutical services, becoming perhaps the earliest practitioners of pharmacy north of the Rio Grande.

More of a threat to the public pharmacists were the shops opened by orders to provide free medicines to the poor. In 1559 the secular pharmacists of Barcelona, incensed by the competition presented by the Dominican friars of Saint Catharine, sought redress from the town council and church authorities. The matter went as far as the pope; the conflict was resolved—and the decline of monastic pharmacy assured— only when the religious orders lost their wealth and power at the hands of the absolute monarchs in the eighteenth century.

Cosmas and Damian

The church, which dominated the life of Western Europe for almost a millennium, could not help but affect medicine and pharmacy. Christian hagiography names some seventy saints connected with medicine—among them Anthony, Luke, Michael, Pantaleon, Eusebius, Diomedes, and Zenobia. Local guilds of physicians and pharmacists might have their particular patron saints, but across Europe the twin martyrs Cosmas and Damian came to be recognized as the patron saints of medicine and pharmacy. Cosmas and Damian were Arab Christians from Aegea, in Asia Minor, who were martyred during Diocletian's persecutions (303–313). They were practitioners of medicine and surgery who

Christ as Apothecary. Swiss, c. 1701. Typical of the genre, this painting depicts Christ preparing remedies to cure the ills of mankind. The inscriptions on the jars have religious themes, and the scales are for weighing sins as well as medicines. Schweizerisches Pharmazie-Historisches Museum, Basel
Overleaf, left

Painting of Christ the Healer, with religious symbols and medicinal plants, including gentian, hemlock, and cowslip. German, c. 1700. Germanisches Nationalmuseum, Nuremberg
Overleaf, right

Pharmacia. Engraving by Wolfgang Kilian in Malachias Geiger, *Microcosmos hypochondriacus,* Munich, 1652. This baroque pharmacy, large enough to house the multifarious materia medica of the time, apparently was associated with a hospital. Three categories of drugs are displayed: galenicals, chemicals (the acids in the foreground suggest an emphasis on Paracelsian remedies), and "preciosa," the last well out of reach. National Library of Medicine, Bethesda

accepted no fees, and their feats of healing were legendary. The most famous of these feats—and the one frequently illustrated— was the grafting of a black leg onto a white patient to replace a diseased leg that had been amputated.

The cult venerating Cosmas and Damian, which began in the fourth century with the dedication to them of churches in Jerusalem, Egypt, and Mesopotamia, spread rapidly in Europe. In the sixth century Pope Felix established a church dedicated to Cosmas and Damian at the Forum of Vespasian in Rome. In succeeding centuries, churches and chapels dedicated to these two saints were established throughout Christendom. In the Piedmont there were at least nine, and even in England, where the cult made comparatively little headway, five churches were dedicated to the sainted brothers.

As might be expected, saints so closely associated with the healing arts had wide popular appeal, attracting veneration far beyond that accorded them by physicians and pharmacists. The widespread relics of Cosmas and Damian (skulls purported to be theirs can be found in Madrid, Vienna, and Munich) and their iconography in statues, carvings, frescoes, paintings, prints, mosaics, icons, medallions, and even embroideries attest to their enormous popularity. Perhaps most impressive is the fact that figures of Saints Cosmas and Damian are among the decorations on the famous crown of King Stephen I of Hungary in the National Museum in Budapest.

The choice of twin saints for medicine and pharmacy was symbolic of the closeness of the two professions. Cosmas, usually associated with medicine, was commonly depicted holding a glass urine-inspection vessel. Damian, who was associated with surgery as well as pharmacy, was depicted holding a spatula and an apothecary jar or pot. Cosmas and Damian were patron saints of the medical faculty of the University of Vienna, and annually throughout the Renaissance a celebration was held on September 29, Cosmas and Damian's Day.

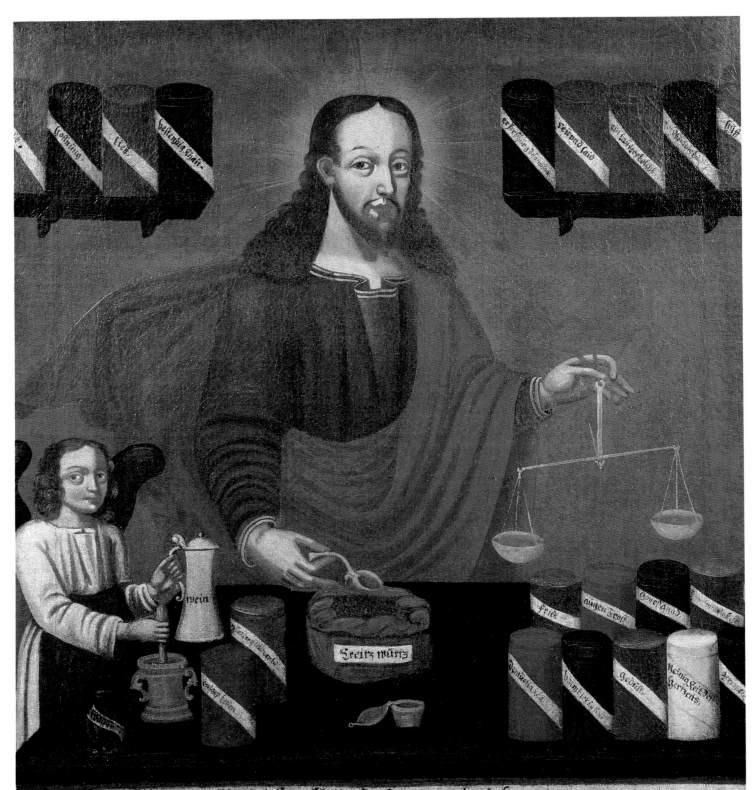

Ein guete Köstliche artzney für alley Kranckhaiten der seelen Zu gebrauchen
Erstlich schicke ein botten deines andechtigen gebets in die Apothecken der h: h: dreyfaltigkait, und bitte den Apothecker, daß ist den hei-
ligen gaist, daß er dir gabe 1 loth, sanft muetig Khait, 2 loth, demuetig khait, 3 loth, barmhertzig khait, 4 loth, gedult und Reinigkhait des hertzens, gem-
einschaft des leibs, dises stoß alles an ein ander, 6 loth Zuckher göttlicher lieb, stoß alles mit einer Innerlichen lieb, betrachtung deß unschuldigen blue-
et vergiessens unsers lieben Herren Jesu Christi, dar nach gieß darein, 7 mal lebentiges wasser, auß den Bäkhen deiner augen, und Trinck
deßelbigen 5 tag nach ein ander, den Ersten Erforschung deß gewissens und sihe wie du dich ver sündiget hast, den anderen tag, hab
ein wahres laid über deine sündt, den driten hab ein lautere beicht, den vierten Thue eine pol khomerie Buesz, den fünff-
ten hab ein starckhen fürsatz hinfue an nit mehr Zu sündigen, und huet dich vor sünden, alß dem fahe an die artzney Zu Trinckhen p: erden hernach sonemb auch ein krafftiges Confect welches dich
Apotheckher daß ist das Haillige Hoch wirdige Sacrament deß altars, die artzney ist bewerth und über Er ist aller arti-
khel wie aber dise köstliche artzney Recht brauchen solleff uns dar Zu der himelische Doctor, daß ist gott de-
ser sohn der ander ist gott der Haylig gaist, und die Haylig Zungfraw maria sey unser Trost

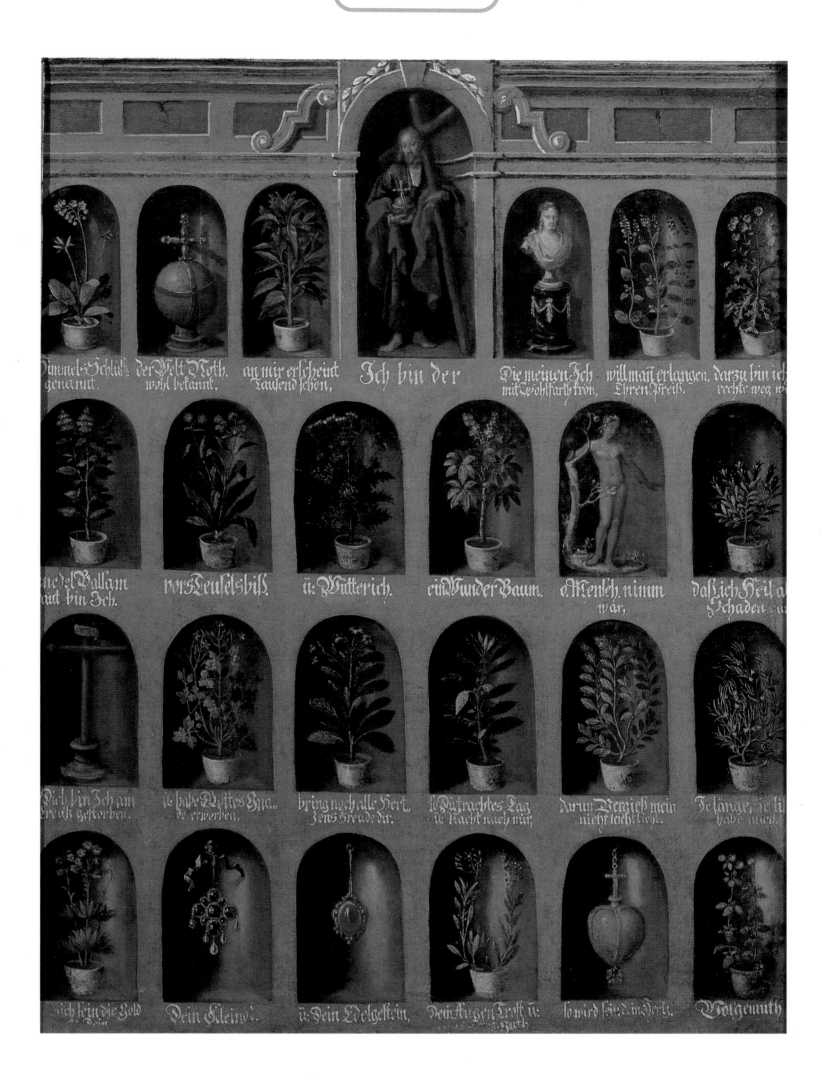

Members of all the health professions were involved—physicians, surgeons, pharmacists, midwives. An imperial ordinance of 1644, and later ordinances, required pharmacists to participate in the celebration.

Christ as Pharmacist

Always in the background of the healing power of the patron saints were references to the many scenes in the New Testament of Christ as the miraculous healer. It was not until the Renaissance, however, that an overt association of Jesus with medicine and pharmacy found its place in the graphic arts. The first known representation of Jesus

An early 17th-century pharmacy. Engraving by Jaspar Isaac from Jean Renou, *Institutionum pharmaceuticarum*, Paris, 1608. Collection Bouvet, Paris

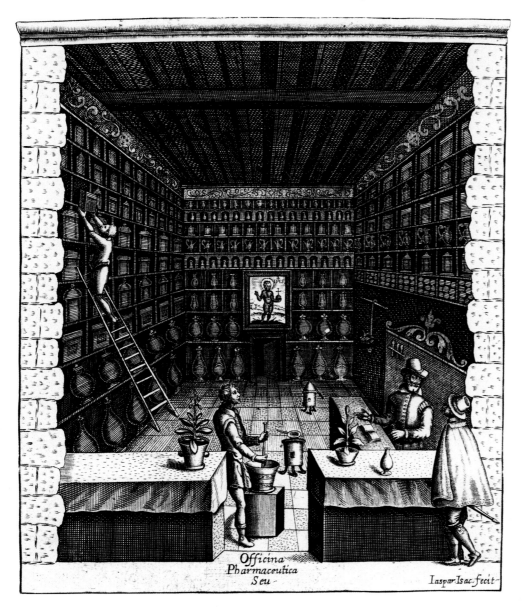

as a heavenly physician appears in a manuscript written between 1519 and 1528, and the first depiction of Christ as pharmacist, holding a set of hand scales, is dated 1619.

More than one hundred such representations of Jesus as physician or pharmacist were produced in the next two centuries. For the most part, these paintings are folk art, with an appeal very different from that of the great masterworks of the Renaissance. They were thought of as devotional exercises, and they reflect a homely piety. They generally show a half-figure of Jesus behind a prescription counter. In his hand he holds scales or a container of drugs. Shelves, drawers, and jars behind him contain "spiritual medicines" with such labels as "Roots of the Cross," "Faith," "Ascension to Love," "Key to Heaven," "Consolation," and "Herb of the Grace of God." The central image is usually framed by biblical quotations. These devotional works have a great deal to tell us about the small individual pharmacy shop of the era. They offer a metaphor: the pharmacist performing a godly function, compounding drugs endowed with spiritual qualities and offering spiritual rewards—a connection not lost on the pious folk of the period.

THE PHARMACY SHOP AND ITS EQUIPMENT

The small shops illustrated in pictures of Christ the Pharmacist are thought to be typical of the plain and practical establishments of small-town pharmacists. Fixtures were not particularly noteworthy, drug containers were rather prosaic, and there was little ornamentation except for some religious accouterments. Not so the court, cloister, and municipal pharmacies, which eventually came to reflect both the grandeur and the excesses of the Renaissance.

In Lemgo, Germany, a wing of the town hall was converted into a pharmacy in 1559. Remodeled in 1612, it emerged as a

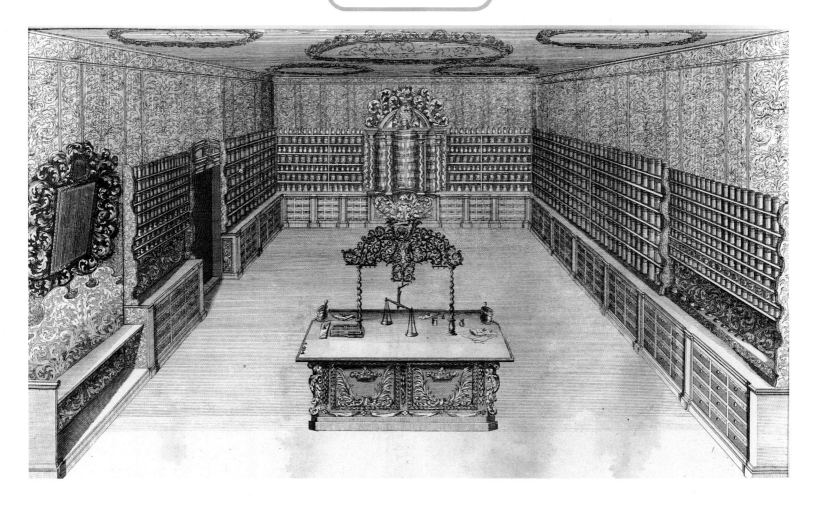

Engraving of a design for the interior of a proposed pharmacy in the city of Rastatt, Germany, c. 1700. Despite the excellence of this baroque design, Johann Leonhard Kellner, the owner of a pharmacy in Nuremberg, who had had it prepared, did not receive permission to proceed with the Rastatt Apotheke.

remarkable example of German architecture of the High Renaissance, with cornices and pilasters, scrollwork and metalwork, busts and obelisks. Five female figures in flowing robes, representing the five senses, adorned the columns. Busts of ten famous philosophers, scientists, and physicians decorated the facade, each with an inscription. Over the windows of the top story was a quotation—refurbished or of a later time—summing up a passage of Ecclesiasticus (38:11–15): "When you are sick, pray to the Lord and cease to sin. Then let the doctor come to you, for he was created by the Lord. Medicines come from the Lord, and it is the apothecary who prepares them."

In a description of the pharmacy of the Hieronymite monks at San Lorenzo del Escorial, written in 1664 by Lady Fanshawe, wife of the English ambassador to Spain, she states that "the apothecary's shop is large, very richly adorned with paint, and gilding, and marble; there is an inward

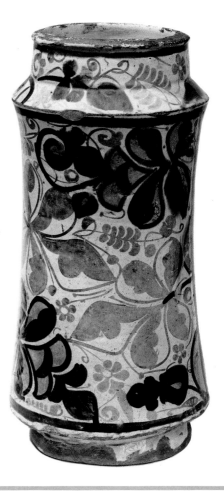

Lusterware albarello with flower and fern spray decoration. Spanish, 15th century. National Museum of American History, Smithsonian Institution, Washington, D.C.

room in which the medicines are made, as finely furnished and beautiful as the shop." The interiors of such pharmacies increasingly manifested a heretofore uncommon grandeur, both in their construction and in their appointments. This was true as well of the containers for drugs and the mortars and pestles that were used.

Containers for drugs are as old as the use of drugs. Excavations at Nippur in Mesopotamia have unearthed pottery jars from about 3000 BC that may have been used to store drugs. The alabaster ointment pots of ancient Egypt, the lekythoi that the Greeks used for unguents and oil, and the glass medication vessels of the Romans are well known.

The need to make earthenware jars impervious, especially those intended to hold liquids and viscous substances, led to the development of tin glazing. This technique probably had its origin between 600 and 400 BC in Mesopotamia. From Persia, where it flourished perhaps as early as the eighth century AD, it spread across North Africa to Spain in the thirteenth century and then to the rest of Europe. Pigments from natural substances were used in the ornamentation: blue, purple, yellow, brown, and green were all obtainable. Processes were developed in the twelfth and thirteenth centuries that made it possible to add to the surface of the pottery an iridescent sheen, a feature that was to distinguish the jars, known as Hispano-Moresque lusterware, manufactured on the Iberian peninsula.

A considerable trade in jars intended for use in the pharmacy (now variously called the "apothecary jar," "pharmacy jar," and "drug jar") developed. They were exported from Persia and Syria to Europe in considerable quantities in the thirteenth and fourteenth centuries. The Moors, who had set up potteries in Spain very early, began exporting tin-glazed earthenware, including jars, in the fourteenth century via the island of Majorca—hence the name "majolica." Some of this majolica ware reached Italy and led to the development of potteries there; one of the sites of manufacture in Italy was Faenza—hence the term "faience."

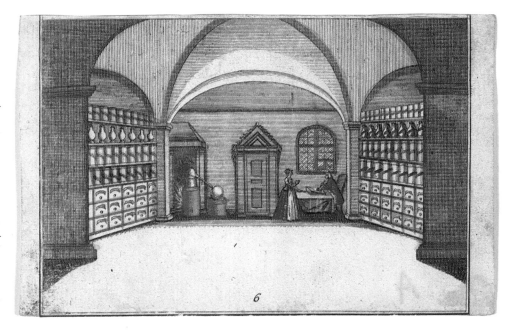

Interior of a Renaissance pharmacy. Color lithograph. German, c. 1840. This small scene was the backdrop for a cardboard peep show.

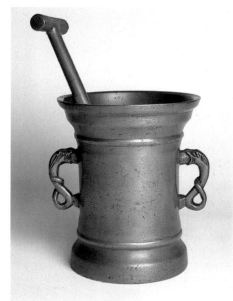

Bronze mortar and pestle. German, 1533. National Museum of American History, Smithsonian Institution, Washington, D.C.

Trade sign of the Löwenapotheke (Lion Pharmacy), carved from soft wood and painted gold and silver. Canton Thurgau, Switzerland, c. 1785. Kunsthaus Lempertz, Cologne

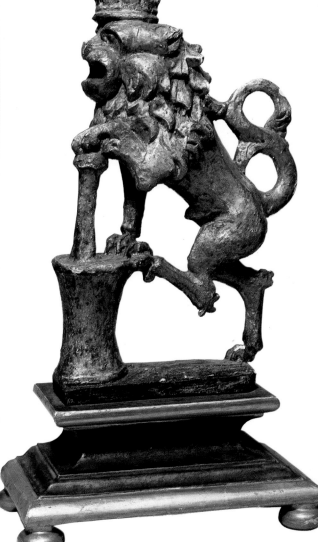

Interior of an Italian pharmacy. Painting by Giuseppe Zais. Italian, c. 1780. The artist has depicted this Venetian pharmacy as a social center as well as a source of medicines. Collection Dorr, Waldenbuch, near Stuttgart

Le Pileur (The Pounder). Color lithograph by Pibou after a painting by Antoine Rivalz. French, c. 1850. The portrait of the boy with the large mortar, the apothecary's servant at the Convent of the Cordeliers in Toulouse, was originally painted on the door of the convent. Collection Bouvet, Paris

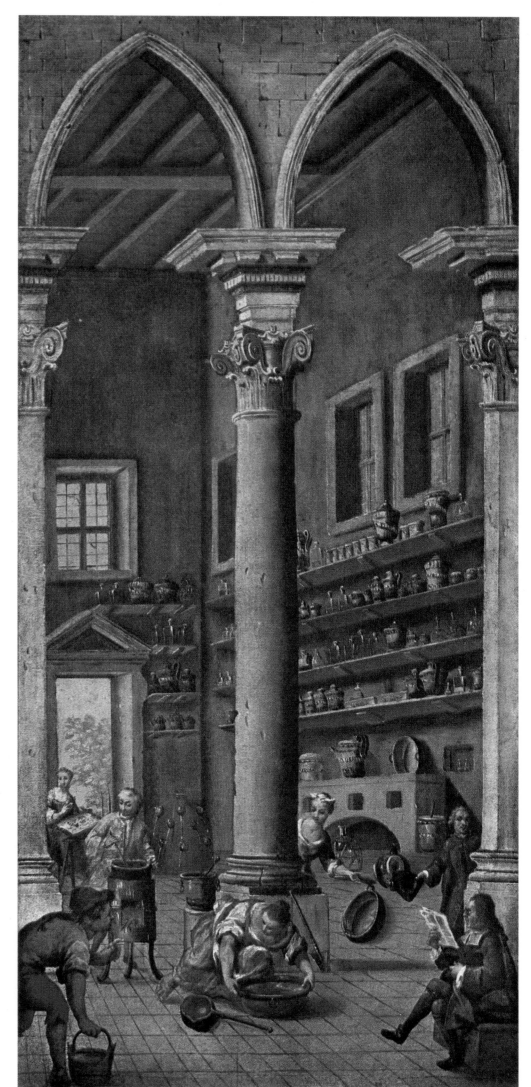

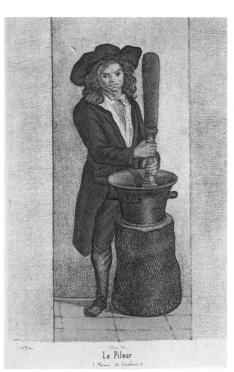

Le Pileur

From Italy the industry spread to France and the Netherlands. Dutch potters developed a tin-glazed earthenware, mainly blue and white, known as "delft"—again from the name of the place of manufacture. From the Netherlands the manufacture of delftware spread to England ("English delft," "Lambeth delft," and others) and to Germany and Scandinavia. From the sixteenth to the eighteenth century there were at least seventy sites in Europe—from Marieberg, Sweden, in the north to Caltagirone, Sicily, in the south, and from Lisbon in the west to Warsaw in the east—where drug jars were being manufactured.

The decorative potential of glazing techniques meant that the apothecary jar often became an object of beauty as well as utility. At first, decoration followed the Arab tradition of overall nonfigurative patterns, but later jars depicted religious or secular scenes, pictured scientists or saints, and displayed the symbol or coat of arms of a pharmacist, a hospital, a religious order, or a monastery. With advances in polychrome techniques the shelves of the pharmacy took on new color, opulence, and beauty. To own a splendid collection of decorative drug jars became the ambition of most pharmacists.

Drug jars were made in many shapes and sizes, depending on their function. Jars used for the storage of solid and viscous materials—herbs, spices, candied fruits, ointments, and electuaries—were generally cylindrical (the albarello), or ovoid, that is, convex and rounded. To protect the contents, these jars, sometimes referred to as "dry-drug jars," were usually topped by a flange over which a parchment cover could be tied, or, later, by a lip for a metal or ceramic lid. "Wet-drug jars" for liquids such as syrups and oils were either ovoid flasks or, more frequently, "syrup jars," bulbous jars on a high base with spout and handle.

Originally the apothecary jar was unlabeled so that it could be used and reused for a variety of drugs. The contents of the jar were indicated by a label pasted on it (jars with blank cartouches were still being pro-

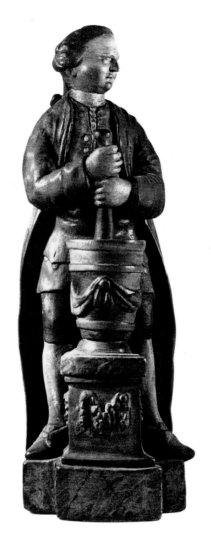

Wooden apothecary figure with mortar and pestle. Swiss, 18th century. Germanisches Nationalmuseum, Nuremberg

duced as late as the eighteenth century). The practice of including the name of the contents in the decoration of drug jars began in the middle of the fifteenth century. Large numbers of jars were needed to store and display the wares of a pharmacy, and pharmacists could have drug containers labeled in accordance with their own systems or in accordance with the local antidotarium, that is, the list of drugs and compositions recommended by the local medical and pharmaceutical establishments.

Pottery was not the only material used for drug storage. Wooden and tin containers were also to be found on the shelves of the pharmacy. Glass was especially important both because it was relatively inexpensive and because it was impervious and usually nonreactive with drugs. Since glass lent itself well to decoration, plain glassware soon gave way to hand-painted glassware, which in turn gave way to glassware onto which the decoration and label had been baked or enameled. Glass containers came in a variety of shapes, round, square, square-shouldered, round-shouldered, glass-stoppered, flange-topped, long-necked, short-necked. Labels were decorated with garlands, crowns, cherubs, Moors, birds, symbols, and coats of arms—all in vivid color.

Just as the pharmacist took pride in his collection of containers, he took pride in his mortars and pestles. First used by prehistoric food gatherers to crush seeds and kernels, the mortar and pestle became a pharmaceutical instrument in ancient times and from the thirteenth century on was recognized as a symbol of pharmacy. In Egypt the mortar and pestle were made of stone; in later centuries and later cultures they were made also of wood, lead, bronze, iron, tin, brass, ivory, porcelain, agate, glass, and gold. By the time of the Renaissance, mortars and pestles used by pharmacists were fabricated mainly of bronze, or bell metal, and were larger than those, usually made of brass, that were used domestically. Philbert Guibert, the physician author of the 1625 manual *Le Médecin charitable,* listed as being "necessary to furnish an Apothecary...a great Morter of Brasse weighing fifty or sixty pound or more, with a pestle of iron. A little Morter weighing five or six pound, with a pestle of the same matter. A middle sized Morter of Marble, and a pestle of wood, and a stone morter with the same pestle."

The working-counter mortar took two major shapes: the earlier, Gothic, type was tall and narrow; the type that became popular in the later Renaissance and the baroque era was shorter and wider. It became fashionable for the pharmacist to display a large and highly decorated mortar and pestle meant for show rather than use. However, this showpiece was sometimes put to use, and there are many representations of a boy apprentice struggling with a huge pestle over a large mortar (sometimes the pestle was so heavy that it was suspended by a chain from a large wooden spring beam). Decorations of ribbing, knobs, spikes, and studs, as well as natural motifs such as lizards and sage leaves were applied to both small and large mortars. Some bore religious representations: among these the Crucifixion and the Christ Child were favored. Inscriptions with pharmaceutical themes, usually naming the pharmacist or the pharmacy, as well as dates, were frequently worked into the decorative scheme. Most mortars had a handle or handles, often ornate. Large mortars stood on pedestals in the form of feet or claws or even a sculpture of a whole animal. The ornamentation—of mortars, pestles, and pedestals—reflected both the creativity of the craftsman and the tastes of the individual pharmacist.

As suggested by the varieties mentioned by Guibert, the choice of materials for mortars and pestles was made perhaps because of considerations of their compatibility or incompatibility with substances to be ground. Definite ideas developed that certain substances were best ground in mortars made of certain materials. In the late 1770s, when the noted chemist Joseph Priestley pointed out that friction created by the constant rubbing of metal pestles created dust that contaminated the drug, his friend Josiah Wedgwood, the potter, was inspired to

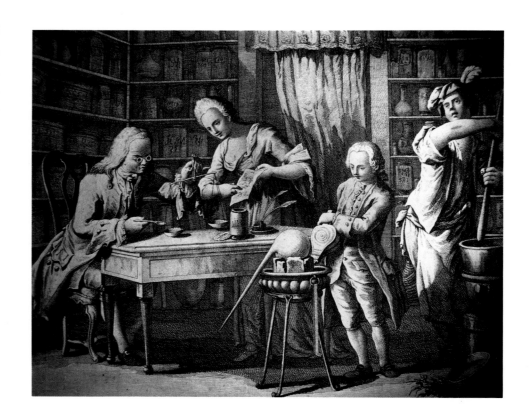

Lo Speziale (The Pharmacist). Engraving. Italian, c. 1750. Wellcome Institute Library, London

develop his ceramic mortar. Thereafter there was some preference given to glass and Wedgwood mortars.

The compounding of prescriptions was done by the pharmacist in his officina, a room or area usually open to the public. Mortars and pestles, balances—usually gold and coin scales, until special scales for pharmacists began to be made, in the seven-

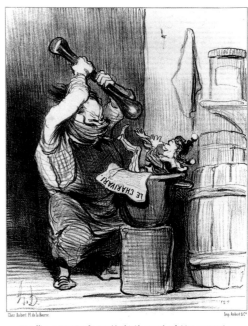

Mimi Véron croit avoir enfin trouvé le véritable moyen de pulvériser son ennemi (Mimi Véron believes he has found the sure way to pulverize his enemy). Lithograph by Honoré Daumier. French, 1850. Louis Désiré Véron, a physician, director of the Opéra, and former marketer of the proprietary medicine Pâte Regnauld, published a journal, *Le Constitutionnel,* which was at the opposite end of the political spectrum from *Le Charivari.* Véron was often depicted as a pharmacist in political caricatures.

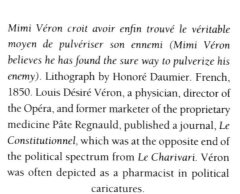

teenth century—pill tiles and spatulas, bowls and pans, bottles and other drug containers, weights, both nested and boxed, all were close at hand.

A special laboratory reflected the pharmacist's role as pharmaceutical chemist. The stills, alembics, condensers, flasks, crucibles, stoves, filters, baths, and other intricate and intriguing apparatus were awesome in their variety. Pharmacists' handbooks, like Antonio de Sgobbis de Montagnana's encyclopedic *Theatro Farmaceutico,* first published in Venice in 1662, described and illustrated the apparatus required and also provided a glossary of the alchemical and chemical symbols that the pharmacist needed to know.

Pharmacy in the Renaissance had come a long way. It had found an independent role to play in the delivery of health care and had attained professional and social status. A combination of self-regulation and government or quasi-government control maintained the integrity and superintended the performance of the profession. An extensive pharmaceutical literature developed, and university education in pharmacy began. The materia medica expanded on two fronts: the importation of larger quantities of known products and of entirely new products from the New World and the Orient, and the introduction of new chemical medicines. The latter, perforce, widened the field of expertise of the pharmacist to include chemical knowledge and operation.

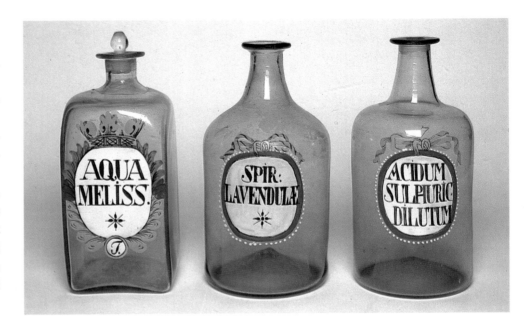

Glass drug bottles with enamel labels. German, 18th century. Schweizerisches Pharmazie-Historisches Museum, Basel

Wooden containers for drugs. 18th century. Schweizerisches Pharmazie-Historisches Museum, Basel

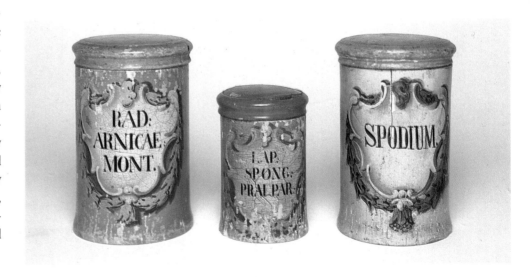

Portable pharmacy in which medications, bottles, pewter canisters, ointment boxes, small syringes, and even reference books were carried. Swiss, c. 1780. Schweizerisches Pharmazie-Historisches Museum, Basel ▶

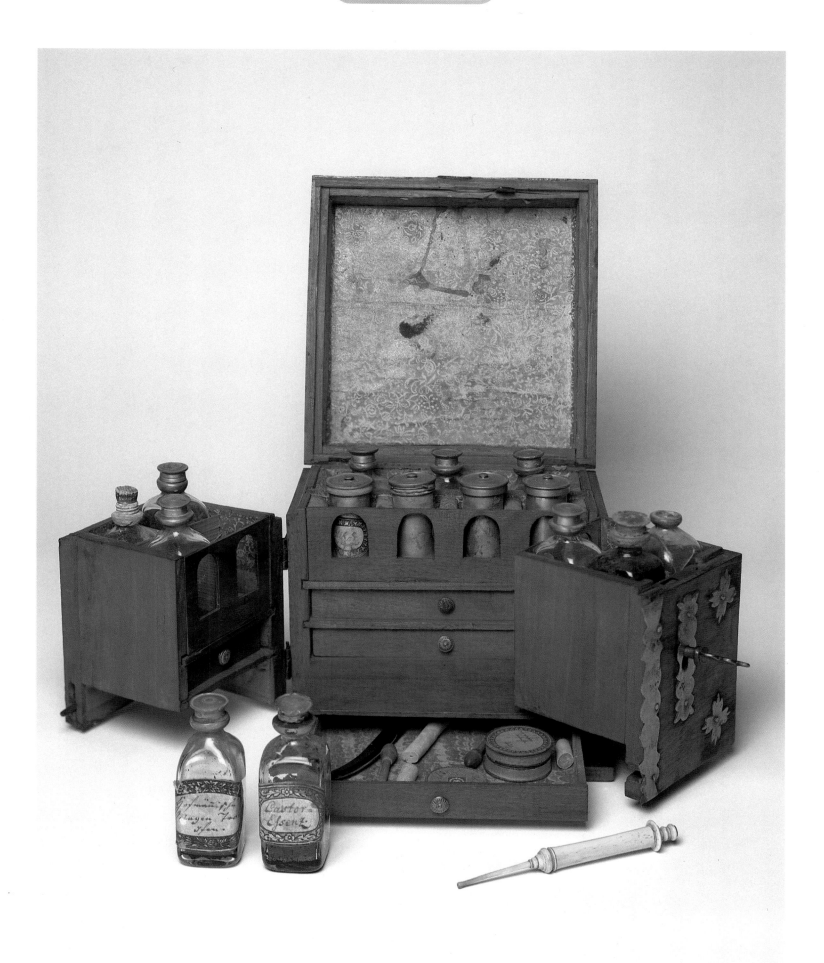

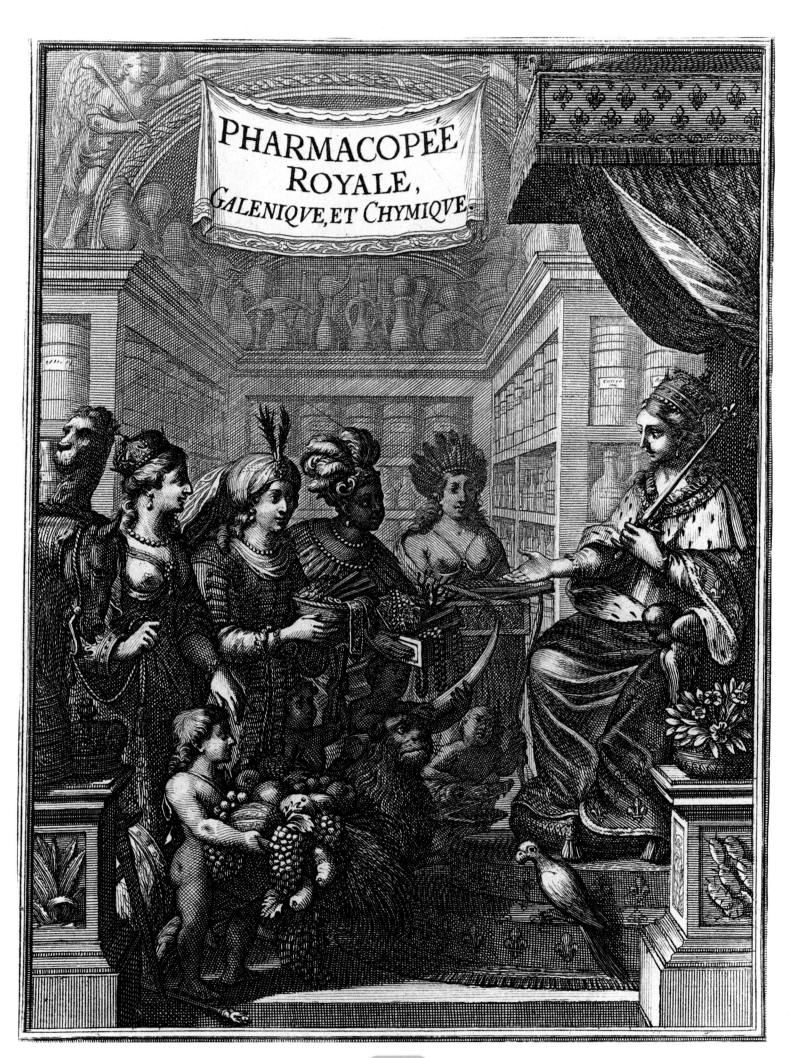

PHARMACOPÉE ROYALE, GALENIQVE, ET CHYMIQVE.

T he modern age begins with the intellectual revolution of the seventeenth century sparked by such momentous contributions as those of René Descartes, Isaac Newton, and John Locke. Their research and enquiries brought about the advances in thought culminating in the eighteenth-century Age of Enlightenment, which had its greatest flowering in France with savants like Voltaire and Rousseau. Scientists such as Isaac Newton, Robert Boyle, Antoine Lavoisier, and Carl von Linné (known as Linnaeus) opened entire new areas of knowledge. The impact of the Enlightenment on pharmacy, as we shall see, did not manifest itself until late in the eighteenth century.

THE UBIQUITOUS PHARMACOPOEIA

The pharmacopoeia came fully into its own in the early modern age. Older pharmacopoeias continued to be revised throughout this period: the Nuremberg *Dispensatorium* until 1666, the Augsburg *Pharmacopoeia Augustana* until 1743, the Venetian *Codice farmaceutico* until 1790, the Amsterdam *Pharmacopoeia* until 1792, and the *Pharmacopoeia Londinensis* as late as 1851. City after city prepared and published its own pharmacopoeia. Between 1638 and 1699, the Low-Country cities of Brussels, Utrecht, The Hague, Antwerp, Ghent, Leeuwarden, and Bruges—in obvious competition—all issued pharmacopoeias. In the next century, Lisbon, Vienna, Madrid, Stuttgart, Stockholm, St. Petersburg, and others followed suit.

The jurisdiction of some of these compilations was not limited to the issuing city. The *Pharmacopoeia Leodiensis* of 1741, for example, was official not only in the city of Liége but also in the regions of Liége and Looz. Vienna, which had issued the *Austraico Viennense* in 1729, issued the *Austraico-provincialis* for the provinces in 1774.

THE EARLY MODERN AGE: THE NEW SCIENCE

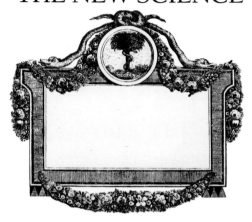

Pharmacists' blank label. French, 18th century. Blank labels were printed in various sizes and were filled in by hand and affixed to bottles, boxes, and other containers.
Collection Bouvet, Paris

Title page of *Pharmacopée royale, galénique, et chymique,* treatise by Moïse Charas, Paris, 1676. The profession of pharmacy, here depicted allegorically as royalty, is receiving the bounty of the vegetable, animal, and mineral kingdoms from representatives of the continents Europe, Asia, Africa, and America.

◄

Sometimes municipal pharmacopoeias gave way to provincial or territorial pharmacopoeias; the *Dispensatorium Brandenburgicum* of 1698 is an early case in point. Indeed, it became the practice for the various German principalities to issue their own pharmacopoeias.

Eventually the scope of the pharmacopoeia was broadened to embrace an entire country. Thus the *Pharmacopoeia Matritensis* of 1739 was considered to be binding on all of Spain. A *Pharmacopoeia Helvetica* appeared in 1771, followed a year later by the *Pharmacopoeia Danica*; these two did not have legal authority behind them. In 1794, the *Pharmacopoeia geral para o reino, e dominios de Portugal* appeared, followed five years later by the Prussian *Pharmacopoeia Borussica*—both harbingers of the nationalization of the pharmacopoeia that was to take place in the nineteenth century.

The pharmacopoeia became a symbol of government involvement in the protection of public health, since it sought not merely to provide standardization of the materia medica but also to guarantee that the pharmacist dispensed what was prescribed. Usually the pharmacopoeia was compiled by the local Collegium medicum, the group of physicians that also served as the medical police for the community. The Collegium seldom condescended to work with pharmacists in compiling a pharmacopoeia; the Liège pharmacopoeia (*Pharmacopoeia Leodiensis*) of 1741—compiled by four physicians and two pharmacists—is a notable exception to the rule. Not until the *Pharmacopoeia Borussica* of 1799 was a pharmacopoeia prepared and influenced largely by pharmacists.

Just as the materia medica of the late seventeenth and the eighteenth century was essentially unchanged from that of earlier times, so the format of the pharmacopoeia changed very little. The first section, *De medicamentis simplicibus,* consisted of a long list of vegetable simples, divided into categories such as roots, barks, herbs, leaves, flowers, fruits, seeds, gums, resins, balsams, tears, and fungi. The list of vegetable

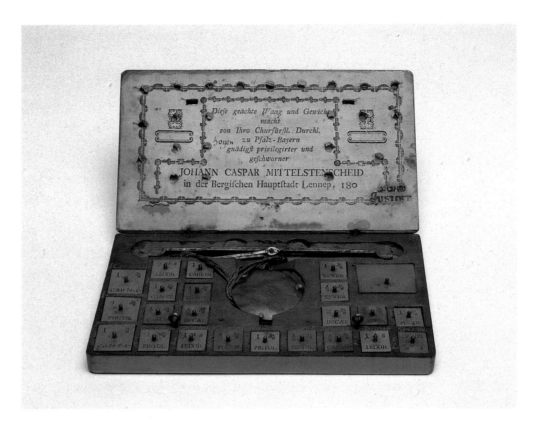

Wooden case containing a scale and twenty-two weights. Bavarian, c. 1820. Schweizerisches Pharmazie-Historisches Museum, Basel

Balance and weights. 18th century. The brass weights were nested in fitted compartments in the drawer. Schweizerisches Pharmazie-Historisches Museum, Basel

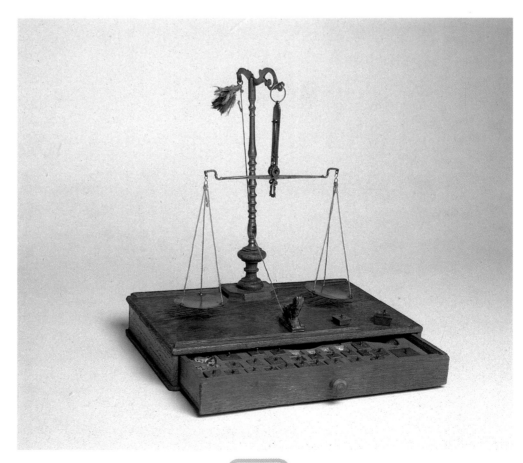

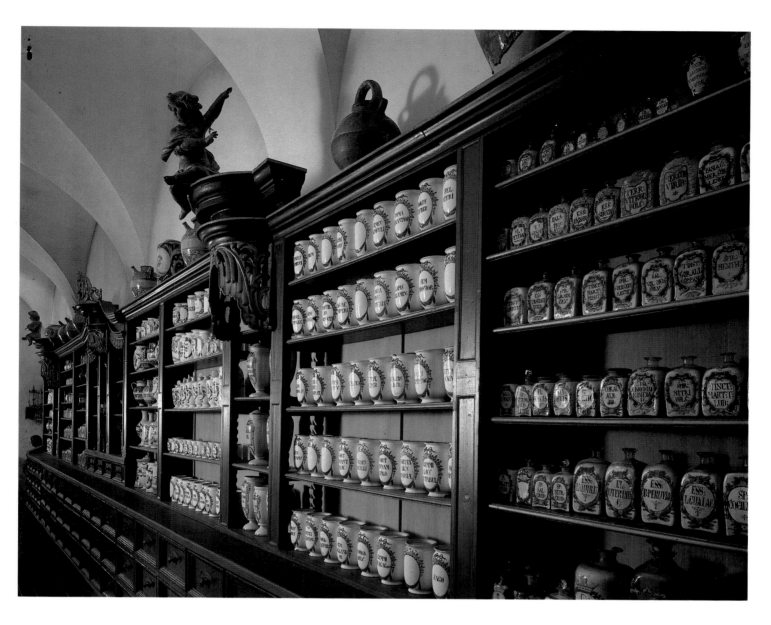

Drug jars and hand-painted glassware on the shelves
of a reconstructed 18th-century German pharmacy.
National Museum of American History,
Smithsonian Institution, Washington, D.C.

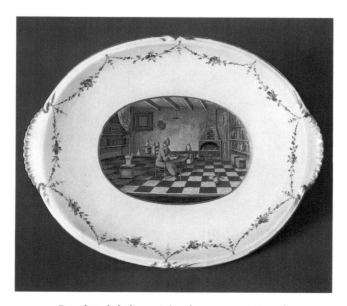

Porcelain dish decorated with a representation of a
pharmacist in his laboratory. It was in such
a private area that the pharmacist and his apprentices
prepared standard products in bulk. Dutch,
c. 1780. Collection Dr. S. Ducret, Zurich

simples was followed by a shorter list, headed *Animalia, Eorum Partes et Excrementa,* which in turn was followed by a list with the heading *Mineralia, Metalla, Lapides et Salia Terrae.* Listed separately were simples from the sea, under the heading *Marina.*

This listing of simples was traditionally followed by *Composita Galencia;* the galenicals included simple distilled waters, composite distilled waters, spirits, distilled vinegars, tinctures, elixirs, decoctions, simple syrups, compound syrups, purging compound syrups, honeys, conserves, electuaries, laxative confections, antidotes and opiates, purging powders, aromatic powders, pills, extracts, troches, expressed oils, distilled oils, balsams, unguents, plasters, and cerates.

The third section of the standard pharmacopoeia consisted of chemical compositions; the great number generally given indicates the influence of iatrochemistry on drug therapy. Among the many substances used in chemical compositions were mercury, antimony, and sulfur.

The pharmacopoeias provided formulas and directions for compounding; specific directions were given for chemical processes. Polypharmaceuticals abounded: in the *Pharmacopoeia Leodiensis* of 1741, the theriaca of Andromachus required sixty-two ingredients; the *mithridatium* of Damocrates required forty-four. Viewed as a whole, the pharmacopoeias pointedly illustrate what it was that the pharmacist was expected to know, what he was expected to do, and what equipment and stock his shop was expected to contain.

CLEANSING THE PHARMACOPOEIA

Tradition and authority illumine the pages of these pharmacopoeias. Not until late in the eighteenth century was there to be any serious questioning of the efficacy of what the compendiums contained or any significant approach to pharmacological

"Room for the Doctor, gentlemen! Room for the Doctor! . . ." Engraving by R. Taylor after a drawing by A. Forestier, from the *Illustrated London News,* 1886. Amid a gathering crowd, an itinerant doctor, mounted on a black steed and engrossed in study, arrives at a fair; on the stage are musicians and entertainers and an open-air pharmacy.

testing. It is not surprising, therefore, to encounter Preparation of Human Cranium in the *Pharmacia Antverpiensis* of 1661 or to find Oil of Earthworms in the *Pharmacopoeia Leodiensis* of 1741, or to learn that in 1696 a noted German physician, Christian Paullini, should have published a volume called *Dreckapotheke (Filth Pharmacy).* Bizarre from the modern point of view but generally included in pharmacopoeias— the *Antidotarium Gandavense* (Ghent) of 1663 and the *Pharmacopoeia Edinburgensis* of 1722, for example—was the bezoar, a concretion, or calculus, found in the ali-

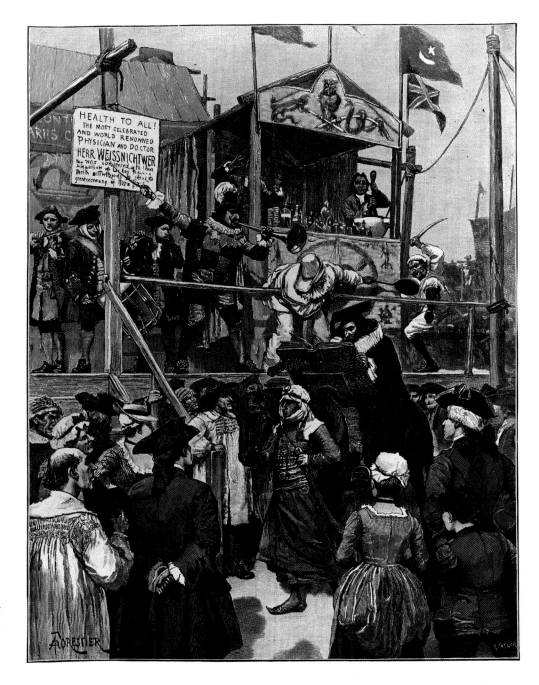

mentary organs of ruminants. The bezoar varied in size, from being as small as a nut to being large enough to be formed into a goblet. The main virtue of the bezoar lay in its detoxifying effect: a drink from a bezoar goblet was sure to have been freed of poison; a drink into which a bezoar had been suspended—usually by a gold chain—was likewise freed of poison. Ownership of one of these costly marvels was a symbol of status; bezoars were not readily found in the shops.

The development of science in the Age of Enlightenment did eventually bring about changes in the materia medica. An event portending these changes was the publication in 1745 of William Heberden's *Antitheriaka: an Essay on Mithridatium and Theriac*, a nineteen-page monograph denying outright that these polypharmaceuticals had antidotal properties against poisons, venoms, or other harmful substances. Doubts about these composites had been raised by others, but Heberden was a scholar and a physician of considerable prestige, and his reasoned arguments against the ingredients, the variations in formulas, and the inefficacy of these compounds were convincing. The *Pharmacopoeia Edinburgensis* dropped theriaca and *mithridatium* in 1756, but pharmacopoeias in France, Spain, and Germany found a place for them well into the nineteenth century, and the last vestige of these ancient remedies did not disappear from the French *Codex* (the *Codex medicamentarius sive pharmacopoeia Gallica*) until 1908.

The persistence in the pharmacopoeias of much that seems to us useless, even during an age that exalted science, demonstrates the tenacity of folk medicine and the power of tradition. Some cleansing and reform of pharmacopoeias did take place during the Enlightenment. Not only did the 1756 Edinburgh pharmacopoeia eliminate theriacs; it also "banished" certain remedies that had been retained through "superstition," "credulity," or "established custom." Furthermore, the number of animal simples listed was reduced from forty-seven to

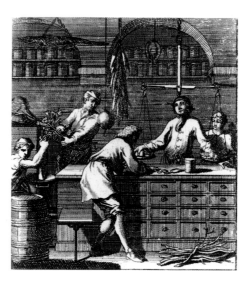

De Drogist and *De Apothecker*. Engravings by Jan Luyken. Dutch, 1758. National Museum of American History, Smithsonian Institution, Washington, D.C.

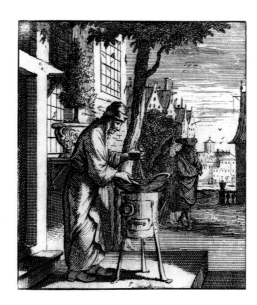

twenty-seven (in the 1774 edition the number was reduced to ten).

The pioneering work in chemistry that the pharmacists of France and Germany undertook in the seventeenth and eighteenth centuries—coupled with advances in pharmaceutical education in the eighteenth century—began to turn pharmacy into a science. Although the new critical attitudes of the age encouraged a more cynical view of the old materia medica, much of the claptrap of the earlier period persisted. But there were some bright spots. One of these was simply practical and utilitarian. In Edinburgh the cleansing of the pharmacopoeia was based on the realization that many substances in the pharmacopoeia were never prescribed and that many just deteriorated on pharmacists' shelves. In Vienna the motivation for change was more subtle—the paternalistic concern of the absolute state for the welfare of the general population, which required the availability of uncomplicated, economical, and effective medicines.

Another bright spot was the awakening interest in testing drugs—the beginnings of modern pharmacology. Most of the interest in experimentation was toxicological, and the significant amount of research that was done on animals was more involved with the study of poisons than with the action of medicines. In Italy, in the eighteenth century, the physiologist Felice Fontana claimed to have made no less than six thousand experiments on viper venom, using three thousand vipers and four thousand animals.

There was, however, a broader concern with the operation of medicines in the human body that spread with the move from Leiden to Vienna of Gerhard van Swieten. In Vienna, the capital of Austria, pharmacological interests were a direct effect of the pressure of a paternalistic state economy that sought self-sufficiency: a search for, and the clinical testing of, native plants and new chemicals that would replace old, imported, and expensive drugs of doubtful efficacy. Van Swieten became Vienna's

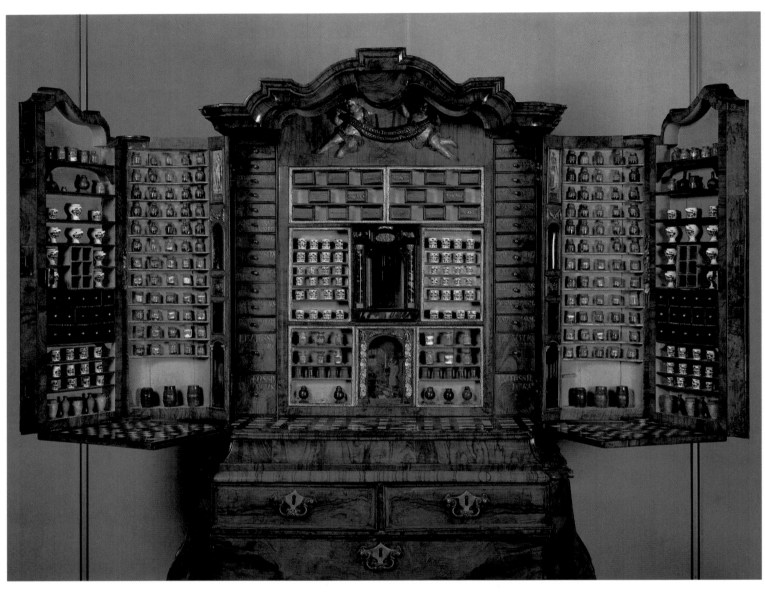

Simplica cabinet. Northern Netherlands, c. 1730. The original simples are still preserved in the miniature delftware jars on the shelves of this oak cabinet, inlaid with walnut, from the Collegium Pharmaceuticum of Delft. Rijksmuseum, Amsterdam

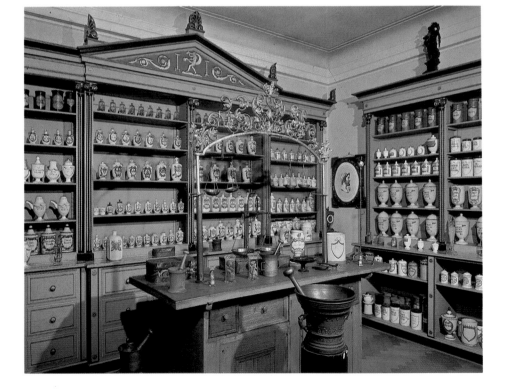

Postcard view of a reconstruction of an 18th-century German pharmacy in the Deutsches Museum, Munich

highest medical official and inaugurated a systematic program of clinical studies of drugs. In 1754 he directed the testing of corrosive sublimate on patients in the syphilitic ward of the Spital St. Marx and then in other Vienna hospitals. The results were so promising, particularly in comparison with the mercury therapy, that the use of corrosive sublimate in syphilis was adopted throughout Europe after 1755.

Under van Swieten's direction, research turned to the testing of native plants for their medicinal properties—the idea being to make Austria as self-sufficient in drugs as in other areas. The process began with the clinical testing of arbutus as a lithontriptic by Anton de Haen, and it flourished in the hands of Anton Störck, who was convinced that plants known to be poisonous could nevertheless be useful, in controlled amounts, as medicines. Störck experimented on animals, on himself, and on his patients with, among other substances, conium and hyoscyamus as anodynes and narcotics, colchicum and aconite as diaphoretics and diuretics, and stramonium as a sedative and antidepressive. Störck's work made a great impression throughout Europe, and both the London and the Edinburgh pharmacopoeias accepted several of his recommendations. Initial enthusiasm waned, however, when his results proved questionable. Even so, his research may have played a role in the popularity in the next century of hyoscyamus, stramonium, and colchicum. Störck not only established the medicinal usefulness of prudent doses of certain substances that are toxic in larger amounts; he also set a pattern for clinical studies and for determining dosage and toxicity.

From this new approach to the clinical testing of drugs came one tremendous boon. In England, William Withering, studying the reputed efficacy of a folk remedy for dropsy, determined that the active ingredient among its twenty-odd herbs was *Digitalis purpurea,* the foxglove, and that its beneficial results came from its diuretic action. After closely investigating digitalis on

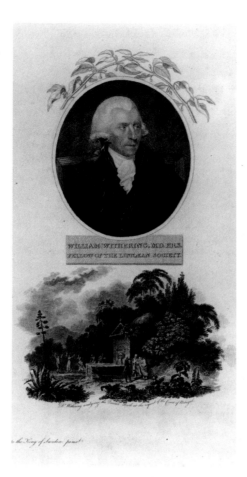

Portrait of William Withering. Stipple engraving by Ridley after Carl-Fredrik van Breda, portrait painter to the King of Sweden. English (London), 1801. Withering (1741–1799), an eminent clinician and botanist, called the attention of the medical profession to the virtues of digitalis in the treatment of dropsy. Below, he is depicted analyzing the Queen's Bath at the request of the Court of Portugal

his own, Withering and his friends at Edinburgh, where he had studied medicine, subjected the drug to clinical trials at the Infirmary there. The results were so favorable that digitalis, which had been removed from the Edinburgh pharmacopoeia as useless, was reinstated—even before Withering published his classic *Account of the Foxglove,* in 1785.

There was interest elsewhere in seeking to verify the "virtues" of plants. In Paris, members of the Académie Royale des Sciences had in the seventeenth century established a program of screening plants, publishing their findings in *Mémoires pour servir à l'histoire des plantes* (1676). The program proved to be of little account, however, probably because the only method used to detect the active ingredients was distillation. (Distillation of organic materials, especially when the ash is discarded, tends to yield the same end products, regardless of the original material.) Other attempts to determine the presence, or proportions, of resin, gum, and salt in a given substance by pharmaceutical-chemical processes of extraction were of little practical value. The breakthrough was not to come until early in the nineteenth century, when chemists—largely pharmacists, as will be seen—succeeded in isolating the vegetable alkaloids.

Two brilliant and momentous scientific developments in the eighteenth century were to influence the cleansing of the pharmacopoeias: the germinal work of Linnaeus, the Swedish naturalist, and the groundbreaking work of the French chemist Antoine Lavoisier. Linnaeus's classifications as set forth in his *Systema naturae* (1735), *Species plantarum* (1753), *Systema naturae, animalia* (1759), and *Systema naturae, vegetablis* (1759) found their way into the pharmacopoeias, as plants and animals alike were identified by their Linnaean characteristics. In the process, duplication and redundancy were eliminated, order was formed out of chaos, and the pharmacopoeia became increasingly scientific as it categorized and described the materia medica with greater specificity.

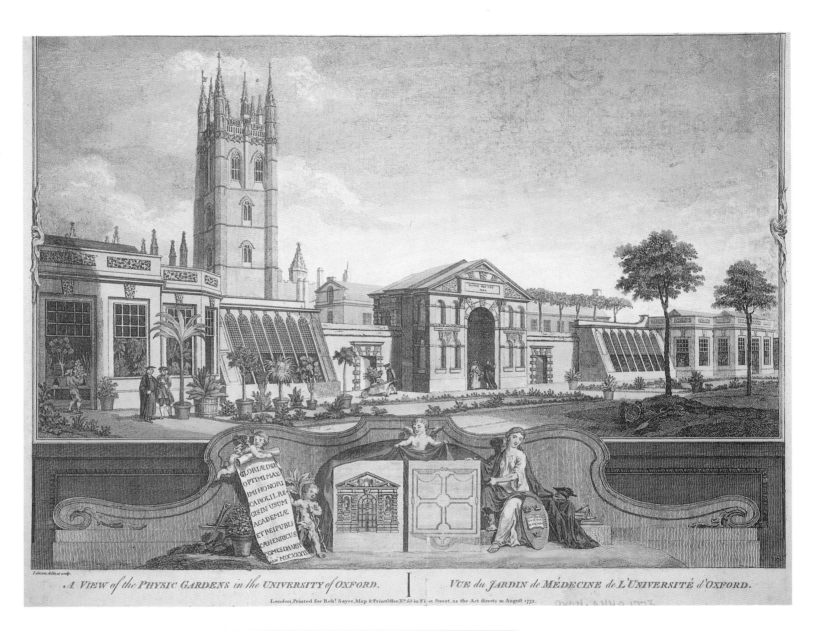

A VIEW of the PHYSIC GARDENS in the UNIVERSITY of OXFORD. | VUE du JARDIN de MÉDECINE de L'UNIVERSITÉ d'OXFORD.

London, Printed for Robt. Sayer, Map & Printseller Nº 53 in Fl. et Street, as the Act directs 10 August 1773.

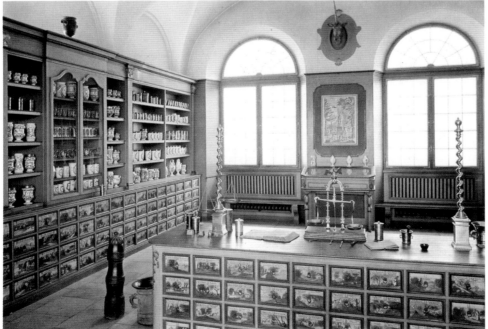

A View of the Physic Garden, University of Oxford. Hand-colored engraving by J. Green. English, 1773

Reconstruction of a Swiss pharmacy interior of about 1830. The collection of drug jars and mortars and pestles includes a large bronze mortar and pestle from 1740 (in the foreground). Schweizerisches Pharmazie-Historisches Museum, Basel

Die Storchen-Apotheke (The Stork Pharmacy). Painting by Carl Spitzweg (1808–1885). German, c. 1865. A qualified pharmacist-turned-artist, Spitzweg painted several works in which a pharmacy is shown. Von der Heydt Museum, Wuppertal, West Germany ▶

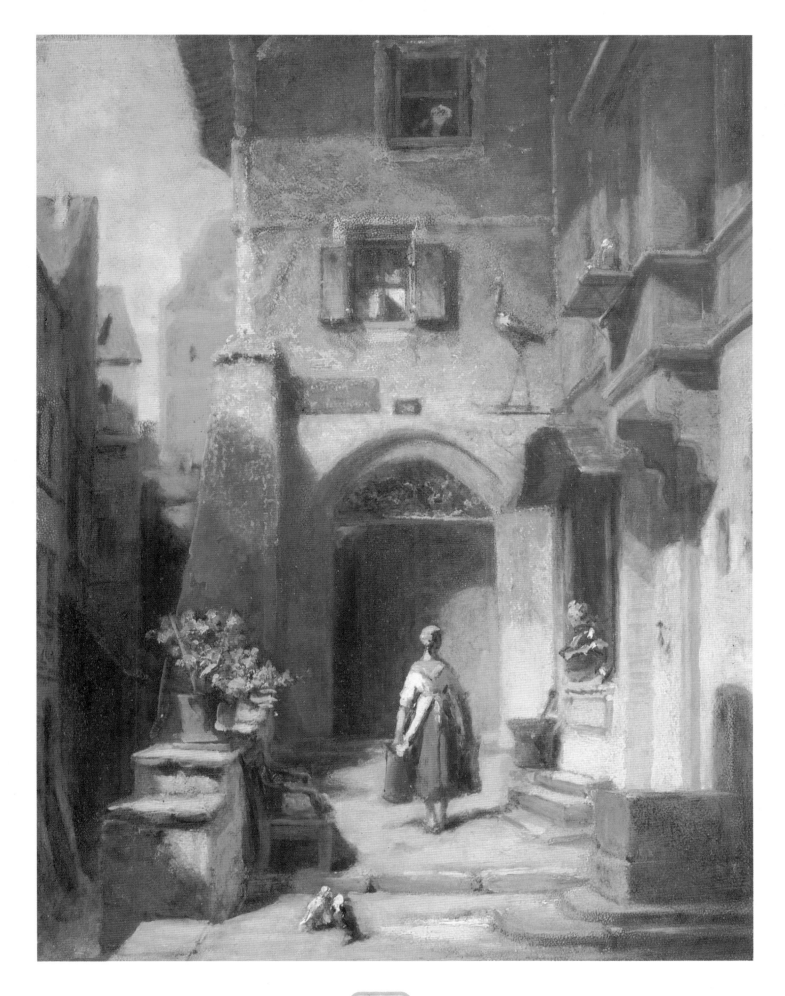

A similar process took place with the chemical compositions in the pharmacopoeias. Lavoisier's *Traité élémentaire de chimie* introduced a new system of nomenclature. It caused complications, for some of the new names were cumbersome and some of the old, familiar names seemed more appropriate. But here too the result was better organization of pharmacopoeias and more scientific identification of chemical compositions.

THE DISPENSATORY AND OTHER PHARMACEUTICAL LITERATURE

Pharmacopoeias were essentially lists of drugs and formulas; they contained little material other than directions for compounding. There was, then, a clear need for a companion publication that would describe drugs, give indications for their use, and provide some account of professional experience with the drugs in question. This kind of book, the dispensatory, became something of a British specialty in the late seventeenth and the eighteenth century.

Among the most noteworthy dispensatories were the *Pharmacopoeia Bateana* of George Bate, the *Pharmacopoeia extemporanea* of Thomas Fuller, and the *Pharmacopoeia officinalis & extemporanea; or, a compleat English dispensatory* of John Quincy. Each was issued in many editions, and Latin, English, Portuguese, Spanish, Dutch, German, and French versions of them appeared frequently in Great Britain and on the Continent. Quincy's work was the prototype of the long series of dispensatories that began with the *New Dispensatory* of William Lewis, which was published in 1753 as a "Correction and Improvement of Quincy." Seven issues of the *New Dispensatory* appeared during Lewis's lifetime and five more after his death, the last in 1799. There was little to distinguish these various issues.

Lewis divided his work into three parts. They were preceded by an introduction, "The Elements of Pharmacy," in which Lewis wrote, "Pharmacy is the art of preparing and compounding natural [the second edition of 1765 added "and artificial"] substances for medicinal purposes in a manner suitable to their respective properties, and the intentions of cure."

Pharmacy, Lewis asserted, was galenical or chemical, and it was made up of theoretical and practical components. Theoretical pharmacy required "the knowledge of medicinal substances themselves, their distinguishing characteristics, the marks of their goodness, genuineness and purity, their several properties and qualities, their relations to one another with regard to miscibility, their fitness or unfitness for different treatments, and their general effects on the human body." Practical pharmacy required "the skilful performance of the several processes, or operations, by which they were fitted for particular purposes." Lewis's introduction also described in some detail pharmaceutical utensils and pharmaceutical operations. The pharmacist was expected to know and use the processes of solution, extraction, depuration (purification), crystallization, precipitation, evaporation, distillation, sublimation, expression, exsiccation, comminution, fusion, and calcination.

The first major section of Lewis's *New Dispensatory* was devoted to the materia medica. The contents were arranged first according to function (diuretics, emetics, cathartics, narcotics, etc.), then on the basis of their "sensible qualities" (acids, astringents, absorbents, etc.), and then alphabetically, by Latin name. The alphabetical list, which covered 164 pages, presented a monograph on each drug that designated whether the drug was to be found in the London or the Edinburgh pharmacopoeia (or both), gave its botanical name, and provided a description of the drug, including its place of origin, its usable parts, its medicinal uses, and, in some instances, the relevant comments of medical authorities.

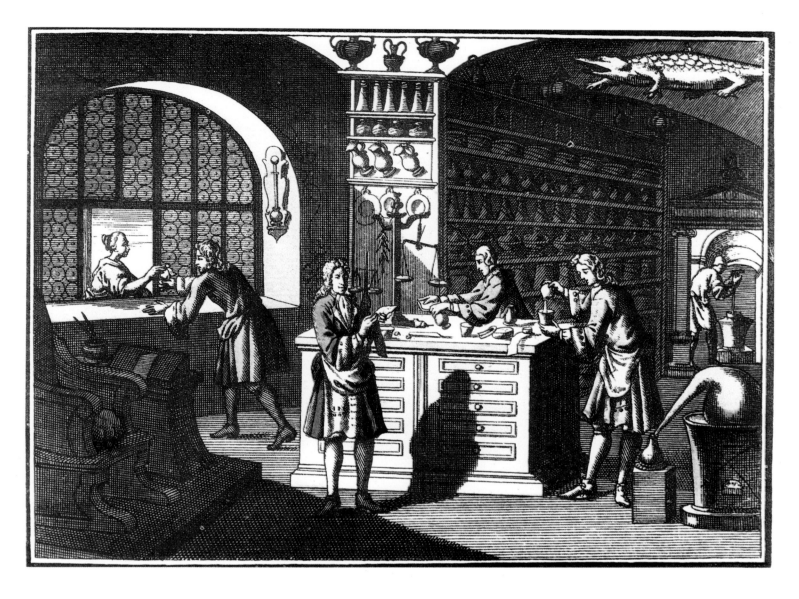

The second part of the *New Dispensatory* offered a "Pharmacopoeia Officinalis," a collection of official compounds in some twenty-six categories (metallic preparations, distilled liquors, syrups, pills, powders, etc.), their formulas, and directions for preparing and compounding. The third part of the *Dispensatory* offered a "Pharmacopoeia Extemporanea," a similar compilation of nonofficial compounds, not officially recognized by either the London or the Edinburgh College of Physicians but that the pharmacist might nevertheless be called upon to make.

A critic writing in 1831 called Lewis's work "the first truly scientific work on pharmacy in the English language." There is much in it that modern commentators would no longer accept as "scientific," yet

Der Apotecker (The Apothecary) Engraving from Franciscus Florinus, *Oeconomus prudens et legalis.* Nuremberg, 1722. National Library of Medicine, Bethesda

for its organization, comprehensiveness, critical attitude, and up-to-date treatment, Lewis's work is a landmark.

In 1786, two "gentlemen of the faculty" at Edinburgh, Charles Webster and Ralph Irving, produced "an improvement" on Lewis, the *Edinburgh New Dispensatory,* which incorporated marked changes. The major change was an emphasis on chemistry. Even galenical forms, they wrote, "are by no means independent of chemistry. . . . this science extends to mixtures of the most simple kind." Thus their work was prefaced with "An Abstract of Dr. Webster's Syllabus of Lectures on Chemistry and Materia Medica," and they converted the first part of the *Dispensatory* into "Elements of Pharmaceutical Chemistry." One of their innovations was the use of Linnaean plant names.

There followed a long series of editions of the *Edinburgh New Dispensatory,* each new edition a genuine revision. From 1786 to 1830 they provide a clear record of the changes taking place in pharmacy and drug therapy. In the lifetime of the *New Dispensatory* and the *Edinburgh New Dispensatory*—1753 to 1830—no fewer than thirty-five British, six American, and twelve foreign language (German, French, Dutch, Italian, Portuguese) printings of them appeared. These dispensatories tell us a great deal about the practice of pharmacy in the period covered.

In both the *New Dispensatory* and the *Edinburgh New Dispensatory* can be found relics of ancient tradition as well as glimmers of progress. By 1794, the *Edinburgh New Dispensatory* noted that from certain drugs "any considerable medical power is not to be expected," and that others "do not possess any remarkable medical properties." The surest mark of progress was the inclusion of a section on "The New Chemical Doctrines Published by Mr. Lavoisier" as noted on the title page of the 1791 and subsequent editions.

MEDICAL SPECULATION

The process of clinical testing of drugs at a time when knowledge of human physiology was limited and biochemistry unknown, was essentially an exercise in trial and error. Because the state of scientific knowledge was so rudimentary at the time, medicine was unable to develop a soundly based critical and scientific empiricism. In its place there developed a speculative, rational approach that was to have an impact on medicine, and on pharmacy, until well into the twentieth century.

A new medical system had already arisen in the late Renaissance to challenge the concepts of iatrochemistry. In this new system, founded by the Italian physician Santorio Santorio and labeled "iatrophysics," the

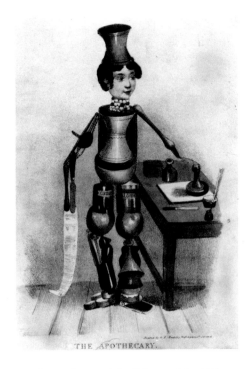

The Apothecary. Color lithograph by G. E. Madeley. English, 1830. The figure is made up of an assortment of pharmaceutical objects and implements, including mortars, pestles, bottles, and a funnel. Wellcome Institute Library, London

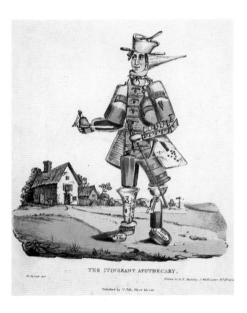

The Itinerant Apothecary. Color lithograph by G. Spratt. English, c. 1810. A figure made of drug bottles, mortars, and other pharmaceutical artifacts. His feet are made of Bilious Pills and Tolu Lozenges.

body was conceived of as a machine. Iatrophysics was followed in turn, about a century later, by the theory of "solidism," which held that in disease the solid parts of the body were either too relaxed or too tense. The armamentarium of the famous German physician who propounded the concept of solidism, Friedrich Hoffmann, consisted therefore largely of sedatives, tonics, alteratives, and evacuants. Hoffmann developed many remedies, one of which, an anodyne and antispasmodic (probably the spirit of sulfuric ether), was long known in pharmacy as "Hoffmann's drops" or "Hoffmann's anodyne."

Other physicians emphatically rejected this materialistic and mechanistic approach to medicine. Hoffmann's colleague Ernst Stahl postulated that the basis of health and illness was the *animus,* the soul, which maintained the rhythm of the body. When this rhythm was disturbed, the body lacked *tonus,* or tone, and it was the function of medication to restore that tone. In the late eighteenth century, Paul-Joseph Barthez and others at the University of Montpellier replaced Stahl's *animus* with a "vital principle," and this "vitalism" prevailed in certain medical centers in Europe well into the nineteenth century.

In Scotland, also in the late eighteenth century, the noted William Cullen varied this theoretical approach by postulating a "nervous principle" that kept the body in tone. Drug therapy should therefore be either irritative, when the body lacked tone, or emollient, when the body was excited.

This theory of *strictum et laxum,* as it was referred to in the medical literature, buttressed by the pioneering work of the Swiss scientist Albrecht von Haller on the physiology of muscle-nerve function, culminated in what became known as Brunonianism, named after its creator, the Scottish physician John Brown, who had been Cullen's pupil in Edinburgh. Brown reduced the causes of disease to two: excessive tension and excessive relaxation. Hence remedies must be relaxing or stimulating; this led Brown's followers to rely, respectively, on opium and brandy. In the United States, another pupil of Cullen's, Benjamin Rush, went still further. All disease had a single cause: irregular or convulsive action in the system due to hypertension of the blood vessels. These ideas supplied a new rationale for purging and bloodletting. Rush's therapeutics—which earned the sobriquet "heroic medicine" because of the strength and the quantity of the measures used—called for calomel, strong emetics, and venesection. Brown's therapeutic ideas are said to have "destroyed more people than the French Revolution." The "heroic medicine" that Rush fathered in the United States accomplished little good and undoubtedly did immeasurable harm. These excesses were to open the way for homeopathy and Thomsonianism in the nineteenth century.

THE PHARMACEUTICAL ESTABLISHMENT

By the end of the Renaissance, pharmacists in Continental Europe had attained both impressive social status and general recognition as providers of health care. However, their activities continued to be closely watched by the health authorities, the medical profession, and their own professional organizations. On the Continent as a whole (to a lesser extent in France) the system that limited the number of pharmacies, established qualifications for the practice of pharmacy, determined who might open a pharmacy and where, fixed prices, and inspected pharmacies prevailed into the early modern period. Inevitably there were differences in the development of pharmacy in different countries. In Italy, which was wracked by political disruption and particularism, the heritage of a highly organized and proud profession seemed to dissipate in the eighteenth century; it was saved by the imposition of Austrian regulations on Lombardy in 1778. Pharmaceuti-

Arlequin Hydropique Comédie. Hand-colored engraving. French, c. 1750. Three commedia dell'arte characters appear in this little medical comedy: M. le docteur Balouard, Harlequin, feigning dropsy, and Pierrot as apothecary (against a backdrop of mortars and pestles and drug jars), wielding a clyster. Harlequin, true to form, makes a mockery of the whole affair with his ridiculous answers to the doctor's questions.

cal legislation soon followed in other Italian jurisdictions.

The German states, in contrast, retained the basic features of the pharmaceutical arrangements they had developed during the Renaissance. The monopoly granted to the pharmacist eventually became more restrictive and limited him more and more to purely pharmaceutical products. One development in eighteenth-century Germany indicated the growth of pharmacy in the public esteem: increasingly, regulations took the inspection of pharmacies out of the hands of physicians and placed it in the hands of the pharmacists themselves. Early in the eighteenth century this became the general rule for all of Prussia.

In France, significant changes did not take place until 1777. In that year a royal decree finally separated the spicers and the pharmacists and turned the Paris pharmacists' guild into the Collège de Pharmacie. Henceforth, the Collège was to be an administrative body overseeing the pharmacists and also an educational institution. The wholesaling of drugs, the selling of crude drugs that required no compounding, and the retailing of a few enumerated drugs were left to the spicers and herbalists. One significant provision, which removed an old thorn from pharmacy's side, was a prohibition on the sale of drugs by religious societies and hospitals.

An interesting French development in this period was a change in title, from *apothicaire* to *pharmacien*—a change that could have come about as it did only in France. Among the duties of the French *apothicaire* was both the preparation of medicated clysters, or enemas, and the administration of these enemas by means of metal syringes. The clyster was a health fad from the fifteenth to the eighteenth century; Louis XIII reportedly had no fewer than 312 clysters in one year. In time the whole idea became an object of jest, and when seventeenth-century French writers began to use the satiric motif of the *apothicaire* administering the clyster, *apothicaires* became uncomfortable. When the great Molière, in *Le Malade*

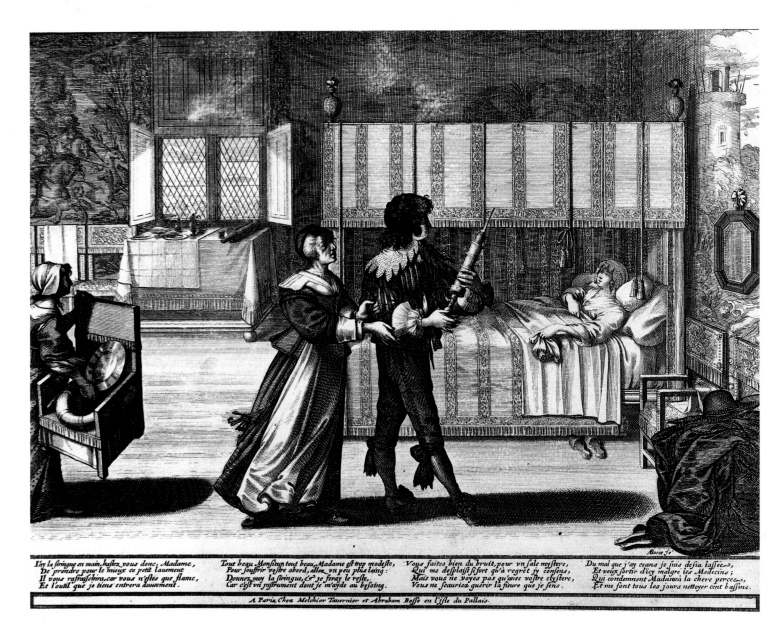

Iey la feringue en main, haftez vous donc, Madame,
De prendre pour le mieux ce petit lauement
Il vous raffraifchira, car vous n'eftes que flame,
Et l'outil que je tiens entrera doucement.

Tout beau Monfieur tout beau, Madame eft trop modefte,
Pour souffrir voftre abord, allez un peu plus loing :
Donnez moy la feringue, & je feray le refte,
Car c'eft un inftrument dont je m'ayde au befoing.

Vous faites bien du bruit, pour un fale myftere,
Qui me deftplaift fi fort qu'à regret j'y confens,
Mais vous ne voyez pas qu'auec voftre clyftere,
Vous ne fcauriez guerir la fieure que je fens.

Du mal que j'ay ceans je fuis defia laffée,
Et veux fortir d'icy malgré les Medecins ;
Qui condemnent Madauva la chere percée,
Et me font tous les jours nettoyer cent baffins.

A Paris, Chez Melchior Tauernier et Abraham Boffe en l'ifle du Pallais.

Apothecary preparing to administer a purge. Engraving by Abraham Bosse. French, 1680. This elegant scene and the accompanying verses reflect a skeptical and satirical view of the clyster. The apothecary is eager to carry out his assignment, the nurse (or maid) thinks she can handle the instrument better, and the patient, annoyed with their arguing, declares she has no faith in the clyster and is already better "malgré les Médecins." Ars Medica Collection, Philadelphia Museum of Art

imaginaire, in pointing up the foibles of both physicians and pharmacists, made the clyster the target of his wit, *apothicaires* were acutely embarrassed. They therefore dropped the term *apothicaire* and adopted *pharmacien.* The change saved face for the *apothicaires,* but their role in the administration of the clyster was not allowed to be forgotten; in the nineteenth century Honoré Daumier and other artists used the clyster-syringe device to poke fun at figures in their caricatures.

The tumultuous political upheaval of the French Revolution did not leave pharmacy untouched. On March 2, 1791, the National Assembly, "in accordance with the revolutionary ideas of freedom of commerce and the professions," suppressed "all of the privileges of the professions," including "the patents and warrants of the masters [and] all the laws governing the admission of masters and wardens of the College of Pharmacy." Almost immediately, in Paris and in the provinces, drug sellers, herbalists, and others took advantage of this new liberty, but the gross abuses that followed lasted only seventeen days—until a pharmacist member succeeded in convincing the National Assembly that it should return pharmacy to its previous status.

In England, pharmacy took on a character peculiar to that country. There apothecaries had increasingly become practitioners of medicine, a development to

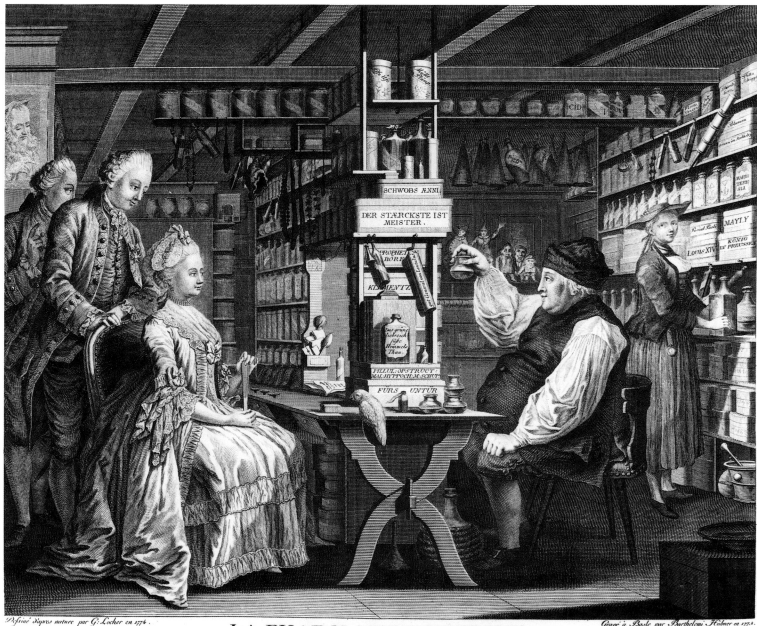

Désiné d'après nature par G. Locher en 1774.   *Gravé à Basle par Barthelemi Hubner en 1775.*

LA PHARMACIE RUSTIQUE

ou Représentation exacte de l'intérieur de la Chambre, où Michel Schuppach connu sous le nom du Médecin de la Montagne, tient ses Consultations.

Cet homme étonnant s'est acquis une célébrité qui fait époque dans l'histoire de l'esprit humain. Il naquit l'an 1707 à Bigle, village du Canton de Berne, et ne fut d'abord que simple Chirurgien de village. Mais une sagacité peu concevable à découvrir les maladies par l'inspection des urines, et nombre de cures surprenantes ont attiré chez lui depuis quelques années de presque toutes les parties de l'Europe, une foule incroyable de Malades la plûpart distingués par la naissance ou par la fortune. C'est surtout à son génie et à sa longue expérience, qu'il doit ses rares lumières, n'étant jamais sorti des environs de Langnan, lieu de sa résidence actuelle. Sa bienfaisance envers les pauvres, la franchise de son caractère et l'originalité de son esprit, ajoutent encore au mérite de ce rustique Hippocrate.

à Basle chez Chrétien de Michel Graveur et à Paris chez Basan et Poignant.

La Pharmacie rustique. Engraving by Barthelemi Hubner after a drawing from life by Gottfried Locher. Swiss, 1775. This engraving shows the "exact interior" of the pharmacy where Michel Schuppach, a simple village doctor who became famous for diagnosing illnesses by the inspection of urine, held his consultations. Well-born and distinguished people from all over Europe flocked here, hoping for one of the spectacular cures effected by this kindly and talented "rustic Hippocrates." Wellcome Institute Library, London

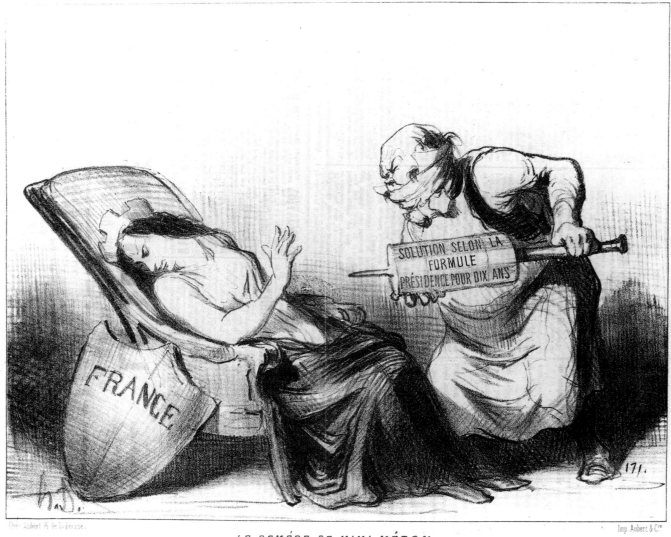

LE REMÉDE DE MIMI VÉRON
apothicaire en chef du Constitutionnel.
— Prenez.........prenez, il n'y a que cela qui puisse vous sauver!

Le Remède de Mimi Véron (The Remedy of Mimi Véron). Lithograph by Honoré Daumier. French, 1850. Again portrayed by Daumier as a pharmacist, the versatile Dr. Véron offers a clyster (extending the president's term to ten years) to France as the only solution of her political problems.

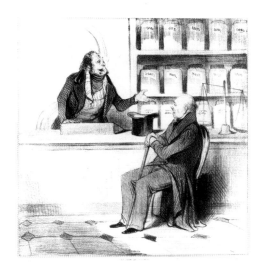

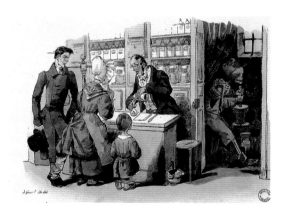

Voyage pour l'éternité. Color lithograph by J. J. Grandville. French, 1830. In this scene, one of a series of ten plates illustrating the Dance of Death, a pharmacist assures the patient's family, *"Soyez tranquille, j'ai un Garçon qui ne se trompe jamais* (Be calm, I have an assistant who never makes a mistake)," while Death, out of sight, prepares his fatal prescription.
Collection Bouvet, Paris

Apothicaire et pharmacien. Lithograph by Honoré Daumier. French, 1837. In a series of caricatures using a central character, Robert Macaire, Daumier lashed out at those who engaged in get-rich-quick schemes. Here the younger *pharmacien,* Macaire, tells the older *apothicaire* how he makes his fortune: he simply takes some tallow, brick, dust, or starch, concocts a gibberish brand name like Onicophane, Racahout, or Osmanaglow, publishes advertisements and circulars, and in ten years makes a fortune.

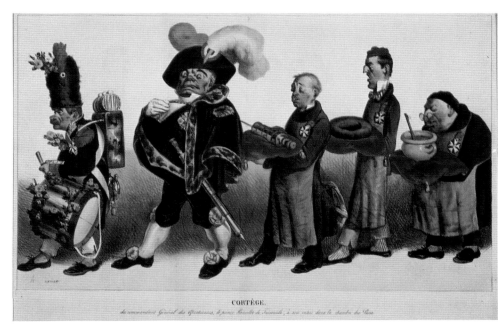

Cortège du Commandant Général des Apothicaires, le prince Lancelot de Tucanule, à son entrée dans la chambre des Pairs. Color lithograph by Honoré Daumier. French, 1833. To quell the riots at the Place Vendôme in Paris in 1831, Marshal Lobau, chief of the Paris police, used high-pressure hoses. Caricaturists immediately dubbed him Commander General of the Apothecaries. Daumier shows him with associates carrying the paraphernalia necessary to this office.

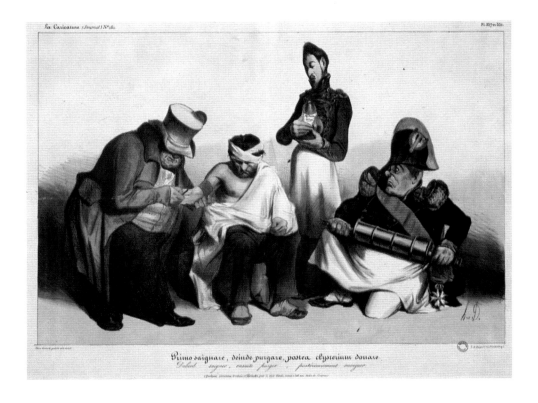

Primo saignare, deinde purgare, postea clysterium donare (First to bleed, then to purge, after that to give a clyster). Color lithograph by Honoré Daumier. French, 1833. The physician attending to the wounds of the nation is King Louis Philippe. Marshal Lobau, the police chief of Paris, waits with his clyster. The title is close to the treatment proposed for all diseases by Molière in his play *Le Malade imaginaire.*

which the Royal College of Physicians had not taken kindly. The physicians' harshest barb, a long poem by Sir Samuel Garth, "The Dispensary," appeared in 1699; the apothecaries' response was the anonymous *Pharmacopolae justificati, Or, apothecaries vindicated from the imputation of ignorance, wherein is shown that an academical education is in no way necessary to qualify a man for the practice of physick.* The quarrel was not of brief duration; Garth's poem went through at least eleven editions, the last appearing in 1768.

This quarrel went well beyond polemics. Members of the Royal College of Physicians took action: they opened dispensaries in London, between 1698 and 1725, where they sold medicines to the poor "in penny doses." However, the impact of these dispensaries is not clear: a proponent claimed, in 1703, that twenty thousand prescriptions had been dispensed, but an opponent claimed that they "were never very successful." In any case, the College of Physicians finally resorted to the courts in their attempt to curtail the medical practice of apothecaries.

In 1703, the critical case of William Rose gave the apothecaries the authority they sought. Rose, an apothecary, was prosecuted for prescribing remedies and was found guilty by the Court of the Queen's Bench. But on appeal to the House of Lords the decision was reversed: the Lords found that the law prohibiting prescribing by apothecaries was not only contrary to custom but also against the public interest, there being hardly a sufficient number of doctors to go around.

The Rose case established the right of the apothecary who had served an apprenticeship to practice medicine as well as to perform his usual pharmaceutical tasks. Over a century later, with the passage of the Apothecaries Act of 1815, the apothecary was finally allowed to charge for his advice as well as for the medication he dispensed. Although he was required by the Act to fill physicians' prescriptions, the apothecary became the general practitioner of medi-

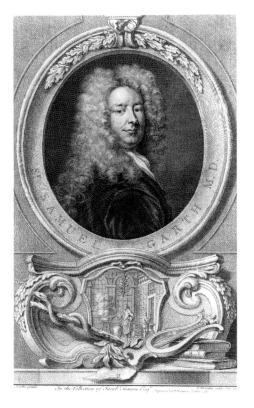

Sir Samuel Garth M.D. Engraving by Jacobus Houbraken after Gottfried Kneller. Dutch (Amsterdam), c. 1748. Garth (1661–1719) was the author of "The Dispensary," a long satirical poem, published in 1699, directed against medical practice by apothecaries. A vignette of a pharmacy interior appears below the portrait.

Apothecary tokens. English, 17th century. Inscribed with the name and address of the tradesman, such tokens were struck at a time when the Royal Mint was not producing sufficient coinage. Apothecaries made much use of them. The reverse of this round token displays the motto and arms of the Worshipful Society of Apothecaries. The British Museum, London

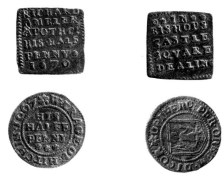

cine. The current Society of Apothecaries in Britain is essentially an examining and licensing agency for general practitioners; it also offers postgraduate medical courses and lectures.

Eighteenth-century apothecaries in England seemed to have had the best of two worlds: they were both physicians and pharmacists. But their hold on pharmacy was challenged by a group that had emerged in mid-century, the functionaries known as chemists-and-druggists. These individuals, who probably started out as chemists and drug wholesalers, did almost everything the apothecaries did. They operated shops in which drugs, compound remedies, and household commodities were sold; they dispensed prescriptions and they counter-prescribed; they made up galenicals and compounded medicines; and they performed minor surgical operations such as extracting teeth and lancing boils. The major difference seems to have been that while the chemist-and-druggist did not leave his shop, the apothecary traveled to a patient's house, at first to administer medicines prescribed by the physician and, after 1815, as a medical practitioner in his own right. As might be expected, apothecaries sought to stop the inroads of chemists-and-druggists into their precincts. This they failed to do, and it is from the ranks of these dispensing chemists-and-druggists that British pharmacy developed in the nineteenth century.

Engraved trade card of I. Taylor, Apothecary and Chemist. English (London), c. 1750. Prior to 1767, London buildings were not numbered, and locations were indicated by landmarks such as St. Dunstan's Church. ▶

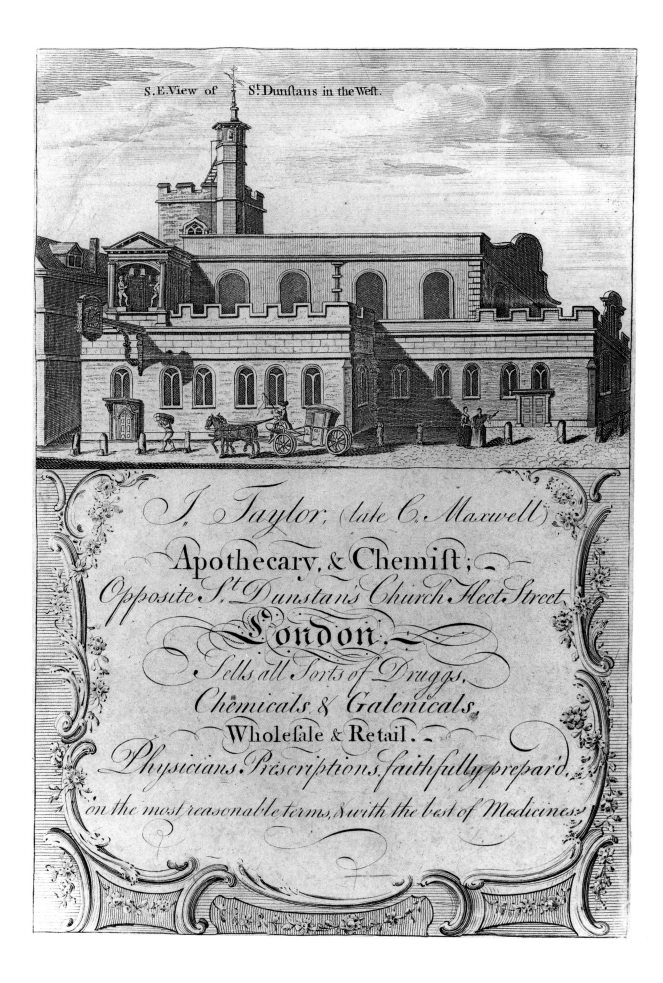

S.E.View of St Dunstans in the West.

J. Taylor, (late C. Maxwell)
Apothecary, & Chemist;
Opposite St Dunstans Church Fleet Street.
London.
Sells all Sorts of Druggs,
Chemicals & Galenicals,
Wholesale & Retail.
Physicians Prescriptions faithfully prepar'd,
on the most reasonable terms, & with the best of Medicines

PHARMACY
IN THE AMERICAS

Pharmacy in the New World reflected both the transfer of European culture across the Atlantic and the impact of geographic realities. In Spanish America there is frequent mention of pharmacists as early as the sixteenth century. Under Spanish law the board of royal physicians—the *proto-medicato*—and other functionaries examined pharmacists and their shops at least as early as 1540. North of Mexico, however, pharmacy did not really take form until the eighteenth century. Only a few pharmacists are known to have participated in the colonization of the Americas. These include Louis Hébert, who left his shop in Paris in 1604 to accompany Champlain to Canada, and John Johnstone, an Edinburgh druggist, who led an expedition that founded the settlement of Perth Amboy, New Jersey, in 1685. By and large, however, there were few pharmacists among the early colonists—a scarcity that, in 1621, caused the Virginia Company, because "of the great want of men of his profession" to be willing to accept the offer of an apothecary and his wife to go to Virginia if the company would pay for the transportation of their two children. There are records of pharmacy shops in Boston as early as 1646 and in New York in 1653. Bartholomew Browne of Salem, Massachusetts, kept an account book (Essex Institute, Salem) which shows that in the late 1600s he charged for both medications and "attendance," in the fashion of the British apothecary.

By the eighteenth century, pharmacy was starting to develop in the British colonies. A printed "Catalogue of Medicine Sold by Mr. Robert Talbot at Burlington" was issued in New Jersey about 1725. According to the inventory of Mr. Talbot's estate, he had been operating a pharmacy reasonably well stocked with European materia medica and well equipped with pharmaceutical apparatus. On the evidence of newspaper adver-

Broadside advertising Shepherd's Medicines. American, c. 1860. The lithograph vignette shows an American schooner being loaded with the specialties manufactured by Bodder & Co., Baltimore.　▶

tisements, it can be stated that there were drugstores in virtually all American cities by the end of the eighteenth century.

During the colonial period and the early years of American independence, there were, as was to be expected in a land so vast and so sparsely settled, virtually no limitations as to where or by whom pharmacy could be practiced. Pharmaceutical services were plainly needed, and the services that were to develop into the separate institution of pharmacy were performed in the eighteenth century by various functionaries. The physician made up his own remedies and, not unlike the British apothecary, probably received most of his income from the medicines he dispensed. There were also individuals who referred to themselves as apothecaries and operated shops; fourteen such shops existed in Boston by the 1720s. There were also individuals who called themselves druggists. Originally they were wholesalers of drugs and might or might not have had a medical or pharmaceutical background; later they not only sold at retail but began to offer pharmaceutical services. There were also merchants and storekeepers who, especially in areas where there were no pharmacies within easy reach, stocked not only crude drugs but packaged drugs and "patent" medicines. Finally, there was the pharmacist whose activities conformed to the modern definition of the term. The lines of demarcation between these various functionaries cannot be clearly drawn; their provinces overlapped, and appellations, which often meant little, frequently changed. But out of their activities pharmacy as we know it emerged in the nineteenth century.

Pharmacy in the Franco-Spanish colony of Louisiana more clearly reflected its development in Continental Europe. As early as 1769, examination of pharmacists and authorization to practice were instituted, and the next year saw the first legal definition issued north of the Rio Grande demarcating pharmacy as a separate branch of medicine. In a proclamation of February 12, 1770, Don Alexandre O'Reilly, the Spanish gover-

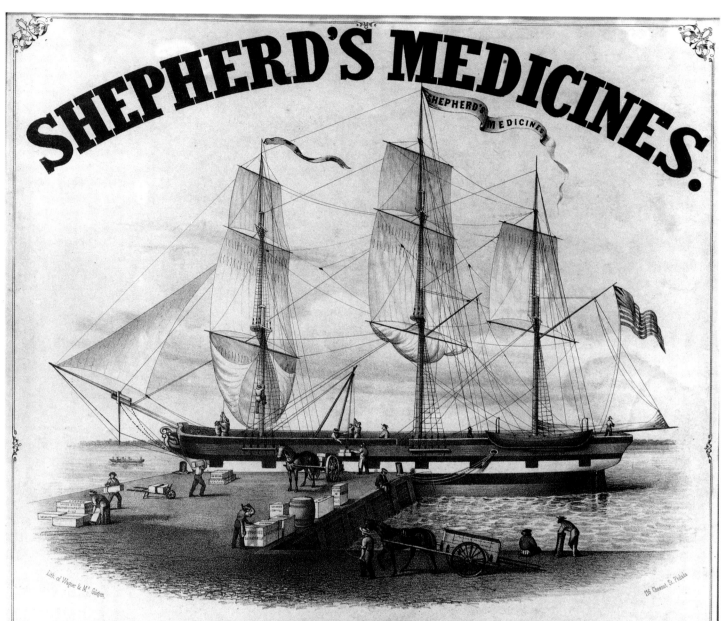

SHEPHERD'S SARSAPARILLA, Price 0.75 cts. per Bottle
SHEPHERD'S VERMIFUGE .... „ 0.25 „ „ „
UNITED STATES VEGETABLE PURGATIVE PILLS „ 0.25 „ „ Box
GREAT WESTERN AGUE SPECIFIC „ 1.00 „ „ Bottle
GERMAN FEVER & AGUE PILLS .... „ 1.00 „ „ Box
FOR SALE HERE.

BODDER & CO. PROPRIETORS, BALTIMORE.

nor of Louisiana, proclaimed that "Medicine…embraces three parts, namely: medicine proper, surgery and pharmacy [that] are its attendants and have their special field….Pharmacy is concerned, generally speaking, with the preparation of remedies."

THE PHARMACIST AND SCIENCE

The scientific aspects of pharmacy had been in the hands of physicians, botanists, and alchemists until the sixteenth century, when pharmacists begin to make contributions to science. It was in the realm of chemistry that this first became evident. The medieval and Renaissance trends that had turned the pharmacist's officina into a chemical laboratory had meant that pharmacists perforce became acquainted with chemistry. By the early seventeenth century, pharmacists had already attained considerable stature as chemists. The first chair in chemistry was held by the pharmacist Johann Hartmann in Marburg in 1609. A series of lectures in chemistry for the public inaugurated at the Jardin des Plantes in Paris in the seventeenth century was delivered by a succession of pharmacists, among them Nicaise LeFebvre, Moïse Charas, Guillaume-François Rouelle, Hilaire-Marin Rouelle, and the Swiss Christophe Glaser.

LeFebvre first published his *Traité de Chymie*, later called the *Cours de chymie*, in Paris in 1660. It was considered the best chemical textbook of the period, even though it was essentially pharmaceutical chemistry. LeFebvre introduced some elementary yet important techniques into chemistry, among them the use of the thermometer, the avoidance of the use of copper utensils when volatile materials were involved in distillation, and the avoidance of metal utensils when acid materials were involved. His text was republished a number of times, and it was translated into both English and German. Charas, who had established his reputation as a master pharmacist, published his *Pharmacopoée royale, galénique, et chymique* in 1672. More pharmaceutical than chemical, it too went through several editions and was translated into Latin and English.

LeFebvre and other pharmacists offered private lessons in chemistry. Also notable among these private teachers of chemistry was Nicolas Lémery, whose *Cours de chymie* was first published in 1675. Over the next century Lémery became one of the most translated authors of the age. His work, which superseded LeFebvre's and was in all probability the world's most widely used chemistry textbook for a century, showed a greater interest in pure chemistry, but the bulk of his treatise concerned the preparation of chemical medications. He has been called the founder of modern phytochemistry (the chemistry of plants.).

Other noted French pharmacist-chemists made significant contributions to chemistry proper. Etienne-François Geoffroy published his tables of chemical relationships in 1718, a pathfinding achievement. His student Antoine Baumé improved the process of distillation and introduced the hydrometer. And Guillaume-François Rouelle, remembered for his chemical definition of the concept of "salt," made a great contribution to chemistry in France as the teacher of Lavoisier.

Three pharmaceutical chemists made direct contributions to pharmacy as well, and they were major forces in turning pharmacy from a technical art toward science. Lémery's *Pharmacopoée universelle* of 1697, and his *Traité universel des drogues simples,* published a year later, went through many editions and many translations. Geoffroy's three-volume *Tractatus de materia medica* (1741) is considered the first book to present pharmacognosy—the identification and description of crude drugs—in a systematic way. Antoine Baumé's *Elémens de pharmacie théorique et pratique,* which first appeared in 1762 and went through at least eight editions, included a review of the work that had been done to date in pharmaceutical chemistry; it also described pharmaceutical apparatus and procedures.

In Germany, the association between pharmacy and chemistry was strengthened by the work of men like Johann Rudolf Glauber, a seventeenth-century physician-chemist who described numerous techniques and produced various compounds, including sodium sulfate (Glauber's salt), ammonium sulfate, and zinc chloride. The first German pharmacist to make a contribution to the literature was Johann Christoph Sommerhoff, whose *Lexicon pharmaceuticum-chemicum,* published in 1701, encapsulated the pharmaceutical knowledge of the time, with special attention to the preparation of chemical remedies. There followed a host of excellent works on pharmacy and pharmaceutical chemistry, culminating in the *Lehrbuch der Apothekerkunst* of Karl Gottfried Hagen, which, after its appearance in 1778, became the most popular textbook in German pharmacy for the next seventy-five years. Hagen was credited with the emancipation of pharmacy—with turning it into an independent scientific discipline.

The end of the eighteenth century saw the publication of the first of the long series of textbooks written by Johann Bartholomeus Trommsdorff, a series that included the *Kurzes Handbuch der Apothekerkunst, zum Gebrauch für Lernende,* issued in 1790, and the first textbook on pharmacognosy, *Handbuch der pharmaceutisches Waarenkunde,* which appeared three years later.

The importance of the role that pharmacy played in the development of chemistry is indicated by the fact that for the last two-thirds of the eighteenth century and the first third of the nineteenth, the professors of chemistry in German universities usually came from the ranks of pharmacy. This trend began in 1724, when Caspar Neumann was called to the professorship of *chymiae practice* (practical chemistry) at the Collegium Medico-Chirurgicum in Berlin. During his tenure Neumann continued to practice pharmacy, and he made his Hof-

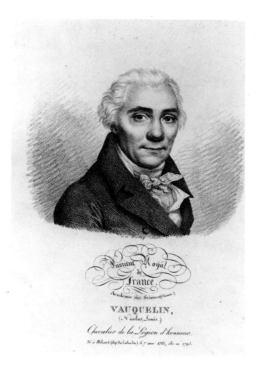

Nicolas Louis Vauquelin (1763–1829). Lithograph by Jules Boilly. French, 1820. Among the discoveries made by this French pharmacist were chromium, nicotine, lecithin, and cyanic acid.

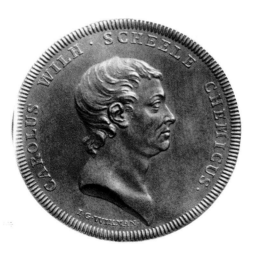

Bronze medal of Carl Wilhelm Scheele (1742–1786) by Johan Gabriel Wickman. Swedish, c. 1790. A practicing Swedish pharmacist, Scheele discovered oxygen (prior to Joseph Priestley), arsenic, citric acid, lactic acid, and many other organic and inorganic compounds. Academy of Science, Stockholm

Apotheke "an exemplary enterprise." Of the five professors of chemistry and pharmacy at the Collegium between 1724 and 1809, three were pharmacists.

The most fundamental of the contributions to pure chemistry by German pharmacist-chemists were made by Andreas Sigismund Marggraf and Martin Heinrich Klaproth. Marggraf, who studied pharmacy and chemistry under Neumann, introduced a number of reagents and discovered sugar in various plants. Klaproth, who became the owner of the Bären-Apotheke in Berlin in 1780, devoted his energies to chemical experiments in the laboratory of his pharmacy. In these cramped surroundings he demonstrated that uranium, zirconium, and cerium were elements, and he verified that tellurium, strontium, titanium, and yttrium were also elements. (In 1797, Louis Nicolas Vauquelin, a French pharmacist, discovered chromium just before Klaproth.) The founder of modern quantitative analysis and modern mineralogical chemistry, Klaproth was called "Europe's greatest analytical chemist" by his contemporary the eminent Swedish chemist Jöns Jacob Berzelius. Klaproth became the first professor of chemistry at the University of Berlin, where he was largely responsible for the *Pharmacopoeia Borussica* of 1799 and for the adoption of the new chemistry of Lavoisier.

Working in St. Petersburg was still another pharmacist-chemist who contributed significantly to analytical chemistry, Johann Tobias Lowitz. He spent his entire career, from apprentice to manager, in the Russian Court Pharmacy. He is credited with, among other accomplishments, discovering the decolorizing and deodorizing property of charcoal and being the first to prepare absolute alcohol and pure ether. Indeed, Lowitz has been called the father of colloidal chemistry and the founder of crystallography; he was one of the first to work on the synthesis of organic chemicals.

There is no better illustration of the dependence of the development of chemistry on pharmacy than the career of Carl Wilhelm Scheele. In the laboratory of his mod-

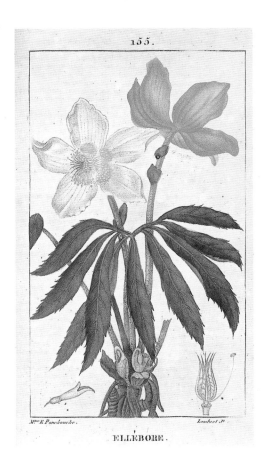

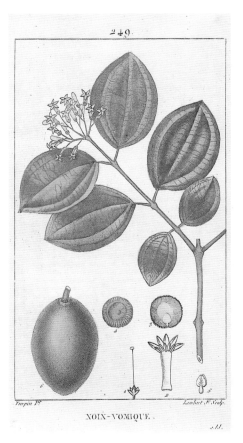

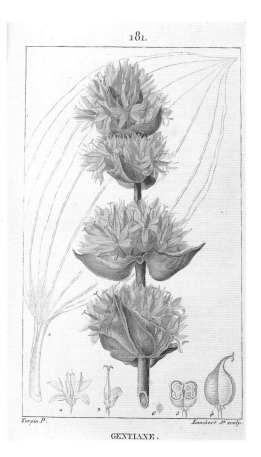

Hellebore, nux vomica, and gentian flowers and seeds. Color engravings from F. P. Chaumeton, *Flore médicale,* vols. 3–5, Paris, 1820. National Library of Medicine, Bethesda

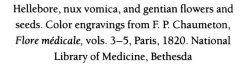

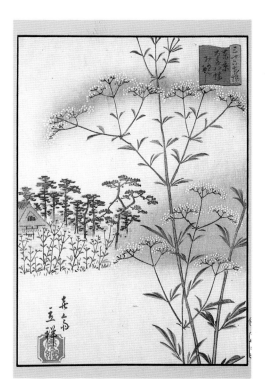

Jalap plant and flower. Color woodcut by Hiroshige II. Japanese, 1867. Collection D. A. Wittop Koning, Amsterdam

Valerian plant and flower. Color woodcut by Hiroshige II. Japanese, 1867. Collection D. A. Wittop Koning, Amsterdam

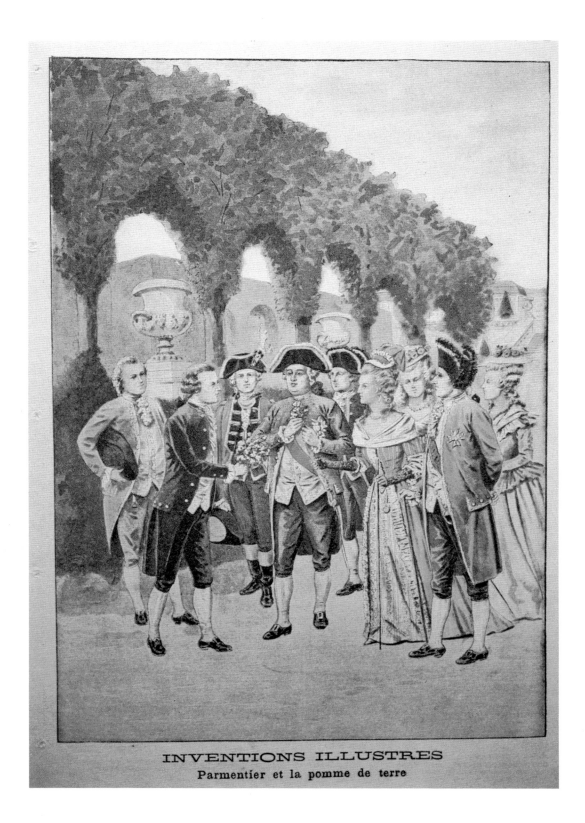

INVENTIONS ILLUSTRES
Parmentier et la pomme de terre

Inventions illustres: Parmentier et la pomme de terre. Color lithograph. French, c. 1901. Jean Antoine Augustin Parmentier spent most of his career as a military pharmacist; he is best known for publicizing the nutritive qualities of potatoes and establishing their value as a food for humans.

est but attractive pharmacy in the out-of-the-way town of Köping, Sweden, Scheele completed the experimentation he had begun during his pharmaceutical apprenticeship and clerkship. The amazing number, quality, and variety of experiments performed by Scheele in his short life suggest that he spent much more time in his laboratory than in attendance at his shop. However, there is little doubt that pharmacy was the basis of Scheele's scientific work. His discoveries were many and varied. To Scheele should properly go credit for the discovery of oxygen, in 1773. Because of a delay in the publication of his findings, and the relative isolation in which Scheele worked, the discovery of "dephlogisticated air" has often been credited to Joseph Priestley. Scheele discovered or identified nitrogen, chlorine (the first of the elements known as halogens), glycerin, manganese, and ammonia, as well as a number of inorganic acids (arsenic, tungstic, molybdic, hydrofluoric, nitrosulfonic) and a number of organic acids (lactic, gallic, pyrogallic, oxalic, citric, tartaric, malic, mucic, uric). He also invented improved processes for preparing calomel, phosphorus, and ether. In all, his accomplishments were gargantuan.

AGRICULTURE AND TECHNOLOGY

The achievements of the pharmacist-chemists had benefits that reached far beyond either pharmacy or pure chemistry. Scheele's discovery of chlorine, for instance, has proved its value in bleaching, disinfection, and water purification. His fruit acids became important to the food and beverage industries. Glycerin found wide use in food, cosmetic, and pharmaceutical preparations, in the manufacture of explosives and resins, and as a preservative, solvent, and lubricant. The chemical researches of Marggraf gave Europe's sugar-beet industry its start, and it was the phar-

macist Jean-Antoine Augustin Parmentier who popularized cultivation of the potato in France. Parmentier did impressive work in food chemistry and nutrition, making chemical analyses of wheat and flour, chestnuts, plant nutrients, milk, and chocolate.

The porcelain industry also owes much to the work of pharmacists. Given the pharmacist's interest in drug jars and involvement in chemistry, this is not a surprising connection. Johann Friedrich Böttger, a German pharmacist with alchemical inclinations, developed a process for making genuine porcelain—first red and then white—in 1709 and 1710. He became director of a ceramic factory in Meissen, a city still renowned for its china. The discovery of the essential ingredient kaolin at Saint-Yrieix in 1757 by the pharmacist Marc-Hilaire Vilaris made the French porcelain industry possible. In England the discovery of a deposit of this "china clay" in Cornwall in 1755 by the prosperous apothecary William Cookworthy led him to establish the country's first porcelain factory, in Plymouth.

BOTANY

It seems strange that the pharmacist, who for centuries had been involved with plant drugs, made less of an impact on scientific botany than on chemistry. It is difficult to explain the paucity of botanical research and writing by pharmacists in the late seventeenth and the early eighteenth century, especially since important work in the field had been done by earlier pharmacists. In Germany, for instance, Basilius Besler, a Nuremberg apothecary who laid out the botanical garden of the bishop of Eichstadt, in 1613 published the *Hortus Eystettensis,* which contained 1,100 copperplates. Similarly monumental were the works of John Parkinson, apothecary to James I and botanist to Charles I; his *Paradisi in sole paradisus terrestris* was published in 1629 and his *Theatrum botanicum* in 1640. The latter contained, in its 1,735 pages, 3,800 plant descriptions and 2,600 woodcuts. In 1673 the Society of Apothecaries of London, which had regularly required its members and apprentices to take part in herborizing expeditions into the countryside, embarked on a new venture when it established a Physic Garden in Chelsea—a garden still in existence.

Any roll call of early pharmacist-botanists must include the Moravian Jesuit George Joseph Kamel, the first European to describe the flora and fauna of the Philippines; the camellia is named for him. Also notable is Arthur Conrad Ernsting, whose work on pollen grains and pollen tubes paved the way for the discovery of cross-fertilization. The Swedish pharmacist Friedrich Erhart, a student of Linnaeus's, is remembered for advances in botanical systemization and for his studies of lichens. David Heinrich Hoppe, one of the founders of the German Botanical Society, was the compiler of a *Botanisches Taschenbuch* that appeared annually for twenty-two years

Ride to Rumford. Colored etching by Thomas Rowlandson. English, 1802. The country apothecary is watched by his wife, and the patient is eyed by the apprentice, as the apothecary places a plaster on the blisters the lady has developed during the ride. Ars Medica Collection, Philadelphia Museum of Art

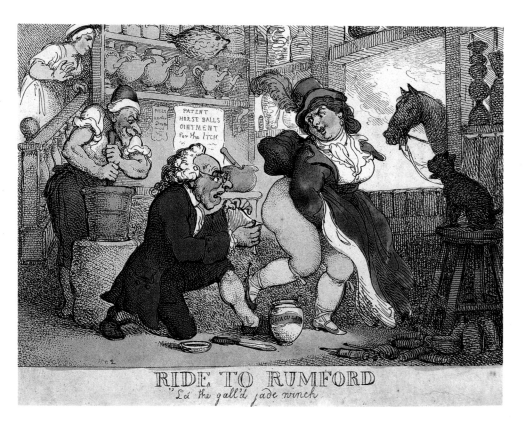

RIDE TO RUMFORD
"Let the gall'd jade winch."

(1790–1811). Carl Ludwig Willdenow, the Berlin pharmacist who became director of the Botanical Garden in Berlin and professor of botany at the University of Berlin, made many outstanding contributions, among them the founding of the study of plant geography. For the English apothecary James Petiver, botany and natural history were consuming passions: upon his death, in 1718, his museum and books were purchased by Sir Hans Sloane and became part of the basic collections of the British Museum; his herbarium eventually went to London's Natural History Museum.

THE EDUCATION OF THE PHARMACIST

Vestiges of the guild system of the Middle Ages remained in the early modern age. The pharmacist guild could become a Colegio, as it did in Valencia in 1441 and in Barcelona in 1445, or a Nobile colegio, as in Rome in 1602, or a Society of Apothecaries, as it did in London in 1617, or a Collegium pharmaceuticum, as it did in Nuremberg in 1632. Although such institutions eventually became involved in formal educational programs, they remained essentially concerned with controlling the training and examination of aspirants and with supervising and disciplining their membership. As a rule, the powers of the pharmacist were circumscribed by the authority of the local or regional Collegium medicum—which was always more than just a medical society, and which became a state agency for the regulation of all matters pertaining to public health.

Formal instruction in pharmacy, as has been noted, goes back to the University of Montpellier in the Renaissance. The Parisian guild of pharmacists made at least two attempts to organize academic programs, but both succumbed to opposition from the faculty of medicine of the University of Paris. Lectures in pharmacy were presented to

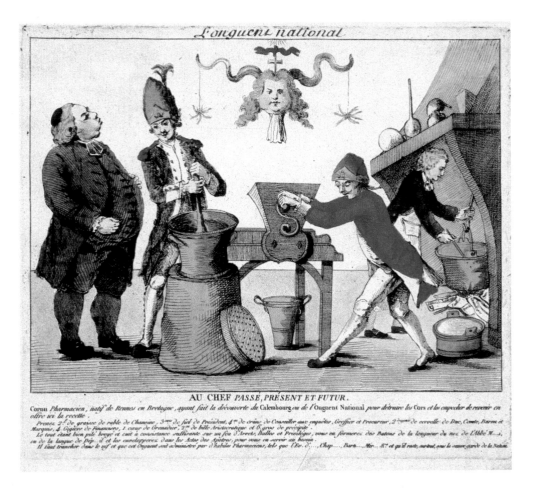

Longuent national

AU CHEF PASSÉ, PRÉSENT ET FUTUR.

Cornu Pharmacien, natif de Rennes en Bretagne, ayant fait la découverte du Calembourg ou de l'Onguent National pour détruire les Cors et les empêcher de revenir en offre ici la recette.

medical and pharmacy students at the Collège Royal de Paris. After the founding of the Collège de Pharmacie in 1777 by royal decree, lectures were presented to pharmacy students in botany, materia medica, chemistry, and pharmacy. During the Revolution the educational function of the Collège became the responsibility of the Ecole Gratuite de Pharmacie, which, in 1803, emerged as the Ecole de Pharmacie.

The medical faculties of the universities cropping up in Europe offered lectures in materia medica, but the evolution of formal education in pharmacy was largely influenced by the rise of centralized political authority under a regional prince or national monarch. The kings of Spain had long since decreed the examination of pharmacists and the inspection of their shops to be a royal prerogative, but the modern convergence of centralized authority and formal pharmaceutical education began in a medical edict issued by Frederick William I, king of Prussia, in 1725. The edict stipulated that in order to practice in a large city a pharmacist had to serve an apprenticeship (usually three to five years), serve as a journeyman for seven years, pursue the

L'Onguent national. Hand-colored engraving. French, c. 1790. Published shortly after the beginning of the French Revolution, the print uses the manufacture of a pharmaceutical product as a metaphor for bringing together the ingredients for a new state. Collection Bouvet, Paris

Scene in a hospital pharmacy. Painting by Philippe-Jacques van Bree. Belgian, c. 1850. Hospital of St. Jean, Bruges ▶

Dispensary of the Hospital of St. Jean in Bruges. Painting by Jef Lambeaux. Belgian, c. 1890. Musée Royal des Beaux-Arts, Antwerp ▶

Processus pharmaceutico-chymicos at the Collegium Medico-Chirurgicum in Berlin, pass an examination before a board consisting of the professor of chemistry, the Royal Apothecary, and two practicing pharmacists, and obtain final approval from the newly established Obercollegium Medicum et Sanitatis. Pharmacists whose practice was restricted to small towns were not required to pursue an academic program. They were, however, required to serve an apprenticeship usually of five years and a clerkship usually of six years, and to pass an examination before the local Collegium medicum.

At the Collegium Medico-Chirurgicum in Berlin, where Caspar Neumann was professor of *chymiae practice,* a 1754 rule required "both the professors of chemistry and pharmacy [the latter was Neumann, the former the professor of general chemistry] shall offer the complete course in Chymico-Pharmaceuticum every year, and in order to better understand the processes and manipulations in the preparation of medicines, those attending the lectures may visit the Royal Hof-Apotheke." Neumann was the Hof-Apotheker and the pharmacy shop to which the students were invited was his.

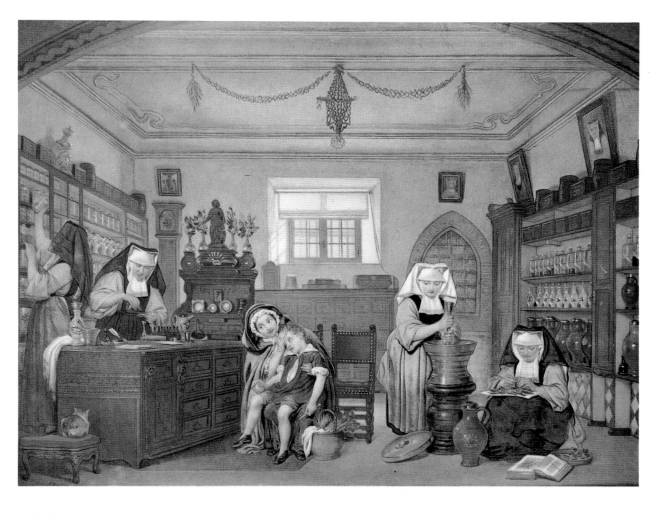

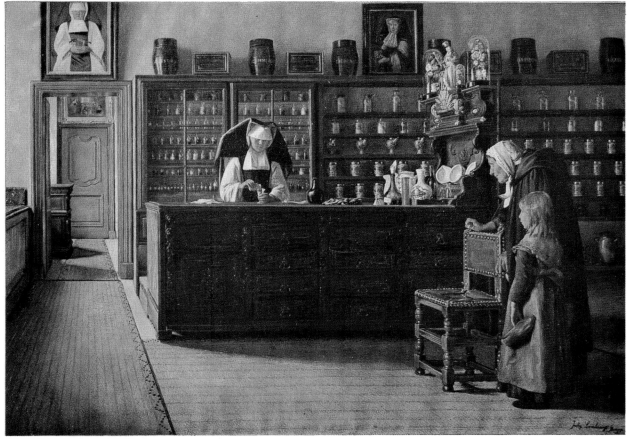

Toward the end of the eighteenth century private institutions for the teaching of pharmacy, established by pharmacists, grew up in Germany. Foremost among them was the Chemisch-physikalische und pharmaceutische Pensionsanstalt set up by Johann Bartholomeus Trommsdorff in Erfurt in 1795, when he had returned to his home city as professor of chemistry and pharmacy at its university. His institute enjoyed a wide reputation, and in 1823 the Prussian government acknowledged that the education provided there met the standards in effect in Berlin.

THE MONASTERIES

Monastic pharmacy continued to be important in the Catholic countries of Europe throughout the eighteenth century. In 1784, in Upper Bavaria alone there were twenty-seven cloisters with complete pharmacies—and this after many cloisters had been shut down or sold off. Benedictines, Benedictine Sisters, Cistercians, Franciscans, Franciscan Sisters, Carmelites, Capuchins, and Englische Fräuleins operated pharmacies. Architectural plans for monasteries built in Austria in the seventeenth and eighteenth centuries invariably included a pharmacy. These shops were sometimes operated by lay pharmacists or journeymen who entered the order as lay brothers. In other cases, pharmacists who retained their secular status were hired by the order to manage the pharmacy.

Competition between cloistered and town pharmacists, and the restrictions placed on the cloisters because of it, are illustrated by the Austrian experience. In Vienna as early as 1569 the religious were forbidden to sell medicines, and cloisters were permitted to operate pharmacies only for their own personnel. Yet public pharmacists were to complain of competition from the cloisters for the next two hundred years. In 1773, cloisters and the religious were enjoined from selling, or giving away

for a consideration, any medicines whatsoever, under pain of severe monetary penalty. Toward the end of the century, cloister pharmacy shops began to disappear. Monastic pharmacy had suffered the fate of the entire monastic system, which was rent by religious and political antagonism and dismantled by monarchs and princes who coveted its immense wealth.

THE PHARMACY SHOP

The urban pharmacy and its cousins the hospital and monastic pharmacies came into full bloom in the late seventeenth century, when the baroque architecture of the age strongly influenced the interior decoration of the pharmacy shop. Such shops might have ceilings of ribbed and vaulted arches supported by slender columns, and these ceilings were often brightly painted in the baroque style. Row on row of matched jars and flasks were housed on shelves that often provided a separate decorated wooden framework for each container. Sometimes jars were placed in little niches, each framed by a small arch and delicate spiral posts or rounded knobs. Where the ceilings were high and the rows of jars, flasks, and drawers reached the ceiling, ladders or steps, fabricated to fit the decor, were provided. Cabinets, chests, shelving, and furniture, all were beautifully crafted, sometimes gilded, and ornately decorated. Paintings and sculptures relevant to pharmacy also adorned the shop, especially statuettes of Cosmas and Damian. There was always an elegant dispensing table that contained the hand apparatus of the pharmacist. There was at least one decorated metal mortar, whose pestle sometimes was so heavy that a mechanical spring device had to be rigged to ease the burden of the apprentice who lifted it.

The baroque pharmacy shop exuded affluence, elegance, and status. As modern visitors to the Köseg Pharmacy at the Budapest Museum of Fine Arts, La Botica de Gi-

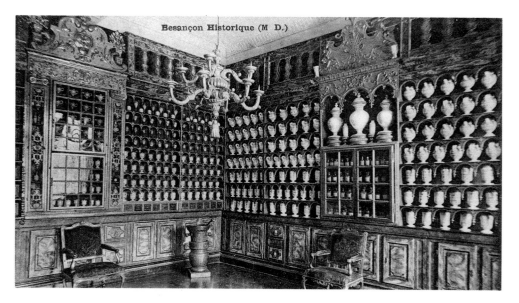

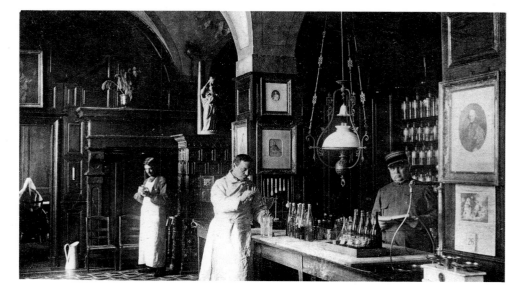

Postcard view (c. 1900) of the pharmacy of the Hôpital St.-Jacques in Besançon, France. The pharmacy, dating from the late 17th century, has elaborately carved shelving in Louis XIV style. The room with arches and carved paneling is still being used as a working dispensary.

bert at the Museo de Farmacia Hispaña in Madrid, the pharmacy of the Ursuline convent in Klagenfurt, Austria, and the Hof-Apotheke of the prince-bishop of Bamberg (now preserved in the Deutsches Apothekenmuseum, Heidelberg) can attest, many of these shops were singularly beautiful.

As if elegance were not enough, the pharmacy shop often sought to instill in patrons a sense of awe and mystery. A stuffed alligator or large serpent might hang from the ceiling, a symbolic "unicorn's horn" might project from a wall, or a sculpture or carving of a griffin might have a place on a table. The Netherlands developed its own symbol of pharmacy—the Gaper. Usually carved out of wood, this was the bust of a man, often dark-skinned and obviously from a faraway place, whose wide-open mouth sometimes had a long tongue drooping from it. The Gaper, the mortar and pestle, and the unicorn horn, prominently displayed on the exterior of the pharmacy shop, became symbols readily identified with the profession.

The Gaper. Polychrome wood figure. Dutch, 18th century. Often ugly and frightening, the Gaper could be found over doorways of Dutch pharmacies and shops selling proprietary remedies. Modern versions can still be seen in some Dutch pharmacies. Medisch-Pharmaceutisch Museum, Amsterdam

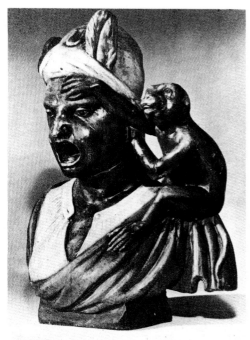

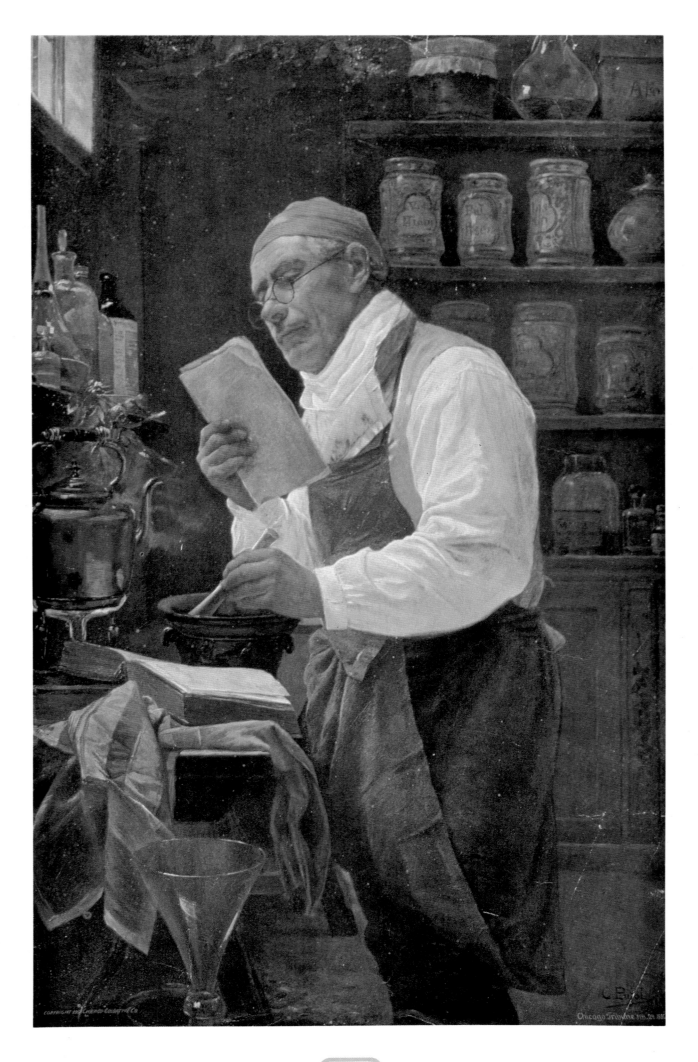

COPYRIGHT BY CHICAGO COLORTYPE CO

The nineteenth century saw a changed world. Absolutism was giving way to democracy and constitutionalism. Nationalism became dominant. Mercantilism had given way to laissez-faire, and the factory system and industrialization had become the basis of a burgeoning productivity. Technological and scientific advances were awesome. Political and economic developments, technology, and science, all had their impact on pharmacy —technology and science most directly.

CHEMISTRY AND PHARMACY

The chemical revolution wrought by Lavoisier—the new nomenclature, his theory of combustion, and his effective demonstration of the law of the conservation of mass in chemistry—helped free chemistry from the limitations of pharmaceutical chemistry. Nevertheless, although certain pharmaceutical circles felt an estrangement from chemistry, pharmacists continued in the nineteenth century to be interested in pure chemistry. Indeed some of the fundamental findings in nineteenth-century chemistry were the results of investigations by pharmacists. For example, important to the development of the atomic theory in chemistry was the work of the French pharmacist Joseph Louis Proust, who, in the first years of the century, propounded the law of definite proportions, which states that the elements in a given compound are always combined in the same proportion by mass. In postulating this law, Proust dared to differ with his contemporary the noted French chemist Claude Louis Bertholet, who maintained that unless some particular factor exerted an influence, the proportion of the elements in a compound varied. It was necessary to build on the law of definite proportions before the nature of complex compounds could be understood.

THE NINETEENTH CENTURY: SCIENCE AND PHARMACY

A pharmacist reading a prescription. Color lithograph, after a painting by French artist C. Pujol, distributed to its readers by *The Chicago Tribune.* 1901

In 1805, the English scientist John Dalton published the first table of atomic weights, and in 1808 the first volume of his *New System of Chemical Philosophy* appeared. His theories presented an atomic explanation of both the law of definite proportions and the law of multiple proportions. A few years later, Dalton's table was improved on by the Swedish chemist Jöns Jacob Berzelius. Such discoveries as the classification of triads in 1829 by the German pharmacist Johann Wolfgang Döbereiner led to the development of the periodic table of the elements in the 1860s and 1870s.

ORGANIC CHEMISTRY

Many of the pharmacist-chemists of the eighteenth and the early nineteenth century were involved in the beginnings of what was to become known as organic chemistry. The discovery of urea in 1773 is credited to H.-M. Rouelle. Milk was an object of chemical analysis by Rouelle, Baumé, Geoffroy, Parmentier, Vauquelin, and Scheele. Lowitz obtained dextrose (grape sugar) in a pure crystallized form from honey in 1792 or earlier; Proust extracted it from grape juice in 1802; and Henri Braconnot developed a relatively uncomplicated method of producing it by treating sawdust with sulfuric acid in 1819. This and other procedures devised by Braconnot proved important to the development of the chemical industry.

Pharmacists also made basic contributions to the understanding of the role of proteins in nutrition. William T. Brande, in England, was the first (1809) to characterize albumin, that is, to delineate its physical and chemical properties. In investigating albumin, Proust discovered the amino acid leucine, in 1819, and the next year Braconnot obtained glycine. In 1878, Camille Méhu, a hospital pharmacist, demonstrated that proteins when saturated with ammonium sulfate precipitate from solution without changing their nature. This discovery was hailed as pivotal in the history of protein investigation. At the end of the century, Charles Joseph Tanret, working in his pharmacy in Troyes, developed the albumin reagent, an acetic solution of mercuric chloride in potassium iodide.

ALKALOIDS, GLYCOSIDES, HALOGENS: A SECOND PHARMACEUTICAL REVOLUTION

Given pharmacists' long tradition of using plant-derived drugs—and given, too, pharmacists' increasing knowledge of chemistry—it was predictable that they would take the lead in discovering the active agents in plants. In the 1770s and 1780s, Scheele had been able to isolate a number of organic acids, but it was not until the nineteenth century that chemists had both the knowledge and the techniques essential to the analysis of plant drugs.

The first steps were taken early in the nineteenth century. The French pharmacist J. F. Derosne, in 1803, and his compatriot Armand Seguin, in 1804, isolated from raw opium a crystalline substance whose chemical nature they could not elucidate. The German pharmacist Friedrich Wilhelm Sertürner showed that this substance, which he called *Morphium* (morphine), was alkaline and could form salts with acids. His discovery was probably made in 1804, but his first note on the subject, in 1805, and two subsequent publications received little attention. However, his classic 1817 paper *Über das Morphium, eine neue salzfähige Grundlage, und die Mekonsäure als Hauptbestandtheil des Opiums* won wide recognition. The term "alkaloid" was coined in 1818 by another German pharmacist, Karl Meissner.

Through alkaloidal chemistry the active principle was extracted from many plants

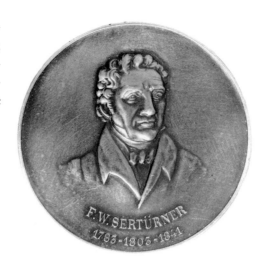

Bronze medal of Friedrich Wilhelm Sertürner (1783–1841). German, 1850. A pharmacist, Sertürner discovered morphine as the active principle of opium and pioneered in the pharmaceutical revolution that introduced vegetable alkaloids. The date 1803 on the medal is sometimes ascribed to this discovery, although 1804 is a more acceptable date. Schweizerisches Pharmazie-Historisches Museum, Basel

that had long been used in pharmacy. The availability of the active principle, now concentrated as a chemical rather than dispersed throughout a crude drug, meant that purity, strength, standardization, and dosage could be controlled as never before. Soon after Sertürner's discovery, other chemists, especially French and German pharmacists, sought out new alkaloids. In 1817, Pierre Joseph Pelletier and the physician François Magendie isolated impure emetine from ipecac, and Pierre Robiquet extracted narcotine from opium. When Pelletier joined forces with another young French pharmacist, Joseph Caventou, they achieved a series of spectacular successes. In 1818 they obtained strychnine, in 1819 brucine and veratrine, in 1820 cinchonine and quinine, and in 1821 caffeine.

Many new alkaloids were brought to light in the course of the nineteenth century. Robiquet introduced codeine in 1832, Philipp Lorenz Geiger discovered coniine and, together with L. Hesse, elucidated aconitine, atropine, colchicine, daturine, and hyoscyamine. Heinrich Emanuel Merck discovered papaverine in 1848. In 1854, Friedrich Georg Gaedcke came close to the discovery of cocaine, but it remained for Albert Niemann to isolate and purify it (1860). Of all the chemists mentioned in connection with alkaloid chemistry, only Magendie and Hesse did not have a pharmaceutical background.

The success of the pharmacist-chemists in extracting alkaloids from plants aided in the discovery of the glycosides, sugar derivatives found in certain plants. The most important of these were derived from digitalis leaves and still are a valuable resource in cardiac medication. In 1869, Claude-Adolphe Nativelle, a French pharmacist, obtained a substance he called "digitalin" from foxglove, and in 1875 Johann Schmiedeberg, the eminent German pharmacologist, produced a similar substance, which he called "digitoxin." These findings triggered more than fifty years of cardiac glycoside chemistry; at least thirteen glycosides derived from the species *Digitalis pur-*

purea and *Digitalis lanata* and from the genus *Strophanthus* have since been made available.

Pharmacist-chemists also played a basic role in the understanding and introduction of halogens into therapeutics, sanitation, medicine, and surgery. First came the discovery of chlorine by Scheele. Then, in 1811, Bernard Courtois, a French pharmacist, discovered iodine in marine algae. Another French pharmacist, Antoine Jérôme Balard, discovered bromine in 1826, the year he graduated from the Ecole de Pharmacie in Montpellier. Balard was also to discover oxamic acid, and he studied and named amyl alcohol. For a time he operated a pharmacy in Montpellier, and his appointments to the faculty of the college of pharmacy and the faculty of sciences of Montpellier were followed by professorships, first at the Sorbonne and then at the Collège de France.

In 1886, the French pharmacist Henri Moissan demonstrated before the Société de Pharmacie de Paris how he obtained free fluorine by electrolytic methods. He also developed an electric-arc furnace and made the first artificial diamonds. In 1907, Moissan was awarded the Nobel Prize in Chemistry, a fitting climax to a great age of French pharmacy.

Alkaloids and glycosides generated a pharmaceutical revolution of far-reaching effect. They provided a precision and a scientific foundation for plant-drug therapy that it had always lacked. The physician and the pharmacist were now presented with a long list of products—products that were to change the prescribing habits of the former and the compounding techniques of the latter. As the list expanded, it eventually included, among others, morphine, codeine, quinine, cocaine, colchicine, ephedrine, atropine, physostigmine, papavarine, reserpine, digoxin, and digitoxin, all potent and effective medicaments.

While the alkaloids and glycosides were essentially old drugs in new, concentrated forms, halogens provided entirely new additions to the materia medica. Chlorine

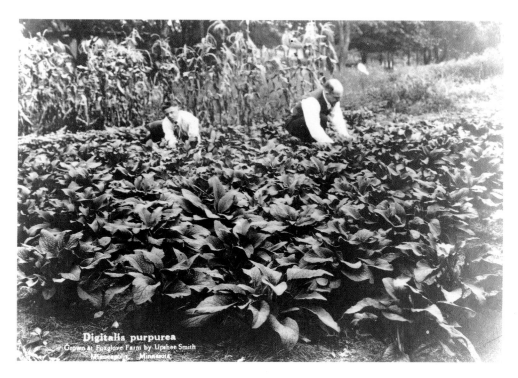

Commercial cultivation of *Digitalis purpurea* at the Foxglove Farm near Minneapolis. c. 1910. National Library of Medicine, Bethesda

Foxglove (*Digitalis purpurea*) plant and seed. Engraving from William Curtis, *Flora Londinensis*, England, 1777–98. Lindley Library, The Royal Horticultural Society, London

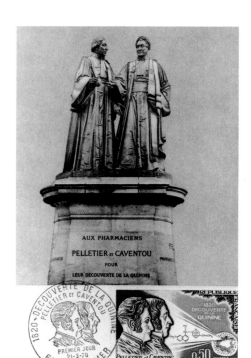

Postcard view of the statue of Pierre Joseph Pelletier and Joseph Caventou, with commemorative stamp and postmark. French, 1970. The two pharmacists were honored on the 150th anniversary of their discovery, in 1820, of quinine, one of a number of vegetable alkaloids they introduced. The bronze statue in Paris has been replaced; the original, shown on the card, was torn down and the metal used for armaments during the Occupation.

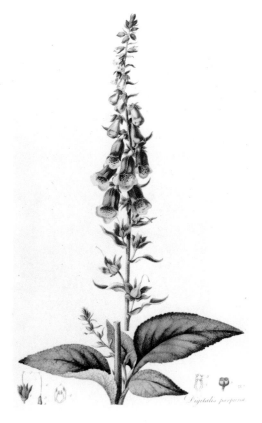

found medical and therapeutic uses in disinfectants such as sodium hypochlorite (for which the pharmacist Antoine-Germain Labarrague was awarded a prize from the French government in 1823), in chloroform, and in chloral. Iodine was used in many compounds: iodoform, developed by the pharmacist Georges-Simon Sérulas in 1822; potassium iodide (Lugol's solution); and tincture of iodine. Aqueous solutions of bromine also found uses in nineteenth-century therapeutics, and by the 1880s inorganic bromides were already being prescribed for their sedative action.

The development of the alkaloids, glycosides, and halogens brought with it a shift from dependence on crude drugs to the availability of chemical entities that made purification and standardization possible. There was no longer need for the pharmacist to know the habitat, the part of the plant used, and the time of gathering. New standards and new knowledge meant new opportunities for precision in prescribing, compounding, and dosing—opportunities pharmacy and medicine had never known before.

It was not only the materia pharmaceutica that changed in the nineteenth-century pharmaceutical revolution; the practice of pharmacy itself went through a radical and consequential change. Increasingly the actual discovery and compounding of remedies moved from the private officina to the industrial laboratory and plant. While the pharmacist continued to isolate active principles and develop new compounds in his own laboratory, research and production were taken over by industry. To a considerable extent the pharmaceutical industry grew out of the pharmacy shop; it also grew out of the chemical industry, which, starting from an interest in dyes, rapidly expanded its activity into pharmaceuticals.

As chemists learned more about organic compounds, the industry—chemical and pharmaceutical, often unified—began to produce synthetics. Synthetic chemistry was to have an overwhelming and worldwide impact on the quality of life; synthetic

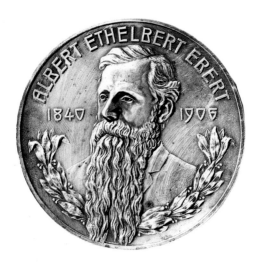

The Ebert Prize silver medal awarded, in 1892, to John Uri Lloyd (1849–1936), a pharmaceutical scientist who made important contributions to plant chemistry and drug extraction. He was also a manufacturer, novelist, and founder of the library in Cincinnati, Ohio, that bears his name. The prize, named in honor of Albert Ethelbert Ebert (1840–1906), professor at the Chicago College of Pharmacy and inventor of the sulfurous process for the manufacture of starch and glucose, is awarded annually by the American Pharmaceutical Association for accomplishment in scientific research. National Museum of American History, Smithsonian Institution, Washington, D.C.

Broadside for alkaloid products of the New York Quinine and Chemical Works (Limited). Color lithograph. American, 1901. Collection Theodore Robinson, Richboro, Pennsylvania ▶

agricultural chemicals, synthetic fibers, and other synthetic products seemed miraculously to provide more food, clothing, and other amenities. In pharmacy there developed a revolution within a revolution as industry became increasingly interested in the creation of therapeutic substances that did not occur in nature. The resulting proliferation of drugs offered the potential of helping in ailments previously relatively untreatable; large-scale production provided these drugs virtually without limit. All this was taking place while Western civilization was going through the process of industrialization; this pharmaceutical revolution was thus but one aspect of the Industrial Revolution.

THE MEDICAL SCIENCES

Medicine made startlingly little progress in the eighteenth century, but one medical advance that significantly affected pharmacy came in the field of pathologic anatomy. Giovanni Battista Morgagni of Padua postulated that disease involved pathologic organs: there were sick organs rather than sick people. Augmented in the nineteenth century by interest in correlating postmortem findings with diagnosis and with clinical indications, Morgagni's theory led to a therapeutic nihilism—that is, to the belief that drugs and other therapy could have no effect on organs. If surgery was not indicated, the patient was left to the healing powers of nature. By the 1830s, moreover, criticism of the heroic drug therapy in vogue in the last decades of the eighteenth and the first decades of the nineteenth century was being heard: not only that the heroic approach was ineffective but that it was downright harmful. Therapeutic nihilism and the disrepute into which heroic medicine had fallen led many to agree with the famous observation of Oliver Wendell Holmes in 1860, that "if the whole of the

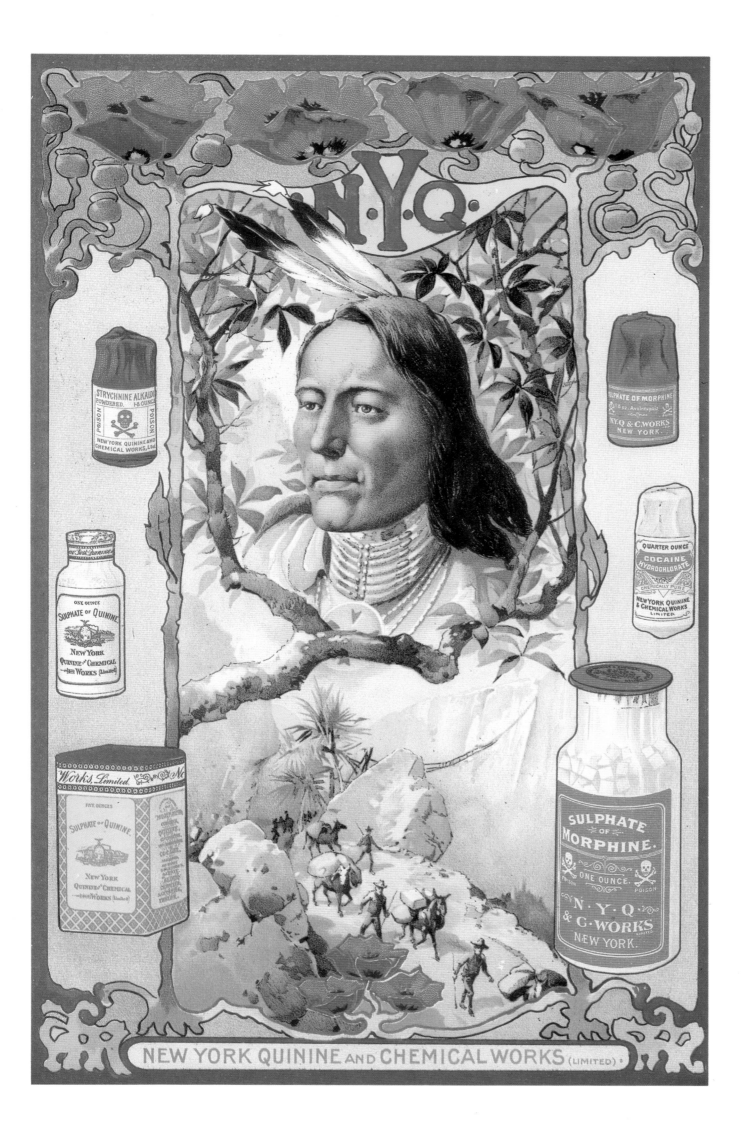

materia medica as now used could be sunk in the bottom of the sea, it would be all the better for mankind—and all the worse for the fishes."

Fortunately for pharmacy, whose professional role in providing drugs was denigrated by such concepts as heroic medicine and therapeutic nihilism, a new understanding of cellular pathology—replacing Morgagni's concept of diseased organs—was introduced in the mid-nineteenth century. In 1858 the German physician Rudolf Virchow, a dominant figure in European medicine, published *Die Cellularpathologie*, postulating that disease involved cells, not organs. The British scientists Thomas Richard Fraser and Alexander Crum Brown next pointed up the need to investigate the relation between a cell's chemical composition and its physiologic action. The outcome was the concept that certain drugs had a particular affinity for certain chemicals, a concept that culminated in the side-chain theory of Paul Ehrlich, a renowned German physician-microbiologist-chemist. A chemical explanation of immunity phenomena, this theory was fundamental to the rationale of drug therapy in general and specifically to the development of twentieth-century chemotherapy.

Pharmacology

The reliance on drug therapy, despite the challenge that therapeutic nihilism posed, was reinforced by the many innovations made by nineteenth-century pharmacists and chemists and by the prestige of the concept of cellular pathology. It was given new impetus by developments in physiology and pharmacology. François Magendie, whose collaboration with Pelletier has been noted, played the dominant role in winning recognition for the alkaloids and halogens. His most noteworthy experiment showed the effect of strychnine in paralysis of the voluntary muscles. His pharmacological studies, published as the *Formulaire pour la*

Plantes dangereuses. Color lithograph by Charles-Henri Bethmont. French, c. 1850. Common poisonous mushrooms and plants are shown above and below three vignettes: the death of Socrates (center), a pharmacist (left), and an herbalist (right).
▶

Advertising card featuring Claude Bernard. Chromolithograph. French, c. 1890. One of "the benefactors of humanity" honored in a series of 84 cards, Bernard (1813–1878) began his career as an apprentice pharmacist and made significant contributions to the understanding of modes of action of poisons and to many aspects of physiology.
▶

préparation et l'emploi de plusieurs nouveaux medicaments, tels que la noix vomique, la morphine, etc. introduced into medical practice not only nux vomica and morphine but also, among others, prussic acid, veratrine, quinine and its salts, and bromine and iodine compounds. The *Formulaire*, first published in France in 1821, was in such great demand that it went through nine editions by 1836 and was translated into several languages. Magendie's early ventures into pharmacology were carried on by his famous student Claude Bernard. Often called Europe's greatest physiologist, Bernard began his career as an apprentice to a pharmacist.

However, the movement that established pharmacology as an independent discipline began in the German universities. Rudolph Buchheim and Oswald Schmiedeberg were its leaders, and their students, among them the American John Jacob Abel, spread the word. But not until the twentieth century did instruction in materia medica in medical schools and schools of pharmacy give way to regular courses in pharmacology.

The major distinction between materia medica and pharmacology is that in the former the efficacy of the drug is generally established empirically, in the nonscientific sense of the term, or is accepted on the basis of tradition, whereas in pharmacology the efficacy of a drug is determined by laboratory and, eventually, clinical testing. Pharmacology provides a scientific rationale for drug therapy; it is essential to the determination of the efficacy and safety of the multiplicity of chemical remedies, and it is basic to the creative development of new drugs to meet particular medical needs.

Pharmacognosy

The nineteenth century saw the development of another essentially pharmaceutical science—pharmacognosy. The description and identification of drugs had been a concern of physicians and pharmacists from ancient times; in the nineteenth century

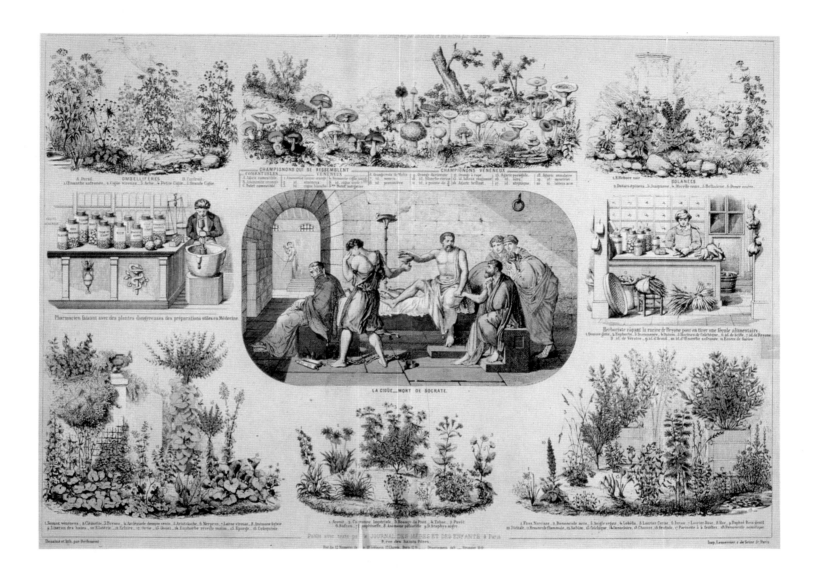

pharmacognosy was given its name, was differentiated from materia medica and pharmacology, and became a distinct science in its own right. Originally it was studied at medical schools as a subdivision of pharmacology and consequently revolved mainly around the actions of drugs. As pharmaceutical education developed at the university level, pharmacognosy was given a more pharmaceutical orientation. Observation and sensory methods of description and identification gave way, under intensive research led primarily by pharmaceutical scientists, to microscopic, morphological, and histological examination—and, eventually, to chemical examination. Since so much of the materia medica was still of plant origin, pharmacognosy became a subdivision of botany.

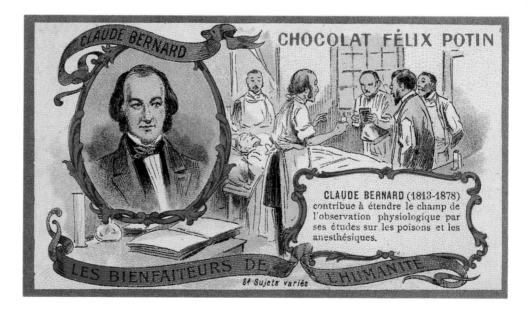

The evolution of pharmacognosy into a pharmaceutical science and a part of pharmaceutical education was a universal phenomenon in nineteenth-century Europe. The process started with the publication in 1820 of the *Histoire naturelle des drogues simples* by Nicolas J. B. G. Guibourt, professor at the Ecole de Pharmacie in Paris. Guibourt was credited with "the separation of pharmacognosy from pharmacology and putting the former on her own feet" by the great doyen of pharmacognosy of the early twentieth century, Alexander Tschirch.

England's Daniel Hanbury gained a reputation as one of Europe's foremost pharmacognosists; he was the author, with the pioneer Swiss pharmacognosist Friedrich August Flückiger, of the definitive *Pharmacographia: A History of the Principal Drugs of Vegetable Origin Met With in Great Britain and British India,* which first appeared in 1874. Typically, the monographs in this work gave for each plant drug—in addition to collection information and the names of the drug in Latin, English, French, and German—its botanical origin, history, description, microscopic structure, chemical composition, commercial importance, and medicinal and other uses. Implications for the progress of pharmacy should be recognized in the fact that Guibourt, Tschirch, Hanbury, and Flückiger had all begun their careers as pharmacists. And, just as the new botanical taxonomy had improved the eighteenth-century pharmacopoeias, so the new exact pharmacognostic studies advanced the scientific caliber of nineteenth-century pharmacopoeias.

Microbiology and the Germ Theory of Disease

Girolamo Fracastoro of Verona, scholar, physician, poet, and professor of philosophy at the University of Padua, wrote in 1546 about "germs of contagion." Some have taken this as a suggestion of the germ theory of disease; others believe that Fracastoro was referring to imperceptible inani-

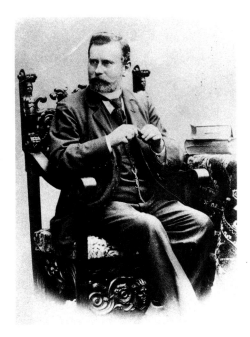

Paul Ehrlich (1854–1915) at the age of twenty-nine. Physician, chemist, bacteriologist, Ehrlich shared the 1908 Nobel Prize in Physiology and Medicine for his work in immunology. His pioneering search for a remedy for syphilis culminated in the discovery of 606 (Salvarsan, or arsphenamine) in 1909 and ushered in the age of chemotherapy.

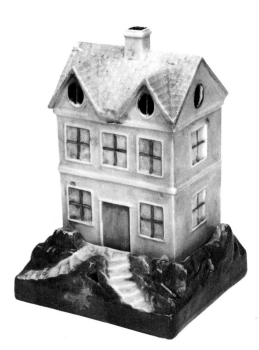

Earthenware pastille burner in the form of a miniature house for deodorizing or fumigating. English, 1820–50. Wellcome Institute Collection, Science Museum, London

mate particles rather than to living organisms. It was over a century later, in 1674, that van Leeuwenhoek saw "animalcules" in lake water. There were a good number of scientists who saw a connection between disease and these little creatures, but two centuries were to pass before the germ theory of disease obtained scientific verification.

The two giants of microbiology who accomplished this feat were the French chemist Louis Pasteur and the German physician Robert Koch. Pasteur's celebrated controlled experiment on anthrax—which used twenty-four sheep, six cows, and one goat and was performed before an audience of officials, doctors, scientists, and journalists at Pouilly-le-Fort in May 1882—gave the coup de grace to the theory of spontaneous generation and to the opposition to the germ theory of disease. Koch's stupendous contribution was the identification of various organisms—most important among them anthrax, tuberculosis, and cholera bacilli—and his incontrovertible proof that each disease was caused by a specific organism.

The immediate effect of the work of Pasteur and Koch was the development of vaccines. Vaccination for smallpox by inoculation with the cowpox virus had become known through the publication of Edward Jenner's *Inquiry into the Cause and Effects of the Variolae Vaccinae,* in 1798. Jenner's boon to mankind, which led in the twentieth century to the eradication of smallpox, was accomplished without his being aware of either microorganisms or the immunity processes of the body. Pasteur, following Jenner's lead, reasoned that an attenuated bacillus might give immunity from the disease caused by that bacillus, and he developed successful vaccines for chicken cholera, anthrax, and rabies.

The next step in this new therapy of vaccination—a term that honors the source of cowpox, the cow—was to determine how the therapy worked. The immune processes of the body began to be unraveled by the studies of Elie Metchnikoff, a Russian zoologist, and Paul Ehrlich, whose side-chain theory was a basic contribution to an understanding of the process.

The search to understand the body's immune responses led to the introduction of yet another class of therapeutic and preventive agents—the antitoxins. In the last decade of the nineteenth century, Emil von Behring, a German physician, and his co-worker Shibasaburo Kitasato developed antitoxins for two of mankind's great scourges, tetanus and diphtheria. The last-named disease was responsible for "the slaughter of the innocents," for its major victims were children—and the nurses and physicians who tended them.

Hormones and Vitamins

These therapeutic advances—vaccines and antitoxins—were nineteenth-century fruits of the new sciences of bacteriology, physiology, and immunology. Old ideas of disease and its treatment—of miasmatic, telluric, and meteoric causes, of heroic medicine and Brunonianism—could not stand up against the findings, and the successes, of the scientific laboratory.

The germ theory was not the only new explanation of the etiology of disease, however. Before the nineteenth century was over, physiologists had found that some disorders resulted from hormonal imbalance. Claude Bernard, whose preeminence as a physiologist has been noted, laid the foundations for modern endocrinology with his mid-century work on glycogen and the pancreatic function. His researches, and those of Charles-Edouard Brown-Séquard, a physician who did most of his work in France, pointed up the correlation between the ductless glands and internal secretions. At mid-century, too, in England, Thomas Addison was studying the suprarenal capsules and describing the disease that bears his name. Both hyper- and hypothyroidism were recognized by mid-century, and thy-

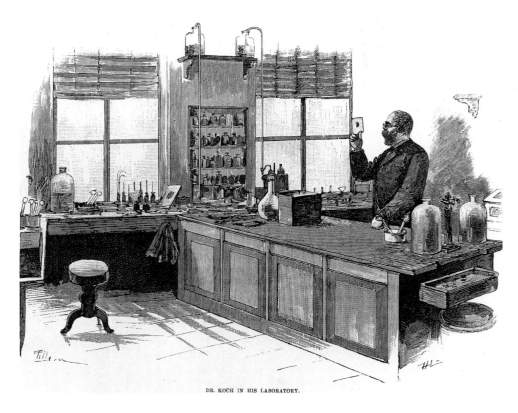

DR. KOCH IN HIS LABORATORY.

Dr. Koch in his laboratory. Engraving from *Frank Leslie's Illustrated Newspaper*, December 13, 1890. Robert Koch identified the tubercle bacillus in 1882 by special techniques of culturing and staining.

An Inoculation for Hydrophobia. Steel engraving from *Harper's Weekly,* December 19, 1885. Louis Pasteur is shown watching an assistant administering his newly developed vaccine.

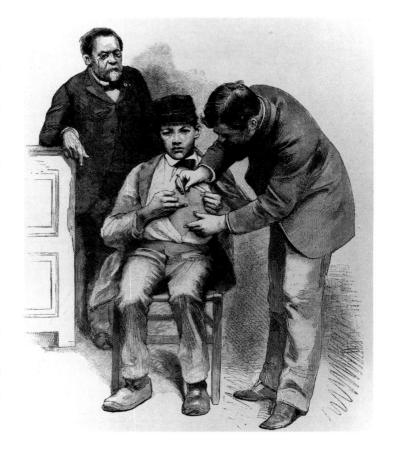

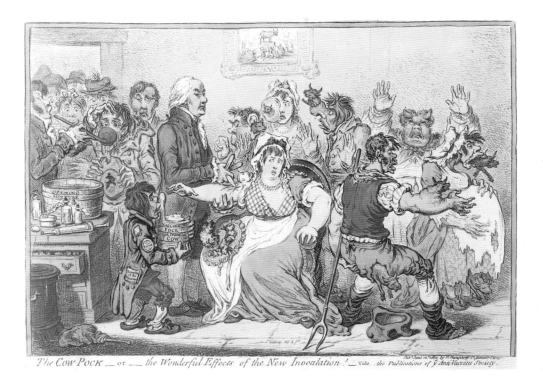

The Cow-Pock — or — the Wonderful Effects of the New Inoculation ! __ vide the Publications of y Anti-Vaccine Society.

The Cow Pock—or—the Wonderful Effects of the New Inoculation! Hand-colored engraving by James Gillray. English, 1802. Burlesquing Edward Jenner's vaccination for smallpox, the artist shows it producing monstrous side effects. Unmoved, Jenner (standing at left center) continues to inoculate.

Les Adieux au Palais Royal. Color engraving published by Martinet. Paris, c. 1815. Soldiers occupying Paris at the end of the Napoleonic Wars being given prophylactics (among them burdock and the root of the strawberry plant) against venereal disease.

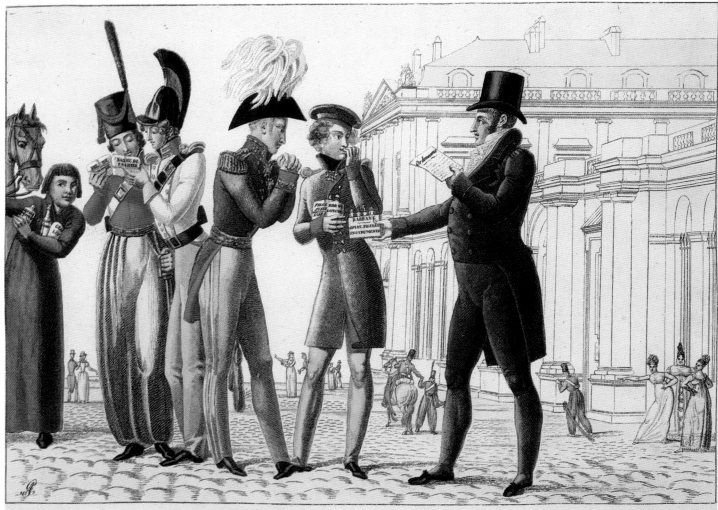

LES ADIEUX AU PALAIS ROYAL
ou Les Suites du Premier Pas.

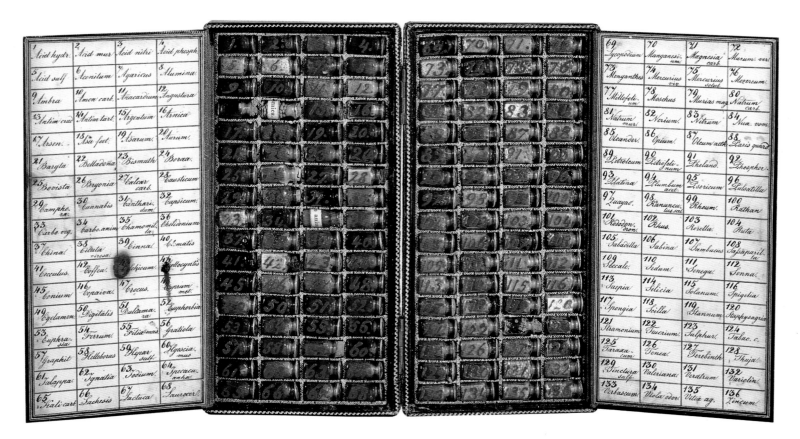

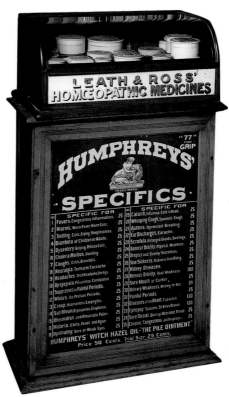

Wooden cabinets for homeopathic medicines. English (Leath and Ross) and American (Humphreys), late 19th century. The cabinet for Humphreys' Specifics lists the products by number on the front; drawers for individual vials opened from the back.

Pocket homeopathic case. Gold-embossed leather. German, c. 1850. Only 10 inches high by 6 inches deep, the case contains 136 numbered miniature medicine flacons; notes on the cover list the contents of each.
Kunsthaus Lempertz, Cologne

Rows of herbal remedies in a modern Chinese pharmacy in Hong Kong

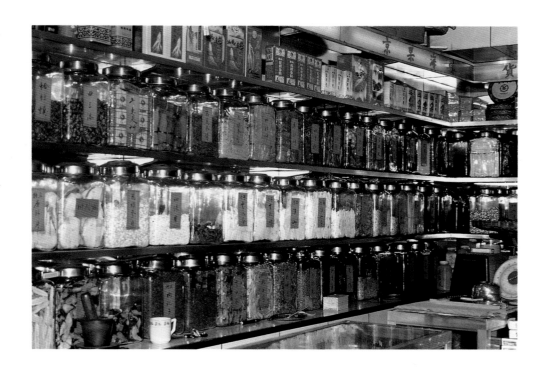

roid extract was introduced into therapeutics before the end of the century.

Vitamin deficiency, or avitaminosis, as a cause of disease was also recognized in the nineteenth century. The experiments of James Lind, an English naval surgeon, had induced the British navy in 1795 to supply seamen with lemon juice as a scurvy preventive. Almost a century later, Christian Eijkman, a Dutch army surgeon in Java, not only recognized beriberi as a deficiency disease but actually induced the disease experimentally.

By the end of the nineteenth century, drug therapy, itself vastly expanded by the addition of many chemical entities, was augmented by new applications of vaccines and the introduction of antitoxins in the conquest of disease. The pharmacist had new products to deal with: these "biologicals" presented what was really a new class of medical agents. And a new piece of equipment, the refrigerator, soon became essential in the pharmacy.

Medical Sectarianism

At various times in the nineteenth century pharmacy felt the effects of the rise of medical sects that challenged the traditional ideas and practices of pharmacy as well as of medicine. Three major medical sects—and many splinter groups—developed in the nineteenth century: homeopaths, Thomsonians and Neo-Thomsonians, and Eclectics, or Reformed Practitioners of Medicine.

The "regular" practice of medicine in the nineteenth century was having its difficulties. Under the influence of Brunonianism and of "heroic" practice, therapy consisted largely of strong cathartics, powerful emetics, enemas, and bleeding—sometimes virtually simultaneously. Calomel, croton oil, veratrum viride, and ipecacuanha were the mainstays of purging and puking therapeutics; opium was the mainstay in dysenteries and as an analgesic and sedative. Results were not salutary, and many of the new

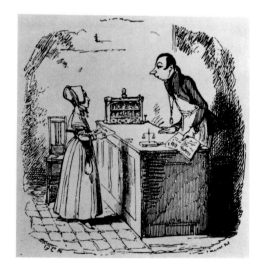

A Caricature of Homeopathy. Engraving by George Cruikshank. English, c. 1840. "Please, sir apothecary, I want a hundred-thousandth part of a grain of magnesia." "Very sorry, miss, but we don't sell anything in such large quantities."

alkaloids and chemical agents were themselves toxic and had to be administered with care.

The first of the medical sects that arose to challenge standard medicine and therapy was homeopathy, the creation of Samuel Hahnemann, a German physician. Hahnemann made a number of cogent criticisms of the drug therapies in general use and of the methods of testing drugs. Drugs could be tested only in the human body, he contended. By testing drugs on himself while he was in good health, he developed one of the basic tenets of homeopathy, the concept of *similia similibus curantur*—like cured by like. According to this concept, disease or its symptoms can be cured by drugs that produce similar symptoms in the healthy body. To this principle he added another: that the effect of a drug can be heightened by giving infinitesimally small doses.

Hahnemann expounded his ideas at length in his *Organon der rationellen Heilkunde,* an 1810 work that was widely reproduced and translated. Homeopathy received quick and wide acceptance throughout Western Europe and North America. In the United States many doctors turned from allopathy—the type of medical practice that cured by contraries rather than by similars—to homeopathy.

Homeopathy directly affected pharmacy, and Hahnemann, who insisted on making up his own tinctures, dilutions, and titrations, encountered opposition not only from the medical establishment but from pharmacists. The homeopathic physician usually compounded his own prescriptions—in disregard of Hahnemann's own preference for using a single active drug at a time—but gradually there emerged, especially in larger cities, homeopathic pharmacists equipped to make up the minute doses that homeopathy required. In addition, regular pharmacists eventually carried a stock of homeopathic remedies that had been prepared and prepackaged by manufacturers of homeopathic drugs.

Homeopaths developed their own medical schools and an abundant literature, including many pharmacopoeias. *The Homeopathic Pharmacopoeia of the United States,* first published in 1876, went through seven editions by 1964. It now enjoys the same official status under American law as *The Pharmacopoeia of the United States.* Homeopathic medical schools gradually lost their sectarian character, mainly under the pressure of advances in medical science and therapeutics, and they eventually joined the medical establishment.

The second medical group whose activities affected pharmacy was the Thomsonians. A botanical practice of medicine, Thomsonianism was the brainchild of Samuel Thomson, a New Hampshire farmer who wanted to become a physician but lacked the requisite education to pursue medical studies. Early in the nineteenth century he established a "system" that was reminiscent of Galen's humoral pathology. It offered plant remedies that were purportedly milder and safer than the harsh, powerful remedies favored by practitioners of heroic medicine. Altogether some seventy plant remedies made up the materia medica of the Thomsonians; lobelia emetics, scalding capsicum, herb teas, medicated enemas, and steam baths were the mainstays of their therapeutics. The tremendous popularity, not to mention promotional success, of Thomsonianism in the United States is attested to by the enormous number of persons—100,000, according to Thomson—who bought the franchise (known as "Family Rights") to practice his system; by the Family Botanic Societies that were established; by the annual conventions of these societies held between 1832 and 1838; and by the frequent republication of Thomson's *New Guide to Health.*

Thomsonians operated infirmaries, depots, and stores where they compounded their medications and dispensed them, in direct competition with the pharmacist. Indeed, those who practiced the system were told to beware of purchasing anything in a regular pharmacy. In Georgia a Botanical-Medical Board of Physicians was created in

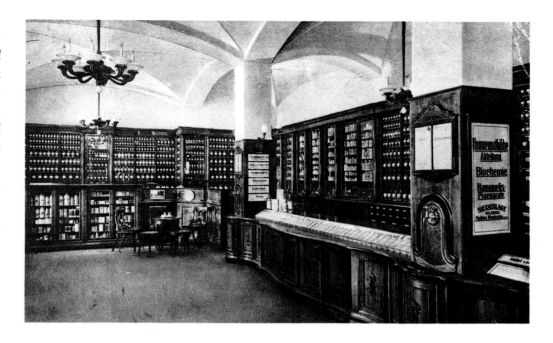

Postcard view of the Löwen-Apotheke in Dresden, Germany. c. 1930. A specialty of the pharmacy was a full line of homeopathic remedies.

1847 with the power to examine and license "Botanic or Thomsonian apothecaries," but it is doubtful that this agency had any significant impact on either medicine or pharmacy.

A movement such as Thomsonianism was certain to find many competitors in a society in which liberal and laissez-faire ideas prevailed, and it soon engendered splinter groups. By the mid-nineteenth century the movement was in decline, its place being taken by so-called Neo-Thomsonians and by two groups almost impossible to distinguish between—the Eclectics and the Reformed Practitioners of Medicine.

The Eclectics were named by the distinguished botanist Constantine S. Rafinesque, who nevertheless regarded himself as belonging to the Reformed Practice. Wooster Beach had given the Reformed Practice its start with the publication in 1836 of his book *The American Practice of Medicine.* The eclecticism of these movements meant that practitioners accepted what they thought useful from any source. As a rule, however, they rejected a large number of mineral drugs, especially calomel.

Reformed Practice, which played an important role in American medicine in the nineteenth century, sought for—and achieved—a high degree of professional respectability. Like the homeopaths, the Reformed Practitioners produced a considerable literature and established their own medical schools. One of these, which opened in Cincinnati in 1837, assumed the name of the Eclectic Medical Institute of Cincinnati in 1845; it did not close down until 1929. Unlike the Thomsonians, the Eclectics and the Reformed Practitioners had a high opinion of the role of the pharmacist. Rafinesque himself maintained that "with the aid of botany and chemistry" pharmacy had become a science.

It is worth noting that the standard practice of medicine was not impervious to the criticisms implicit in the botanical and reformed movements. Heroic medicine gradually gave way to more moderate methods, and the materia medica absorbed what was considered valuable from Thomsonian and Eclectic remedies. Thomson's tincture of capsicum and myrrh was admitted into the *United States Pharmacopoeia* and his Composition Powder (as the Compound Powder of Bayberry) into the *National Formulary.* Many of the plants used by Eclectics, among them *Berberis aquifolium* and *Rhamnus purshiana,* became used in medicine generally. The Eclectics also developed "resinoids," concentrated botanicals that were manufactured and marketed extensively but did not measure up to alkaloids in effectiveness.

Chapter VII

THE NINETEENTH CENTURY: THE PHARMACEUTICAL ESTABLISHMENT

The upsurge of the national state in the nineteenth century, and the concomitant and pervasive cultural nationalism, had a direct influence on pharmacy. The clearest manifestation of this was in the development of the pharmacopoeia.

THE NATIONAL PHARMACOPOEIA

Everywhere, local and regional pharmacopoeias disappeared, to be replaced by national pharmacopoeias. This trend began in the eighteenth century when the pharmacopoeias of Spain, Switzerland, Denmark, Portugal, and Prussia, though not official, became operative countrywide. In France, the *Codex medicamentarius sive pharmacopoeia Gallica* was made official for the entire country in 1818. *The Pharmacopoeia of the United States of America* (usually referred to as the *United States Pharmacopoeia*) appeared in 1820. The pharmacopoeias of London, Edinburgh, and Dublin were replaced by the *British Pharmacopoeia* in 1864. In the new Germany forged by Bismarck, one of the first manifestations of the new national spirit and unity was the publication of the *Pharmacopoea Germanica,* in 1872. Italy was laggard in this respect: although unified by 1870, it did not adopt its *Farmacopoea ufficiale del regno d'Italia* until 1892. The Japanese, for their part, demonstrated how Westernized their pharmacy had become by 1886 with the issuance of a Japanese pharmacopoeia.

These national pharmacopoeias did more than provide standards for a country; they were also vehicles of national pride. Attitudes in the United States, then a relatively new country, bear this out. "A national pharmacopoeia," Dr. James Thacher, a physician of Boston, wrote in 1817, "is highly important to our national character." The new national pride is amply evident in

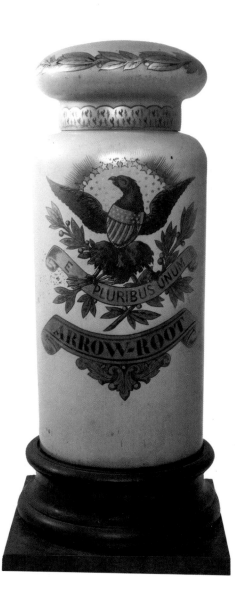

Glass specie jar used for display in windows of American pharmacies. c. 1880. National Museum of American History, Smithsonian Institution, Washington, D.C.

the language of the first edition of the *United States Pharmacopoeia,* which claimed to embody "the whole Corpus Medicum, in these free, independent, and United States" and declared itself "the first performance of the kind,...compiled by the authority of the faculty throughout a nation."

PHARMACY AND SCIENCE: THE UNITED STATES PHARMACOPOEIA

Additions, deletions, and changes in format, in particular, and the approach to pharmacopoeias, in general, tell the story of the progress in pharmacotherapy and the emergence of pharmacy as a modern science in the nineteenth century. The *United States Pharmacopoeia* (U.S.P.) illustrates these advances; decennially revised, it sought to keep abreast of changes and innovations at home and abroad, and it reflected developments in the French *Codex* and the British and German pharmacopoeias.

The first pharmacopoeia of the United States was issued "By the Authority of the Medical Societies and Colleges." In Latin and English, on facing pages, it provided two alphabetical lists of the materia medica: a main list containing simples and some prepared medicines that were to be "kept in the shop of the apothecary," and a secondary list containing substances "of doubtful efficacy," included because they were part of the traditional materia medica. A long list of compositions was arranged alphabetically, mainly by dosage forms; directions for compounding accompanied this list. Except for the melting, fusing, and treating of metals, there was little to suggest the use of chemistry; the directions for compounding were relatively simple.

The gradual displacement of the traditional materia medica can be discerned in the first revisions of the national pharmacopoeia (two competing revisions appeared, in 1830 and 1831). It ceased to be mainly a catalogue of the materia medica. The 1830 issue, for example, described the "properties" and gave a brief description of the "medical operations" of each item. Chemicals appeared among the simples, along with the usual plant, mineral, and animal substances. Quinine sulfate, quinine, morphine sulfate, and iodine sulfate made their debut.

Other new chemicals—alkaloids, glycosides, halogens, and synthetics—slowly made their way into the U.S.P. Bromine was made official in the 1842 revision; chloroform in the 1851 revision; "atropia," cinchonine, chlorine, and strychnine in the 1863 revision; "aconitia" and "digitalin," veratrine, chloral hydrate, and iodoform in the 1873 revision; caffeine, piperine, and codeine in the 1882 revision; cocaine, hyoscyamine, and salicylic acid in the 1893 revision.

Even so, the United States lagged behind Europe in accepting new remedies. The *Pharmacopoea Belgica Nova* of 1854, for instance, had already found a place for aconitine, atropine, strychnine, veratrine, salicylic acid, chloral hydrate, and iodoform. The *Pharmacopoea Germanica* of 1872 included all these and codeine and ethyl chloride as well.

In the latter half of the nineteenth century, a great number of chemical compounds were introduced into the *United States Pharmacopoeia*. Lead nitrate, potassium chlorate, lead iodide, iron iodide, zinc carbonate, and potassium bromide were added in 1851, and solutions of iron citrate, iron subsulfate, iron tersulfate, and nitrate of mercury were added in 1863. Nonetheless, vegetable drugs continued to dominate the materia medica; the U.S.P. eliminated more plant drugs than it added, but it did make additions. Outstanding among them was cascara sagrada, which was brought to the attention of the medical professions in the 1870s and entered the U.S.P. in 1893. Cascara sagrada was to earn the reputation of being the most widely used cathartic.

Portable wooden medicine chest. American, c. 1865. National Museum of American History, Smithsonian Institution, Washington, D.C.
Overleaf, left

Three Japanese military doctors in the Shosheido Pharmacy, Tokyo. Color woodblock print by Shikanobu. Japanese, 1878. From right to left, the doctors are Matsumoto Jun, Sato Naonaka, and Hayashi Yoshi. The posters behind them advertise products of the Shosheido Pharmacy.
Overleaf, right

Already apparent in the 1830 revision of the U.S.P. was its evolving scientific approach to the materia medica. Noted for the first time in that initial revision was the importance of temperature, specific gravity, and solubility in the identification of basic substances. Iodine, for example, was described as vaporizing at 347°F, having a specific gravity of 4.948 at 61½°F, and being soluble in 7,000 parts of water. In the revision of 1842, new tests were introduced that made use of reagents and litmus—evidence of the increasing responsibility taken by pharmacy to assure the genuineness and purity of materials going into medications.

Major advances were made in the U.S.P. issued in 1882. According to the foremost student of the subject, Glenn Sonnedecker, the 1882 edition was noteworthy for several reasons: "Casual mention of a few tests was replaced with detailed tests for identifying and determining the purity of many of the drugs. Detailed processes for assaying the alkaloids appeared for the first time. Drugs from the vegetable and mineral kingdoms were more meaningfully described as to physical characteristics and, where possible, chemical properties. Symbolic formulas and molecular weights were introduced. . . . Nomenclature was revised. . . ."

It is also noteworthy that this 1882 edition, often called the first modern U.S.P., was the first edition whose revision was entirely in the hands of pharmacists rather than physicians.

The evolution of the U.S.P. in the 1800s thus gives evidence of increasing recognition of the scientific and professional status of the pharmacist. Although the first revision noted that it had passed "the examination of pharmacists of acknowledged eminence in their profession," it was not until the revision of 1851 that pharmacy was accorded official representation on the Committee of Revision of the General Convention of Physicians responsible for the U.S.P.

The pharmacists who participated came from the colleges of pharmacy, and as their interest in and influence on the U.S.P. in-

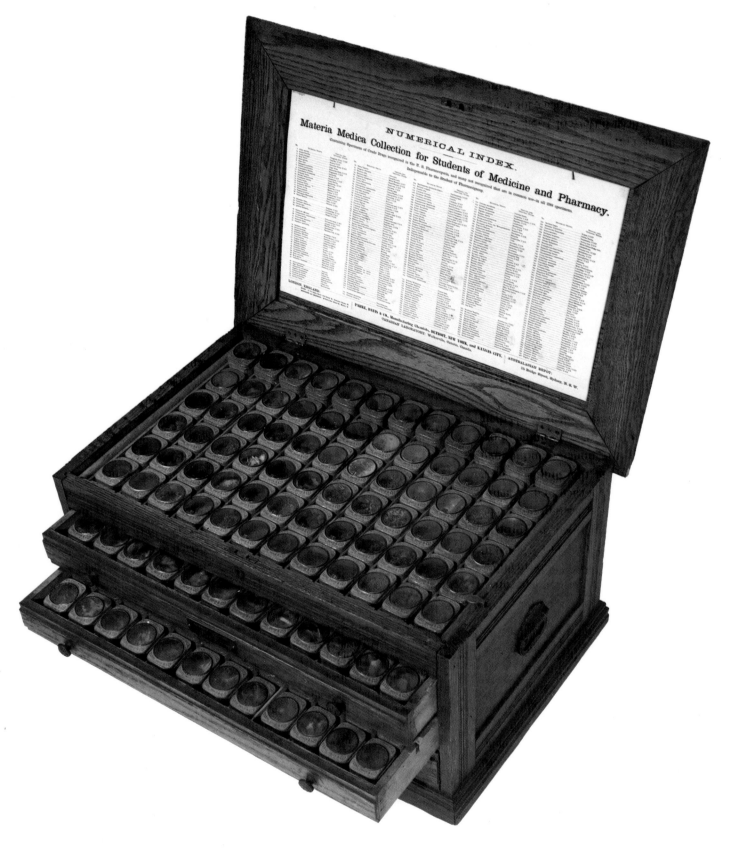

Wooden specimen case, containing a materia
medica collection for students of medicine and
pharmacy, prepared by Parke, Davis & Co.
American, c. 1890. National Museum of
American History, Smithsonian Institution,
Washington, D.C.

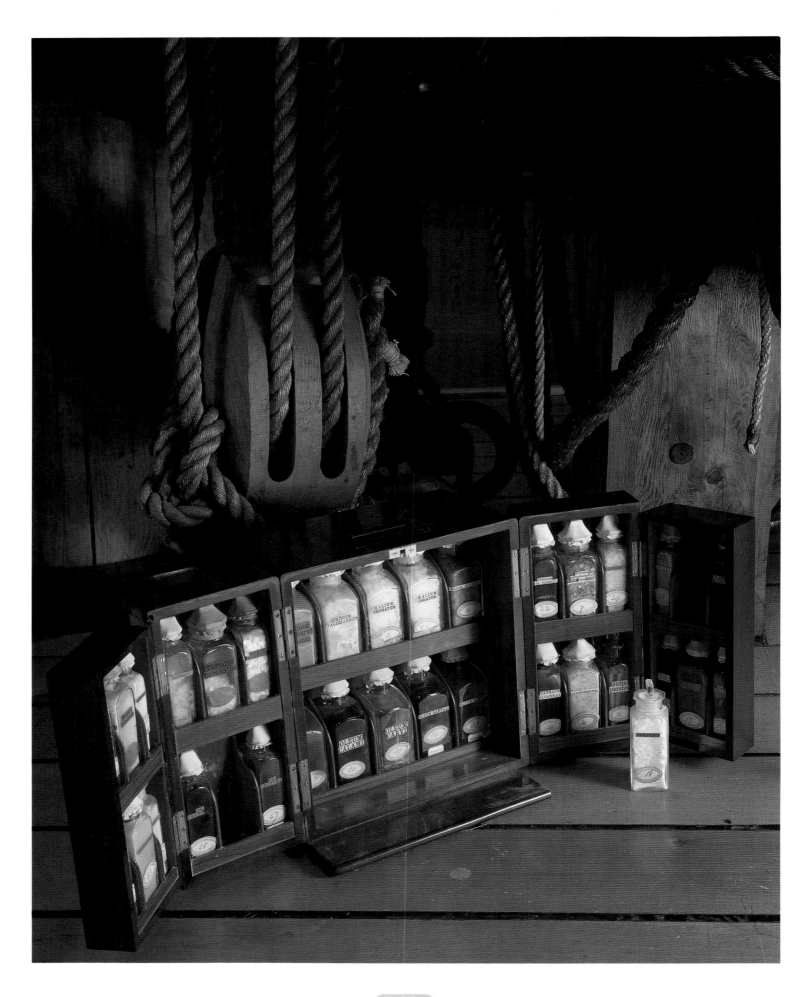

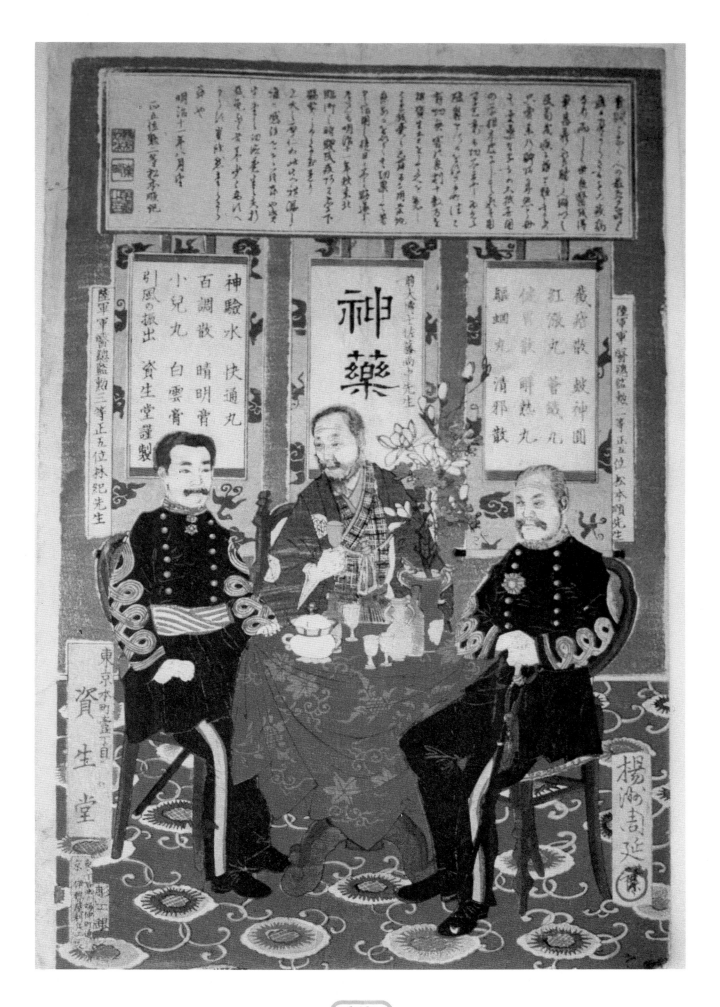

creased, that of physicians decreased. With the increasing complexity of the new drugs, the educated pharmacist had become more knowledgeable about drug specifications than the physician. Moreover, it was to the interest of the pharmacist to maintain a recognized and respected pharmacopoeia, both as a bulwark against the inroads of proprietary medicines into the proper domain of pharmacy and as a reliable standard that enhanced the integrity and reputation of the profession.

By the 1880s, pharmacists formed a majority of the Committee of Revision, and the American Pharmaceutical Association, which had come into existence in 1852, gave the pharmacopoeia a loose kind of sponsorship without actually assuming control. The edition of 1882, which, as has been said, must be credited wholly to pharmacists, and which represented the arrival on the scene of the modern pharmacopoeia, was the basis of all later editions. After 1882, the *United States Pharmacopoeia* was pharmacy's substantial and most significant contribution to the determination and maintenance of drug standards. In 1900, the General Convention of Physicians established the United States Pharmacopoeial Convention as a separate corporate body; thereafter it assumed responsibility for overseeing pharmacopoeial revision.

In 1888, the American Pharmaceutical Association had begun to issue a publication corollary to the U.S.P. that is generally known as the *National Formulary* (N.F.). It contained standards for drugs omitted from the U.S.P. and for drugs that might later be transferred to the national pharmacopoeia. It attained a scientific standing on a par with that of the U.S.P. and became official, along with the U.S.P., in 1906. In 1975, after negotiations with the American Pharmaceutical Association, the United States Pharmacopoeial Convention assumed responsibility for the N.F. as well, and the U.S.P. XX and the N.F. XV, although separate and distinct, were issued in a single volume. The scope of both publications was changed: the contents of the pharmacopoe-

ia were limited to drug substances and dosage forms, while the formulary's contents were limited to pharmaceutical ingredients. This separation, with appropriate cross referencing, eliminated a great deal of duplication.

In Great Britain a similar development produced the *Extra Pharmacopoeia,* known as "Martindale" after its compiler, the pharmacist William Martindale. It has been regularly revised and continues to be issued.

PHARMACEUTICAL LITERATURE

Pharmacy's flowering in the nineteenth century is evident from the plethora of literature that was produced to implement the new science. The *Edinburgh New Dispensatory* last appeared in English in Edinburgh in 1830—a huge volume of more than a thousand pages. But the traditional British dispensatory soon gave way to the conspectus, an overall view of various pharmacopoeias, exemplified by Anthony Todd Thomson's *Conspectus of the Pharmacopoeias of the London, Edinburgh and Dublin Colleges of Physicians.* The conspectus was primarily intended as a physicians' handbook.

American dispensatories took over where the *Edinburgh New Dispensatory* left off. Indeed, the two earliest American examples—John Redman Coxe's *American Dispensatory* and James Thacher's *American New Dispensatory,* published in the first decade of the nineteenth century—were unabashedly based on the Edinburgh work. Both went through several editions. But the work that proved most important to physicians as well as pharmacists was the *Dispensatory of the United States,* first published in 1833. This dispensatory was the work of George Bacon Wood and Franklin Bache, physicians affiliated with the Philadelphia College of Pharmacy who had been dominant figures in the revision of the national pharmacopoeia until pharmacists took over the task.

Wood and Bache's *Dispensatory* was a voluminous work, a veritable encyclopedia of pharmacy. It found a place for old as well as new drugs and contained a monograph on each drug giving synonyms in various languages, describing the drug (including botanical and chemical information where pertinent), giving something of the drug's history and the pertinent literature, detailing methods of preparing the drug, and listing its medicinal properties. The *Dispensatory* was immensely popular in the United States and, to a lesser extent, abroad. While Wood was alive, it sold between 120,000 and 150,000 copies. It was continued by others after Wood's death and retained its encyclopedic character until the twenty-sixth edition, issued in 1967, when its contents became more selective.

In Germany encyclopedias of pharmacy, as distinguished from texts and handbooks, date from the 1790s, when Samuel Hahnemann, of homeopathic fame, issued a two-volume *Apothekerlexicon* (1793–98). The trend culminated with the publication of the fourteen-volume *Realenzyklopädie der gesamten Pharmazie,* in the early 1900s by Hermann Thoms and Josef Moeller.

The increasingly scientific basis for pharmacy—and the growing need for pharmacists educated in the new developments—led logically to the expansion of textbook literature in the nineteenth century. In Germany, the textbooks of Karl Gottfried Hagen and Johann Trommsdorff retained their popularity through the first half of the century. In 1847 a book was published that was not only widely used in Germany but almost immediately translated into English: the *Lehrbuch der pharmazeutischen Technik* of Carl Friedrich Mohr, a professor of pharmacy and chemistry at the University of Bonn.

In 1848 the British pharmacist Theophilus Redwood, professor of chemistry and pharmacy at the School of the Pharmaceutical Society of Great Britain, issued a translation called *Practical Pharmacy Founded on Mohr's Manual,* and the next year William Procter, Jr., professor of pharmacy at the

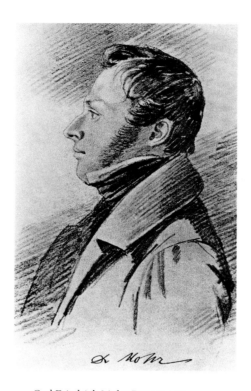

Carl Friedrich Mohr. Drawing. German, c. 1870. Mohr (1806–1879) made contributions to volumetric analysis, invented many instruments and pieces of auxiliary apparatus used in technical analysis, and was the author of a textbook on pharmacy that was popular in Germany, Great Britain, and the United States. Collection Dr. W. Schneider, Brunswick, West Germany

Philadelphia College of Pharmacy, published an American edition. Procter acknowledged the work done by Mohr and Redwood, but he edited and augmented the volume, increasing its size considerably. The title that Procter gave his book indicates its nature and thrust: *Practical Pharmacy: the Arrangements, Apparatus and Manipulations of the Pharmaceutical Shop and Laboratory.*

Mohr's work was supplanted in Germany by Hermann Hager's *Handbuch der pharmazeutischen Praxis,* first issued in 1880; it continued to be published and enlarged by others and is still available in an impressive illustrated eight-volume edition. In Great Britain and the United States, John Attfield's *Chemistry, General, Medical and Pharmaceutical,* first published as *An Introduction to Pharmaceutical Chemistry* in 1867, was very popular. Attfield, professor of practical chemistry at the School of the Pharmaceutical Society of Great Britain, assured himself of an American audience by taking into account the chemistry and preparations of the *United States Pharmacopoeia.* By 1906 his work had gone through nineteen editions.

The first textbook on pharmacy to originate in America was Edward Parrish's *Introduction to Practical Pharmacy.* As this book, which appeared in at least seven editions between 1856 and 1884, became increasingly directed toward pharmacists, its title changed—first to *Practical Pharmacy,* then to *Treatise on Pharmacy.* In 1885, Joseph Remington's *Practice of Pharmacy* appeared; it was destined to become immensely popular, and under the editorship of various successors to the author it is still issued as an encyclopedic work of reference and instruction under the title *Remington's Pharmaceutical Sciences.*

In France, *L'Officine ou Répertoire général de Pharmacie pratique* by François-Laurent-Marie Dorvault was first issued in 1844. Its twenty-first edition appeared in 1982 and was revised in 1985. A comprehensive and voluminous reference work in pharmacy, it is the French equivalent of the American *Remington.*

The end of the nineteenth century saw the appearance also of two texts that sought to present the theory and art of pharmacy in a concise fashion—primarily as study tools rather than as reference works: *Handbook of Pharmacy* by Virgil Coblentz, published in 1894, and *Treatise on Pharmacy for Students and Pharmacists* by Charles Caspari, Jr., issued the next year. Caspari's book proved the more popular and went through eight editions, the last in 1939.

Pharmaceutical Journals

The transformation of pharmacy through its interaction with the expanding medical, chemical, and biological sciences—so evident in the professional literature of the nineteenth century—made the updating provided by periodical literature a necessity. Until the end of the eighteenth century, pharmaceutical studies had been published in medical and scientific journals, and the first journals that covered pharmacy had usually covered chemistry as well. For the most part, these journals were private enterprises, edited and published by individual scientists. As the century progressed, pharmaceutical associations assumed greater responsibility for such publications.

The first journal with a largely pharmaceutical orientation, the *Taschenbuch für Scheidekünstler und Apotheker,* had appeared in Weimar in 1779. Its editor was Johann F. A. Göttling, a pharmacist and a professor at Jena. The *Taschenbuch* eventually became the responsibility of Johann Trommsdorff, who had been issuing his own *Journal der Pharmacie für Aerzte und Apotheker* since 1793. In 1834, Trommsdorff's publication merged with the *Annalen der Pharmacie,* established two years earlier by Justus von Liebig. In 1840 this became the *Annalen der Chemie und Pharmacie,* and since 1875 it has been published under the title *Liebigs Annalen der Chemie.*

Other such journals were published in Germany; some continue to be published.

These include the *Archiv der Pharmacie,* whose origins go back to 1820; the *Pharmazeutische Zeitung,* first published in 1856; and the *Deutsche Apotheker-Zeitung,* first published in 1861.

A close connection between pharmacy and chemistry in the periodical literature also obtained in France. The *Journal de la Société Libre des Pharmaciens de Paris* was started by the Société in 1797. Two years later it was merged with the *Annales de Chimie,* a journal in existence since 1789, whose staff included several noted pharmacists. In 1809 the *Bulletin de Pharmacie* was founded; it became the voice of scientific pharmacy in France. In 1942 it was one of two journals that merged to become the *Annales Pharmaceutiques Français.*

The first successful British journal in the field was the *Pharmaceutical Journal,* launched in 1841 by Jacob Bell, the dominant figure in British pharmacy at the time. In 1859, Bell turned its ownership over to the Pharmaceutical Society of Great Britain, which has continued to publish the journal as its organ. In 1859, too, *The Chemist and Druggist* first appeared. Introduced as a trade journal, it still continues to fulfill that function.

Interestingly enough, the first pharmaceutical journal in the English language appeared not in London but in Philadelphia. The *Journal of the Philadelphia College of Pharmacy,* founded by the college in 1825 in a burst of pride and aspiration, in 1835 became *The American Journal of Pharmacy.* Highly esteemed in the United States and abroad, the *Journal* is still being published, as an annual. It can lay claim to being the oldest journal dedicated entirely to pharmacy.

Except for the annual *Proceedings of the American Pharmaceutical Association,* which began publication in 1852, in the nineteenth century only the *American Journal of Pharmacy* emanated from professional sources and had a national audience in the United States. However, there developed a number of private journals devoted to practical pharmacy and to the economics of the drugstore as well as to the scientific aspects of the profession. The *American Druggist's Circular and Chemical Gazette* first appeared in 1857 and continued to be published (with an intervening change of name) until 1940, when it merged with *Drug Topics.* The *Pharmaceutical Era,* a similar journal, was published from 1888 to 1933. A number of these journals were addressed to local or regional audiences and continue to be published in various American cities.

THE EDUCATION OF THE PHARMACIST

The burgeoning of pharmaceutical sciences and pharmaceutical literature in the 1800s necessitated advances in pharmaceutical education. These sciences were changing and growing dynamically, and pharmacy was obligated to provide institutions capable of educating practitioners in a profession that was becoming increasingly closer to being a science than to being an art.

In the German states, private pharmaceutical teaching institutes, usually run by pharmacists, had developed in the late eighteenth century and flourished in the first decades of the nineteenth. Opportunities for education also increased in the German universities and polytechnics, where students in pharmacy selected their courses, more or less independently, with a view to preparing for state examinations. From 1800 to 1830, almost 1,500 students matriculated in pharmacy in eight German universities.

Pharmacy continued to be taught in association with medicine, but separate institutes with an orientation toward pharmacy and chemistry began to appear at German universities. The curriculum of Justus von Liebig's Institute at Giessen, first offered in 1826, was heavily weighted toward chemistry, and it included study in mathematics, physics, and botany. The only purely

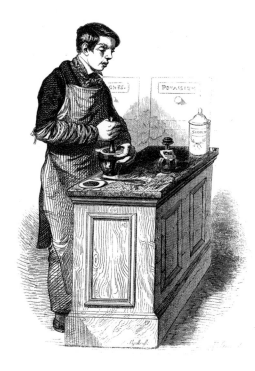

Le Pharmacien and *L'Elève en pharmacie. (The Pharmacist* and *The Student of Pharmacy).* Lithographs by J. J. Grandville. French, 1840

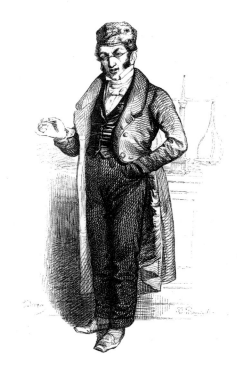

pharmaceutical course was a course in pharmacognosy.

In France, the educational structure of pharmacy was established in the Law of Germinal an XI (April 11, 1803), the "organic" law of nineteenth-century French pharmacy. The law not only set up the Ecole de Pharmacie in Paris as successor to the Revolution-sponsored Ecole Gratuite de Pharmacie, but also provided for the establishment of five additional schools. Only two of these materialized, at Montpellier (where the long tradition in pharmaceutical education continued, though disturbed by the Revolution) and at Strasbourg. The law required the schools to provide instruction in materia medica, pharmacy, and chemistry.

In 1840, the schools of pharmacy in Paris, Montpellier, and Strasbourg were incorporated into the universities in those cities and a baccalaureate was required of entering students. Between 1874 and 1890, mixed faculties of medicine and pharmacy were established at Bordeaux, Lyons, Lille, and Toulouse. The pharmacy schools at Paris, Montpellier, Strasbourg, and Nancy were to develop into the present pharmacy faculties.

France also established, in 1803, the rank of second-class pharmacist. Apprenticeship and course work were required of candidates, and, to aid in educating them, new pharmaceutical training institutions were created over the years. These included *écoles préparatoires,* of which twenty-one were set up in 1849, and *écoles de plein exercice,* of which four were created in 1875. The category of the second-class pharmacist, whose practice was limited geographically and for whom a localized system of examination was developed, was eliminated in 1906.

Modern pharmaceutical education in Spain began at the outset of the nineteenth century, first in Madrid and then in Barcelona and Granada, with the establishment of schools of pharmacy. Degrees of bachelor of pharmacy and doctor of chemistry were awarded. A three-year baccalaureate curriculum that included courses in natural history, chemistry, and pharmacy gave way at mid-century to a five-year program that included mineralogy, zoology, applied botany, and inorganic, organic, and applied chemistry as well as pharmacy.

In Great Britain, where the status of apothecaries as general practitioners of medicine had been assured by the Apothecaries Act of 1815, pharmacists (usually called "chemist-and-druggist," or "pharmaceutical chemist," or just "the chemist") had no educational tradition to fall back on. In addition, English concern with liberty of the individual and freedom of trade had left pharmacy virtually unregulated. Even after laws were passed providing for the examination and registration of those seeking certification as pharmacists, any individuals could make and sell drugs (except, after 1868, certain poisons), so long as they did not claim to be chemists, druggists, or pharmacists.

The chemists-and-druggists succeeded in establishing the Pharmaceutical Society of Great Britain in 1841. They were aware of the progress of pharmacy and recognized that the apprenticeship system would not meet the needs of the profession. They were aware also that the Apothecaries' Society was seeking to gain control over them. Lectures in materia medica and botany were available at Apothecaries' Hall, and chemistry and physics were being taught at some London hospitals and at the Royal Institution in London, but these hardly provided a systematic education.

In 1842, a year after its founding, the Pharmaceutical Society of Great Britain established its School of Pharmacy in London. Attracted to the faculty were such scientists of note as A. T. Thomson, Theophilus Redwood, and Jonathan Pereira. The program was directed to the practicing pharmacist: courses and laboratory work were offered in chemistry, botany, materia medica, and practical pharmacy. With professors who were leaders in their fields, a high level of scientific instruction was maintained. In 1844 the Society's School of

Pharmacy became the first in Britain to supplement lectures in chemistry with instruction in its own teaching laboratory, and its laboratory became a model for others.

Despite this auspicious beginning, the absence of a specified curriculum required for examination (none was specified until 1918) led to a mushrooming of "cram schools"—private proprietary pharmacy schools and polytechnic schools that gave instruction in pharmacy. By the end of the century there were forty-five institutions offering total or partial instruction in pharmacy. The caliber of the instruction was not high, and eventually they all disappeared; in the twentieth century the demands of new pharmaceutical knowledge were beyond the resources of the proprietary school. The School of Pharmacy of the Pharmaceutical Society became a constituent college of the University of London in 1949, and the School of Pharmacy at the Chelsea Polytechnic became Chelsea College and is part of King's College of the University of London. In addition, eight university schools of pharmacy in Great Britain grant degrees in pharmacy. The degree of bachelor of pharmacy or bachelor of science in pharmacy and one year of postgraduate training in a pharmacy are required for registration.

Pharmaceutical education in the United States ran a not dissimilar course. As in Great Britain, concepts of personal freedom and free trade prevailed, and for most of the nineteenth century in all but a few jurisdictions anyone could set up shop as a pharmacist—or a physician. This absence of restriction reflected the frontier conditions that prevailed in the great expanses of the United States and the political organization of the country, a decentralized federation of states.

These economic, geographic, and political considerations—and the example of the British apothecary—played a role in the development of the dispensing physician, one who both compounded and dispensed medications. The first medical school in the country, the Medical College of Philadel-

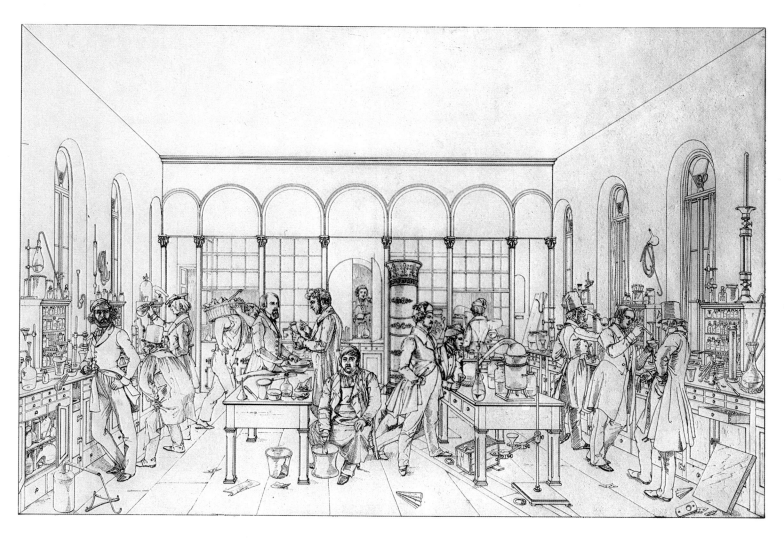

phia, included in its original offerings, in 1765, lectures on the theory and practice of pharmacy, and throughout the nineteenth century the curricula of medical schools continued to provide instruction in pharmacy. Indeed, vestiges of the teaching of pharmacy to medical students were still to be found as late as 1950. This instruction was important to the dispensing physician because a good portion of his income was derived from the medicines he dispensed. As a result, the "doctor shop," a pharmacy operated by a physician who might or might not also practice medicine, was a rather common phenomenon in the United States until the early twentieth century.

When, in 1820, the University of Pennsylvania, of which the Medical College of Philadelphia had become a part, seemed about to initiate a program of pharmaceutical education, the pharmacists of Philadelphia, disturbed by the prospect of the

View of the interior of the laboratory at Liebig's institute at Giessen. Drawing by Wilhelm Trautschold. German, 1842. Justus von Liebig (1803–1873) had been a pharmacy apprentice and an inspector of pharmacies in Hesse, Germany, and did important work in pharmaceutical chemistry. His laboratory style of instruction was instrumental in shaping modern teaching methods. Shown at work in the laboratory are eleven identifiable students of Liebig's. Deutsches Museum, Munich

education of the pharmacist falling completely into the hands of the medical profession, formed a local association called the Philadelphia College of Apothecaries (1821). Its name was soon changed to the Philadelphia College of Pharmacy, perhaps in recognition of the fact that the American pharmacist's role differed from the dual role of the British apothecary. The College offered lectures on Materia medica, Pharmacy, and Pharmaceutical Chemistry and granted diplomas to those who completed "two courses of each of the lectures."

Not surprisingly, the College was involved in activities other than education. One interest of its sixty-eight founding druggists and apothecaries was evidenced by the publication, in 1824, of formulas for the imitation of patent medicines being imported at the time from England. In 1826 the College published a *Druggist's Manual* that was a price-current of drugs, medi-

Administration militaire et service de santé.
Lithograph by G.David after a painting by
Alfred de Marbot. French, c. 1840. The
Pharmacist Second Class stands between the
Chief Surgeon (on a white horse) and a
physician.

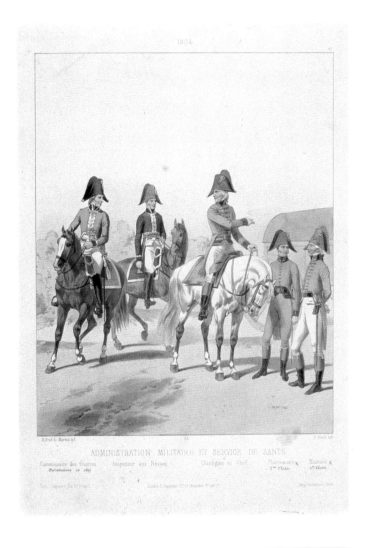

Anonymous 18th-century painting of a
pharmaceutical scene—an examination at the
Faculté de Pharmacie in Paris. In the
foreground, various pharmaceutical activities
are in progress. Faculté de Pharmacie, Paris

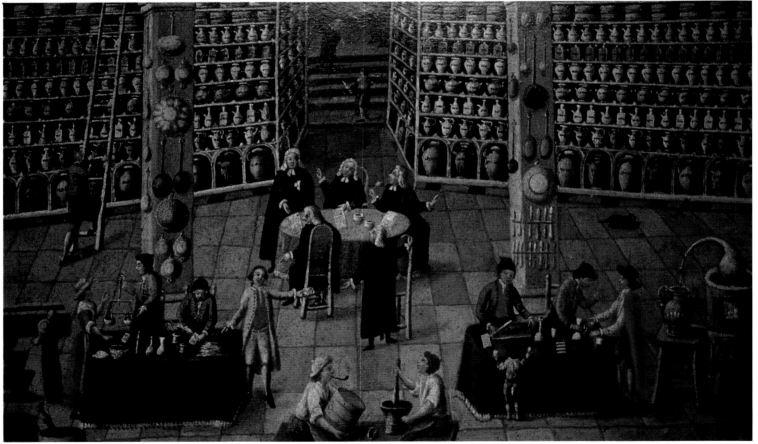

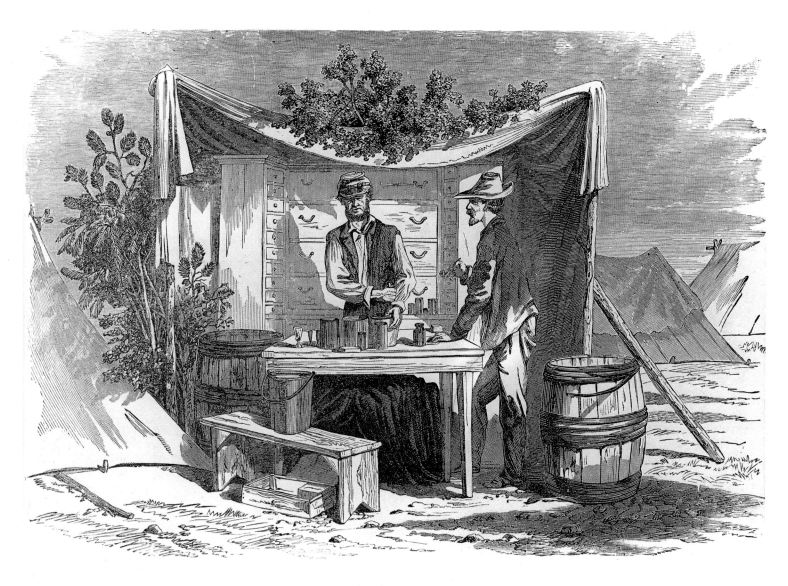

Hospital Steward Filling Surgeons' Orders at the Army Drug Store. Wood engraving after a drawing by Joseph Becker from *Frank Leslie's Illustrated Newspaper,* 1864. The scene is a temporary field pharmacy during the Civil War.

cines, and various products then sold by the pharmacist; it also contained drug synonyms and lists of foreign drugs.

By the time of the Civil War, pharmacists in six other American cities had followed the lead of the Philadelphia pharmacists. However, these other pioneer educational ventures did not meet with the quick success of the Philadelphia project. For example, the Massachusetts College of Pharmacy, although it offered occasional lectures after its founding, in 1823, did not mount a regular program of instruction until 1867. The Philadelphia College of Pharmacy had a regular flow of students and graduates from the beginning but did not open a pharmaceutical and chemical laboratory for individual instruction until 1870.

The post–Civil War period in the United States saw a great proliferation of schools and programs offering education in pharmacy. By 1900, more than sixty had been set up. For the most part, these were proprietary institutions interested in making a profit. (In this, pharmacists were following the example of physicians.) But various universities did create departments or schools of pharmacy in this period. A few medical schools even sought to add pharmacy departments, Tulane University as early as 1838. But these ventures were successful only in the case of the Medical College of the State of South Carolina and the Medical College of Virginia, where early pharmacy programs evolved into the present schools of pharmacy.

Much more significant was the introduction of pharmacy programs into the new, publicly supported state universities. This step was taken by the University of Michi-

Certificate of membership in the Maryland College of Pharmacy. Lithograph published by A. Hoen & Co., Baltimore, c. 1860. In the vignette, the alchemist of old is contrasted with the scientific pharmacist.

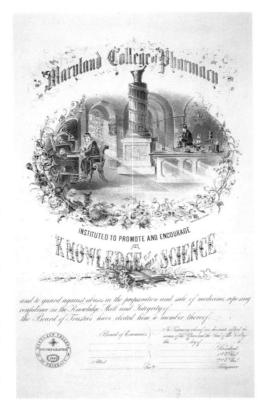

gan in 1868 and in 1883 by the University of Wisconsin. Before 1900, eight state universities had programs in pharmacy. This development had highly significant consequences for American pharmaceutical education: it took the education of pharmacists out of the hands of practical-minded proprietors; it provided both for a regularized program of studies and for a wider exposure of students to a variety of sciences; it contributed greatly to the developing pharmaceutical sciences; and it led, eventually, to graduate programs in pharmacy. The proprietary colleges—with the exceptions of the Philadelphia College of Pharmacy (now the Philadelphia College of Pharmacy and Science), the Massachusetts College of Pharmacy, and the St. Louis College of Pharmacy—have now either disappeared or found a haven within a university.

Pharmaceutical education, even at the university level, did not put an end to the apprenticeship system, under which fledgling pharmacists were expected to spend a given period of time actually working in a pharmacy under the supervision of a pharmacist. This was true in Europe as well as the United States. In Prussia, for example, an apprenticeship of three years was re-

quired prior to enrollment in a university program. In France, from 1803 to 1854, eight years of apprenticeship—without formal education in pharmacy—qualified one for an examination. Graduates of one of the *écoles supérieures*, as the schools in Paris, Montpellier, and Strasbourg were known after 1854, were still required to serve a three-year practicum. In the United States in 1868 the Philadelphia College of Pharmacy required its students to have "served out" at least four years under a qualified pharmacist. It was possible until the 1920s, at least in certain jurisdictions in the United States, to take qualifying examinations for licensure on the basis of apprenticeship alone, without having had any formal pharmaceutical education.

THE PRACTICE OF PHARMACY: LEGAL REQUIREMENTS

On the Continent, and even in the United States, with its more laissez-faire outlook, pharmacists sought formal education long before state licensing laws came into effect. But formal pharmaceutical education required the support of law to become compulsory and universal. Legal requirements for the practice of pharmacy derived from two sources. They were a continuation of the self-regulation and monopoly that pharmacists had experienced under the guild system, and they were set in motion by the realization that they were necessary for the protection and preservation of public health.

It was not accidental that the imposition of legal requirements for the education, examination, and licensing of pharmacists had its early modern beginnings in countries with benevolent paternalistic rulers. The outstanding examplar of this sort of paternalism was Frederick William I of Prussia, whose concern for the health of his people led him to issue the edict of 1725.

Title page of a booklet of formulas published for pharmacists by the Philadelphia College of Pharmacy in 1824. The eight formulas were for leading imported proprietary medicines, including Turlington's Balsam of Life, Hooper's Female Pills, and Dalby's Carminative. This information enabled American pharmacists to prepare equivalent remedies. Library, Philadelphia College of Pharmacy and Science

FORMULÆ

FOR THE

PREPARATION OF EIGHT

PATENT MEDICINES,

ADOPTED BY THE

PHILADELPHIA COLLEGE

OF

PHARMACY.

MAY 4th, 1824.

SOLOMON W. CONRAD, PRINTER,
No. 32, Church Alley.

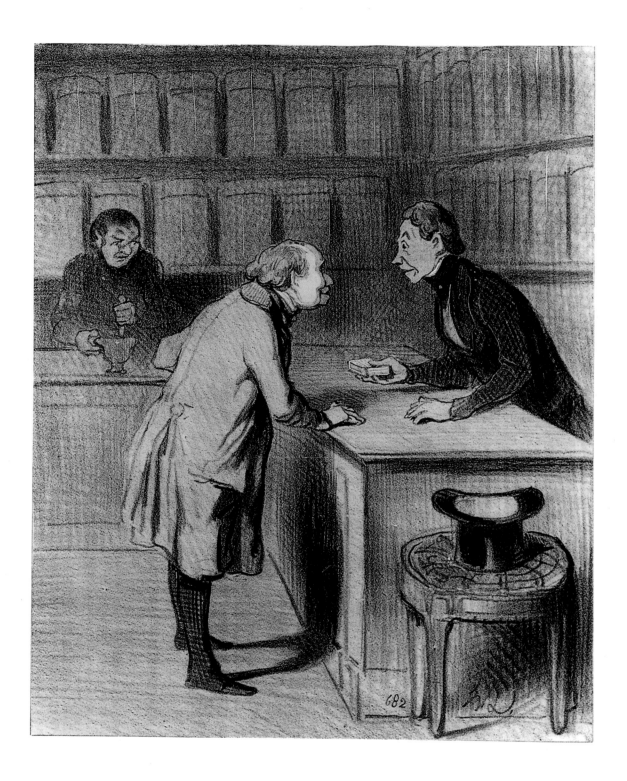

Les Philanthropes du Jour (The Philanthropists of the Day) was the title that Honoré Daumier gave to a series of about 35 lithographs he made between 1844 and 1846. Here a pharmacist who describes himself as "dedicated by circumstance and by feeling to the purest philanthropy" is discoursing to a gullible client on the merits of a lozenge he has compounded out of wood lice and snails. French, 1844

The edict gave considerable power to the Obercollegium Medicum et Sanitatis and its subordinate *collegii* and, as has been noted, established the basic rules for the training and examination of pharmacists.

The nineteenth century saw the imposition of requirements for the practice of pharmacy developing everywhere in the West. On the Continent, where there was a tradition of education and examination, and where the state had long controlled matters of health, this was a predictable evolutionary process. In Germany, examining boards were established at all universities in 1875, soon after unification. In France, the basic pharmacy law, enacted in 1803, took the control of the pharmacy out of the hands of practitioners and placed it in the hands of the state. Second-class pharmacists were examined under the administration of the appropriate departments by a board made up of two physicians or surgeons. Prospective first-class pharmacists were examined at their schools by a board that included pharmacists who had themselves studied at the schools. The role of the medical profession in these examining bodies rankled pharmacists, but not until 1878 were examinations placed solely in the hands of pharmacists.

In Spain, where examination and licensing of pharmacists went back to the Renaissance, state control gave way, under a royal decree of 1800, to a Junta Superior Gobernativa de Farmacia. This, in turn, gave way, some forty years later, to a new series of governmental boards. Complete control of pharmacy—including the issuance of degrees in pharmacy, the issuance of licenses to practice, and the inspection of pharmacies—rested in such boards. Early in the nineteenth century a degree in pharmacy

Reconstruction of the interior of a 19th-century American pharmacy. National Museum of American History, Smithsonian Institution, Washington, D.C.

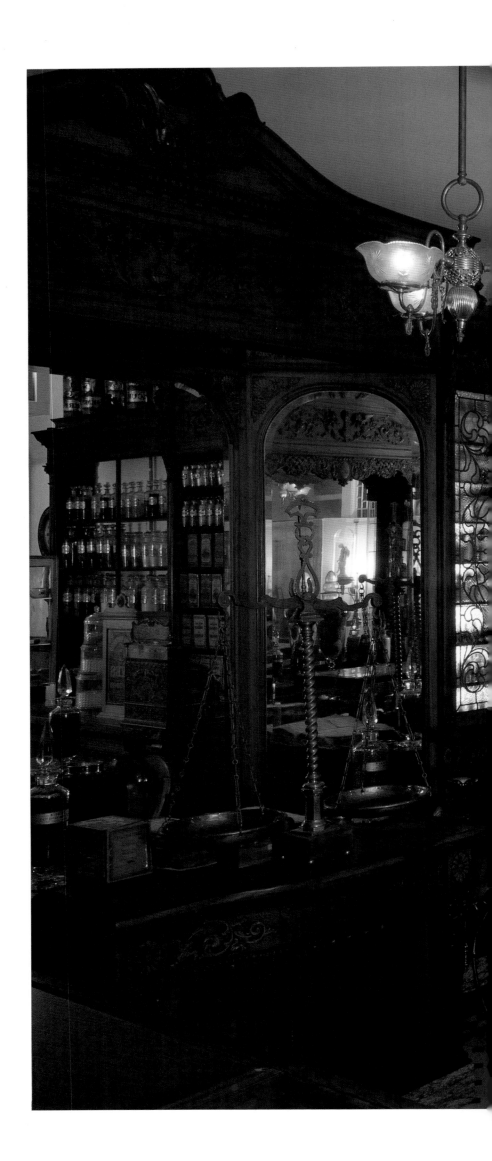

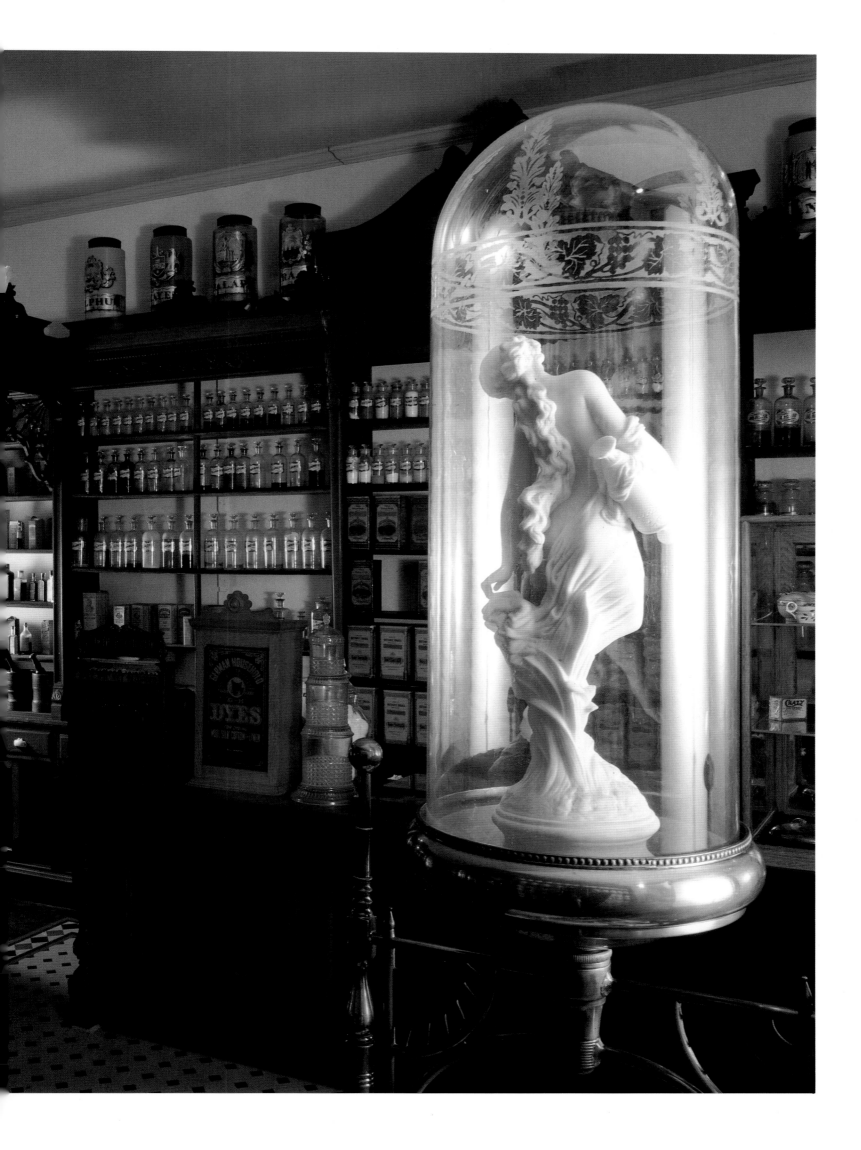

earned the same privileges as a degree in medicine or surgery.

As already noted, the United States was far behind the Continent in both the regulation of pharmacy and the education of the pharmacists. The social and political conditions in the United States responsible for this were compounded by the American system of federalism. There was no single political jurisdiction to govern pharmacy. In 1800 there were sixteen states, and by 1900 there were forty-five—each having the power to regulate pharmacy independently.

A few attempts were made to require the licensing of pharmacists before the Civil War, but it was not until the last third of the century that the American society was mature enough to accept governmental regulation. The impetus for regulation came from the American Pharmaceutical Association, particularly its secretary, John Maisch. At his urging, state pharmaceutical associations were established, and they sought legislation requiring the examination and licensing of pharmacists.

The first modern law was passed in 1870 in Rhode Island; by 1900, government regulation was in effect in all but one state. The legislation created state boards of pharmacy that were given the major responsibilities for establishing requirements for examining and licensing, for inspecting pharmacy shops, and for oversight of pharmacy in general. These state boards were composed entirely of pharmacists, and members were usually selected from panels recommended to the governor by the state pharmaceutical association. This meant that the profession was in some measure self-regulating—at least as self-regulating as the new governmental involvement allowed.

As in other countries, state pharmacy laws in the United States provided for a subordinate class of pharmacists. Arrangements varied, but, in general, "registered assistant pharmacists" or "qualified assistants" were those who had passed an examination on the basis of apprenticeship but had not met formal educational require-

ments. The assistant, who was not entitled to own or manage a pharmacy, disappeared as a legally recognized functionary in the first half of the twentieth century.

The British experience was, once again, different from that of other countries. Originally chemists-and-druggists had resisted any attempt to regulate pharmacy as an infringement upon their rights, but they came to realize the seriousness of the need for education, qualification, public recognition, and public support. Thus the charter of the Pharmaceutical Society of Great Britain, obtained in 1843, provided for the certification of chemists-and-druggists and assistants and apprentices already in practice, and for the examination of any who presented themselves thereafter. The Society effected the passage of a Pharmacy Act in 1852 that established a Register maintained by the Society under the direction of a Registrar. "Pharmaceutical chemists, assistants, and apprentices or students" were to be placed on the Register either through acceptable affidavits attesting to their having been actively engaged in the calling for stated periods or through an examination by the Society's examiners. Nothing in this law, or in subsequent laws, prohibited the practice of pharmacy by an unregistered individual. What was prohibited was the use of the titles of Pharmaceutical Chemist, Chemist-and-Druggist, Chemist, Druggist, Pharmaceutist, or Pharmacist by anyone not in the Register. Likewise, a shop that was not owned or managed by a pharmacist in the Register could not be designated a Chemist-and-Druggist shop or a Pharmacy.

In Great Britain, then, control was exercised by definition. Theoretically the laws did not grant a restrictive monopoly to the pharmacist; in the nineteenth century, after 1868, as noted, only the dispensing of certain poisons was prohibited to an unregistered individual. (After 1968, prescription drugs and "pharmacy only" drugs could be dispensed only by registered pharmacists; this in effect supplanted the traditional control by definition. There was also developed a General Sales List that could be sold by nonpharmacists. It included only drugs that carried little risk.)

The General Sales List in Great Britain had its antecedents on the Continent. The shop (*Drogerie*) of the German *Drogist* was distinct from the shop (*Apotheke*) of the *Apotheker*. Germany's *Drogisten* (who established themselves in the nineteenth century) are still an avenue for the distribution of a limited number of "harmless" pharmaceuticals. The modern *Drogist* is essentially a merchant, dealing in cosmetics, spices, dyes, toiletries, candies, dietetic aids, and technical chemicals and permitted to sell only drugs that are not restricted by law to the *Apotheker*. France saw the emergence of a similar functionary, the *droguiste*. But although there still exist French shops called *drogueries,* which carry a variety of merchandise and many items one might expect to find in a drugstore, they do not carry drugs or prescription items.

With the advances in education and licensing requirements in the nineteenth century, changes took place that affected the legal status of pharmacists and the pharmacy shop. In Germany, attempts were made to establish new freedom for pharmacies, a broader freedom that would allow the pharmacist to establish himself wherever he wished. These attempts came to naught. In fact, the Business Law of 1869, which established freedom of trade for the individual, specifically excluded pharmacy.

The proposed changes were undoubtedly too liberal for Germany, but change took place nevertheless. To the old system of the *privilegium* was added a new system of concessions granted by governmental authority. These were either *Real-Konzessionen,* which carried with them the right of a widow to continue in business, or *Personal-konzessionen,* which ceased with the death of the recipient and reverted to the state. Such privileges and concessions were valuable properties, and they were to endure until 1958. (A new pharmacy law of 1960 provided for *Niederlassungsfreiheit,* the right of pharmacists to establish themselves wherever they wished.)

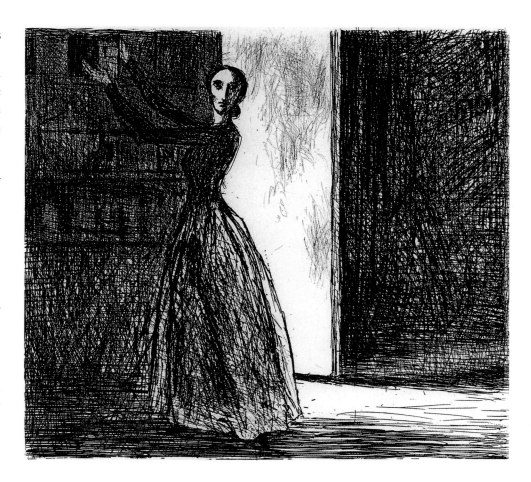

Madame Bovary. Lithograph by Michel Ciry. French, c. 1950. Pictured is the grim moment in Flaubert's novel when Emma, seeing no other way out, reaches for the blue bottle containing the white powder that she will swallow to end her life.

Finland, Russia, Austria, and the Scandinavian countries followed the German model rather closely. Various Italian states followed a similar pattern, but the new kingdom of Italy in 1888 sought to bring uniformity to the country by permitting qualified pharmacists to open pharmacies wherever they chose. The result was severe competition in the cities and a shortage of pharmacies in the country. Italy therefore went back to regulation in 1913.

In France, where the limitations placed on pharmacists and pharmacies reflected old guild practices, there was, however, considerable freedom throughout the nineteenth century. Not until the 1940s did ordinances once more limit (by setting proportions) the number of pharmacies. One pharmacist was allowed for every 3,000 people in cities of over 30,000 population, one for every 2,500 people in communities of 5,000 to 30,000, and one for every 2,000 in communities under 5,000.

In 1954, a study covering fifty-six countries indicated that thirty restricted the

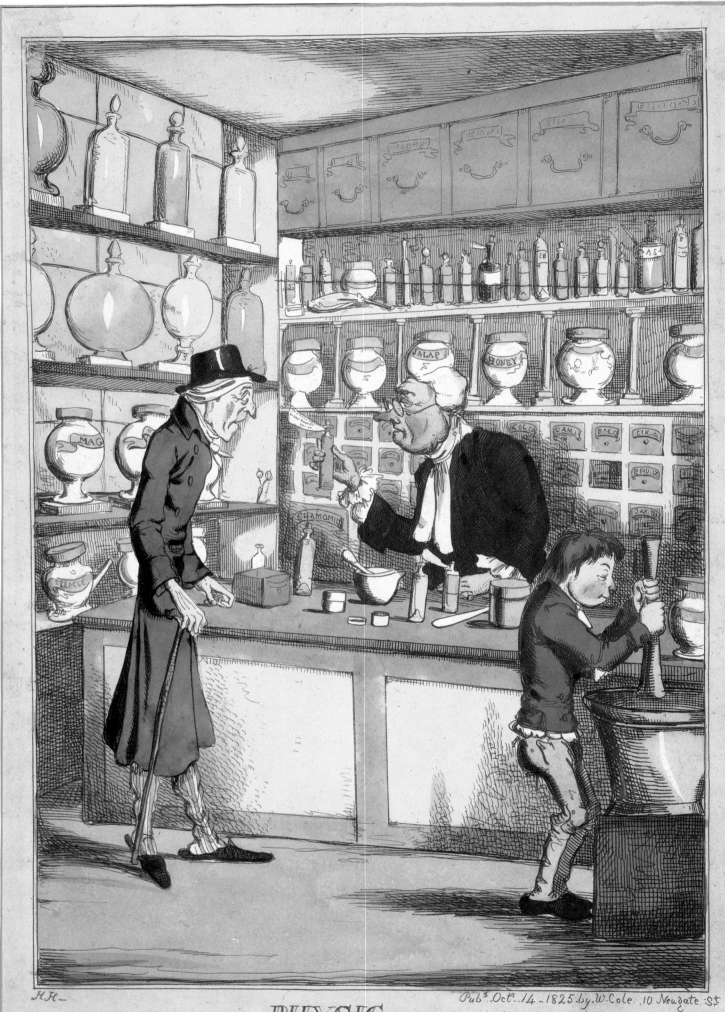

PHYSIC.

Pub.d Oct.r 14 - 1825 by W.Cole. 10 Newgate St.

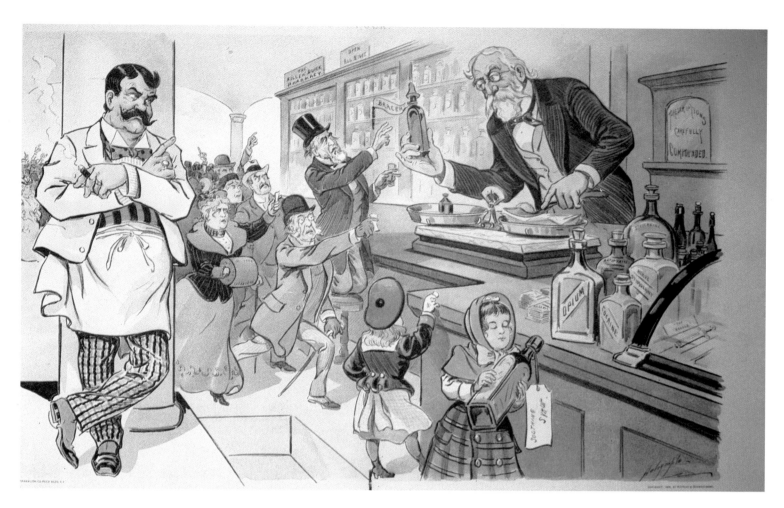

The Age of Drugs. Color lithograph (from *Puck*) by Louis Dalrymple. American, 1900. The saloon keeper, casting a baleful glance at the druggist, says, "The kind of drunkard I make is going out of fashion. I can't begin to compete with this fellow." Meanwhile, contented customers are walking out of the shop with medicines labeled BRACER and SOOTHING SYRUP.

The Prohibition Movement—The Drug Store of the Future. Lithograph by F. Graetz. American, 1882. The cartoon suggests the possible effects on the pharmacy of prohibition legislation, under which alcohol could be obtained only with a physician's prescription.

Physic. Color engraving by H. Heath. English, 1825. The medicine bottle that the apothecary is dispensing to his dyspeptic customer has the label attached to the cork. This method of labeling was common practice until the middle of the 19th century and continued until the end of the century in Scandinavia and the East European countries.

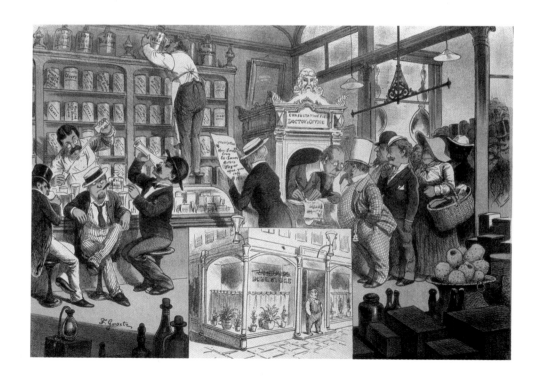

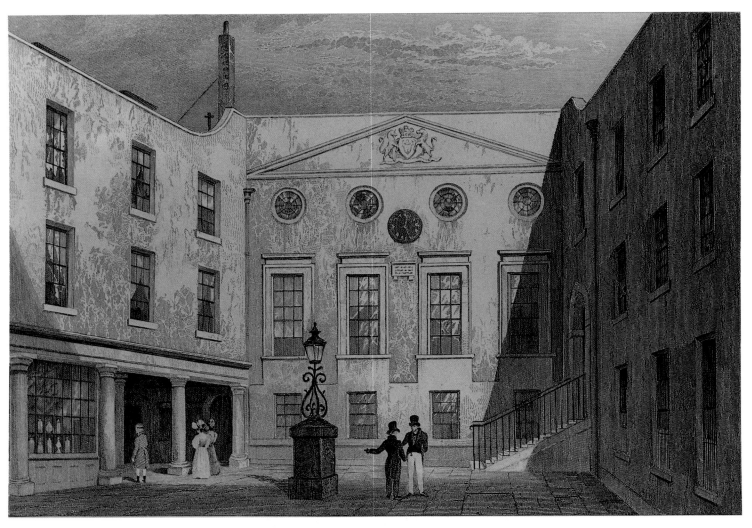

Apothecaries' Hall, Pilgrim Street, London. Engraving by John James Hinchliff after a drawing by Thomas H. Shepherd. English, 1831. One of the two guildhalls that survived the bombing raids of World War II, this building still houses the Worshipful Society of Apothecaries of London.

number of pharmacies in accordance with population at various ratios, while twenty-six—including the United States, Great Britain, Canada, Holland, and Spain—did not.

THE ORGANIZATION OF PHARMACY

In the nineteenth century the right of a duly qualified pharmacist to open a shop was not absolute even in the countries with liberal regulations. In a throwback to the days of the guilds, the pharmacist was often required to be a member of the organization of pharmacists of the country or region. Thus, the development of pharmaceutical organizations in the nineteenth century played a basic role in the institutions that arose.

Associations of pharmacists, organized for economic, social, professional, and scientific purposes, had their origins in the guild system. Local associations in the cities were known in the eighteenth century, but it was the nineteenth century that saw the development of organizations of pharmacists on a larger territorial or political scale. Perhaps the earliest of these was the Pharmazeutischer Verein of Bavaria, founded in 1816. Thereafter the organization of pharmacy reflected political changes taking place in the German states, and after the unification of Germany a national organization, the Deutscher Apotheker-Verein, came into existence. In 1890, the Deutsche Pharmazeutische Gesellschaft, founded by Hermann Thoms, professor of pharmaceutical chemistry at the University of Berlin, became an exclusively scientific society. Both the Verein and the Gesellschaft fell prey to National Socialism, but both were revived after World War II. These were voluntary societies.

There also developed in Germany an organization that owners of pharmacies in a particular jurisdiction were obligated to join—the *Gremium*. This was a quasi-public administrative body that helped the state regulate pharmacy and also provided social welfare programs for its members. The *Gremiumen,* which first appeared in Bavaria in 1842, gave way in the twentieth century to the *Kammern,* associations with greater disciplinary power.

In France, with the dissolution of the royal Collège de Pharmacie, there were set up, in 1796, the Ecole Gratuite de Pharmacie, as already noted, and a Société Libre des Pharmaciens de Paris. In 1803 the latter became the Société de Pharmacie de Paris and was transformed into an elitist scientific society with a limited membership. The Société gained an enviable scientific reputation, and similar societies were founded in several other French cities. (The Paris Société became the Académie de Pharmacie in 1946 by presidential decree.) The organization of pharmacists in France did not become nationwide until 1876, however, with the establishment of the Fédération Génerale des Syndicats Pharmaceutiques. This was an association devoted to the economic interests of pharmacy: scientific activities remained in the hands of local organizations.

In the United States the organization of pharmacy, for all that it reflected a desire to promote recognition of the professional aspects of pharmacy, had as its immediate motivation the improvement of conditions in the drug trade. The United States was considerably dependent upon imports for

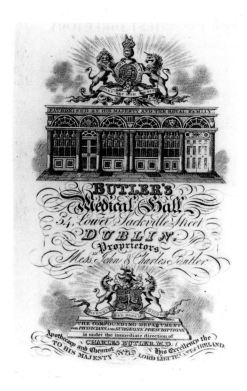

Advertisement for Butler's Medical Hall. Engraving. Irish, 1832. This was used as the frontispiece to *Butler's Medicine Chest Directory,* a catalogue of the drugs and chemicals offered by the proprietors of a Dublin pharmacy. (In Ireland the term "medical hall" is frequently used instead of "pharmacy.")

its drug supply, and too much of what was arriving was of poor quality or adulterated. A federal law of 1848, which sought to examine all drugs at the port of entry, had proven ineffective. In 1851 the College of Pharmacy of the City of New York issued a call for a meeting of all five colleges of pharmacy to discuss ways of combating the problem of drug adulteration, but the Philadelphia College broadened the scope of this meeting to cover "all the important questions bearing on the profession."

These were the circumstances under which the American Pharmaceutical Association came into existence, in 1852. State pharmaceutical associations, established in the last thirty years of the century, were called the "children" of the national association. The American Pharmaceutical Association, in recognition of both the economic and the social pressures on community pharmacy—and in recognition of the reality of the American federal system, which made action on the state level imperative—encouraged the establishment of state pharmaceutical associations and their sponsorship of state pharmacy laws. Although the national body was not oblivious to the economic problems of the pharmacist, it was mainly oriented toward professional and scientific aspects of pharmacy. To fill the need, there developed, in 1883, the short-lived National Retail Druggists' Association. Its successor, the National Association of Retail Druggists, was founded in 1898, and both it and the American Pharmaceutical Association have been active organizations ever since. They symbolize pharmacy's split personality in the United States—part profession, part business.

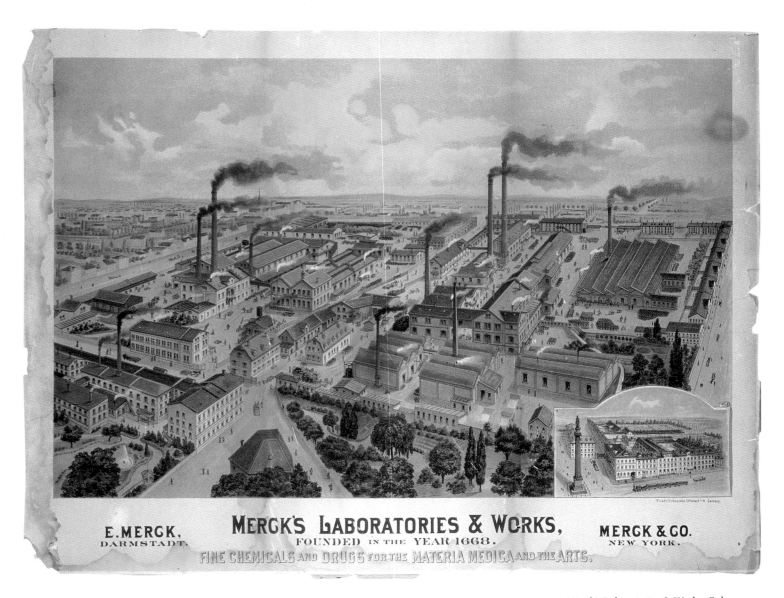

Containers, mostly of tin, for 19th-century proprietary medicines from various countries.

Merck's Laboratories & Works. Color lithograph. German, c. 1900. The main view shows the manufacturing plant of E. Merck in Darmstadt, Germany. The company began its United States manufacturing operations in 1895.

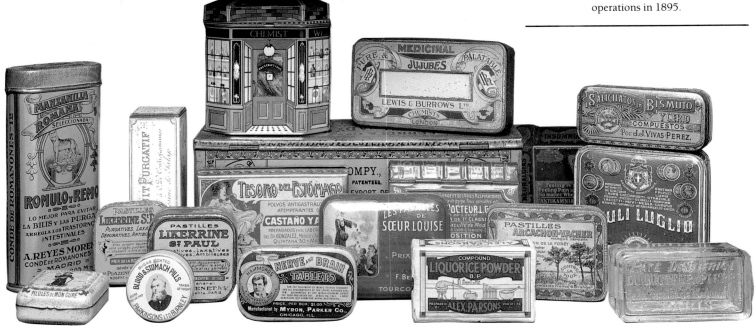

Chapter VIII

PHARMACY AND THE INDUSTRIAL REVOLUTION

The rapid change from hand methods to machine methods of production that characterized the Industrial Revolution found a ready application in pharmacy, especially under the impact of the scientific developments of the nineteenth century. Phytochemistry and synthetic chemistry created new derivatives of old drugs and new chemical entities of medicinal value that strained the capacity of the individual pharmacy.

The Industrial Revolution depended on the development of capitalistic institutions based on the principle of production for profit and belief in the salutary effects of competition and the protection of property rights. Production for profit laid to rest the medieval ideal of production for use that made the medieval guild monopolies workable. Protection of property rights led in pharmacy to the development of "patent," or proprietary, medicines.

Large-scale drug manufacture was not a new phenomenon; it had begun at least as early as the fourteenth century, when Ven-

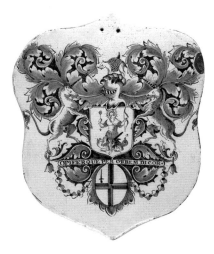

Decorated pill tile. Museum of the Pharmaceutical Society of Great Britain, London

Ceramic lids and containers for medicines and related products sold in pharmacies. Chiefly English, 19th century

ice manufactured, and sold throughout Europe, such products as troches of viper and Venice treacle, or theriac. In Amsterdam, Glauber was producing medical chemicals on a large scale in the seventeenth century, and in London the Worshipful Society of Apothecaries established a joint stock company in 1672 that operated a chemical laboratory with great success. (Indeed, this laboratory did not cease manufacturing fine chemicals until 1922.) The Society's chemical laboratory and its Navy Stock Company—a company established on the basis of a monopoly granted by Queen Anne to provide medicines for the royal navy—supplied medicines profitably to the navy, the army, the East India Company, and the Crown Colonies until the mid-nineteenth century.

In France, individual pharmacists went into large-scale manufacturing in the eighteenth and nineteenth centuries. In 1775, Antoine Baumé offered some 2,400 preparations, of which about 400 were chemicals, produced in his manufacturing laboratories.

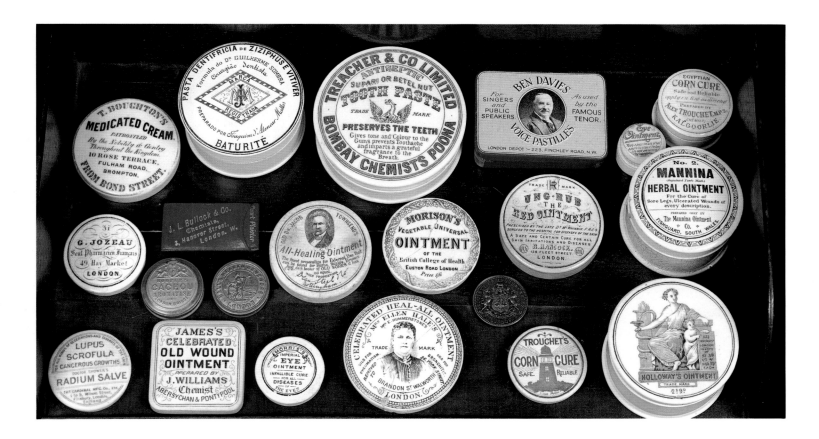

THE PHARMACEUTICAL INDUSTRY

It was the alkaloids, introduced early in the nineteenth century, that especially lent themselves to large-scale production. While some of the new agents could readily be prepared in the individual pharmacist's own laboratory, there were some that could not. Powerful and often toxic, alkaloids could not be isolated readily by everyday techniques and equipment. It soon became clear that these new drugs probably could be produced on a large scale more economically, and with greater assurance of purity, by the growing pharmaceutical industry. Many pharmacists in France and Germany became manufacturers of drugs, particularly of alkaloids. Among them were the pioneers in alkaloid research Caventou and Pelletier, who made the manufacture of quinine their specialty, and Heinrich Emanuel Merck, who discovered papaverine.

It was not only alkaloids that lent themselves to industrial manufacture. Galenicals, especially in the form of fluid extracts—which could readily be prepared by the pharmacist—were also appropriate for industrial production, since industry could provide this class of drugs more economically and in a quality and uniformity superior to that which the individual pharmacist was capable of achieving. Thus the pharmacist Eugen G. H. W. Dieterich, who founded the Chemische Fabrik bearing his name in Helfenberg, Germany, in 1869, devised the necessary manufacturing processes, built appropriate machinery, and found effective means of critically evaluating both raw materials and finished products.

Dieterich's success was attributable to his efficient production of medicinals scientifically superior to what the individual laboratory could produce. As early as 1800, W. E. Stüve und Kompagnie of Bremen was offering ten extracts, including those of arnica, cinchona, and rhubarb. In the United States, Tilden & Co., of Lebanon, New York, was by 1856 offering twenty-four fluid extracts and twenty-one "inspissated alcoholic and hydro-alcoholic extracts," some of which were original with them. Parke, Davis & Company, in Detroit, began the manufacture of fluid extracts in 1869, and they laid claim to attaining a uniformity and standardization new to this dosage form.

The progress made by this new industry is demonstrated by the catalogue of the American firm G. D. Searle, which by the late 1880s listed 400 fluid extracts, 150 elixirs, 100 syrups, 75 powdered extracts, and 25 tinctures and other drug forms. Searle, too, claimed uniformity of potency for its products.

The pharmaceutical industry undertook another function that the individual pharmacist could not perform—the search for new plant drugs. By 1880, Parke, Davis had made up forty-eight fluid extracts from plants that had been collected by its field agents. These plants came from many parts of North and South America and even from places as far away as the Fiji Islands.

What was true of alkaloids and galenicals was also true of medicinals that derived from halogens—iodoform, chloral hydrate, and ethyl chloride, for example. Industry was increasingly taking over the role of producer of substances created or developed in the pharmacy. To be sure, the pharmaceutical industry had another parent, the chemical industry: the interest of the synthetic chemical industry, especially in Germany, in organic compounds, coal-tar derivatives, and dyes soon spilled over into synthetic chemicals useful in medicine, among them carbolic acid, salicylic acid, phenacetin, and the antipyretics.

Such drugs had neither a traditional nor an empirical basis for use, and they presented problems of both safety and efficacy. The new science of pharmacology provided some help in this regard, but although Parke, Davis in the United States had a rudimentary pharmacology laboratory in 1894, other pharmaceutical houses did not estab-

American and British pharmacists' labels. Round labels were used for circular containers and were affixed to the corks on small bottles. Late 19th century ▶

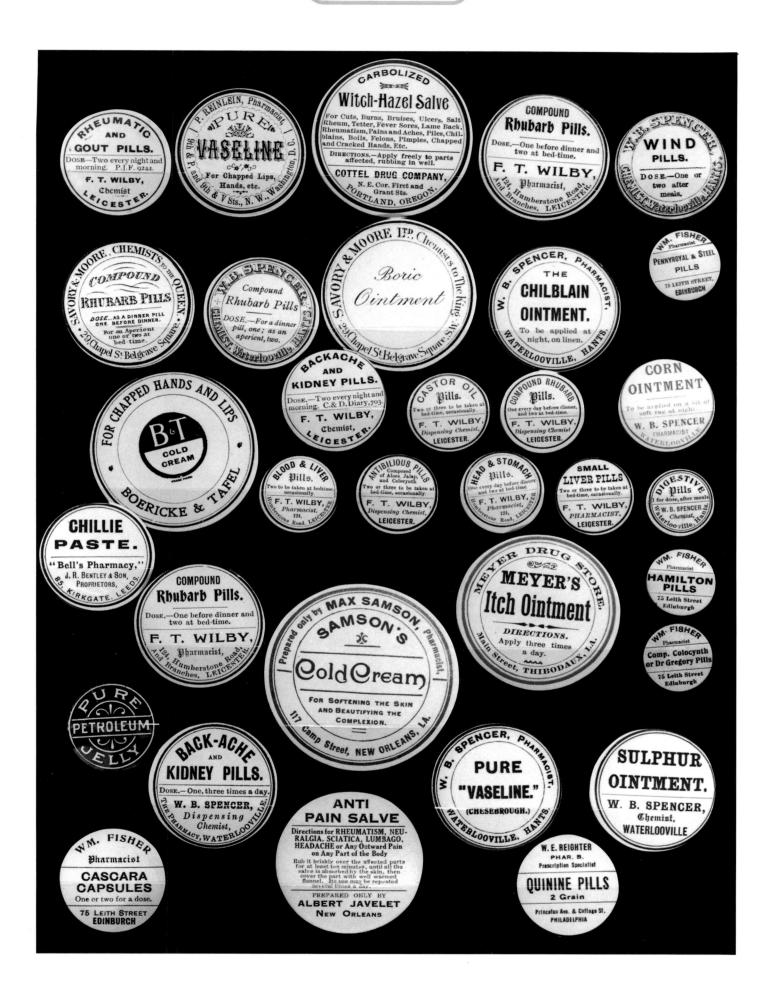

lish such laboratories until well into the twentieth century (Eli Lilly & Co. in Indianapolis in 1929 and Merck & Co. in Rahway, New Jersey in 1933). Farbwerke Hoechst in Germany, for instance, apparently had no pharmacological resources to help Ehrlich and von Behring, two of the foremost scientists of the time, in their efforts to standardize diphtheria antitoxin; as late as 1891 both men had to purchase their own experimental animals. There was, however, some clinical testing of the new entities in the 1880s. Hoechst's work with antipyretics began after Wilhelm Filehne had put kairine, the first synthetic in this class, through a series of tests on healthy persons and had investigated dosages for sick persons.

The processes involved indicate the way new drugs were introduced in the nineteenth century. Kairine had been synthesized by the chemist Otto Fischer at the Munich Hochschule; its medical potential was recognized by Filehne, then professor of materia medica at Erlangen; and it was eventually put into production by Hoechst. The sequence was: chemist—pharmacologist—industry. But the great role the industry was to play in pharmacological and clinical research would not come about until the twentieth century.

MASS PRODUCTION: DOSAGE FORMS

The same inexorable march of industrialization that took the preparation of drugs out of the officina and put it into the laboratory and factory also affected the forms in which drugs were dispensed. Again, basic developments were made by individuals, usually pharmacists, and again industry took advantage of these developments and improved upon them, making them more practical and more economical. The pill, for example, had for ages been handmade. Eighteenth-century pill tiles made of delft, Wedgwood, or plate glass marked with graduations give evidence of the process. The rolled pill mass was placed alongside

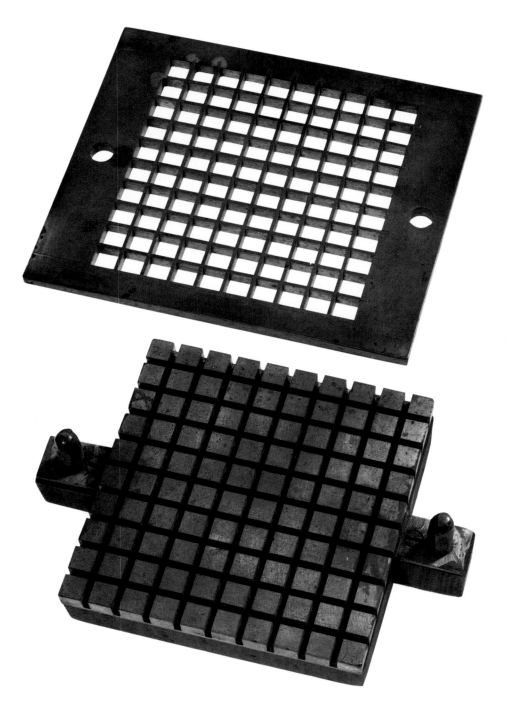

Hard-rubber mold for making tablet triturates. American, c. 1920. Mixed powders were moistened into a pastelike consistency and applied to the upper form so that the holes were completely filled. When the mixture had dried, the lower form pressed out the finished tablets. National Museum of American History, Smithsonian Institution, Washington, D.C.

the graduations and cut with a knife or spatula. Other devices that worked similarly included brass or bone combs with regularly spaced teeth and wooden boards with corrugated metal plates. Each segment of the pill mass then needed to be rolled into a globular pill. This was done by hand, one at a time, or by the use of a "pill-finisher," a circular disk of wood that was rotated over the segments with increasing velocity until the pills were rounded. These simple tools were readily adaptable to the factory setting. At first large numbers of handworkers

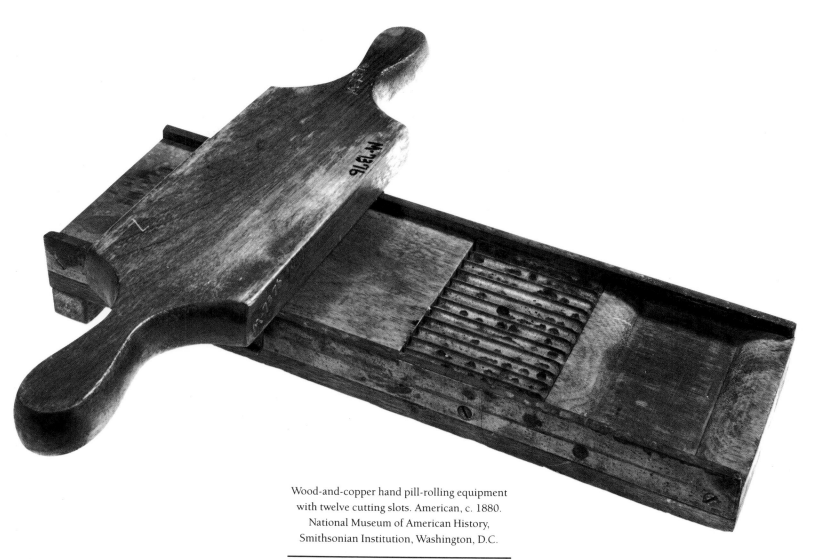

Wood-and-copper hand pill-rolling equipment
with twelve cutting slots. American, c. 1880.
National Museum of American History,
Smithsonian Institution, Washington, D.C.

were used, and then power-driven machinery was devised to cut, round, and sort pills by the thousands. This development pushed the art of hand pill-rolling into obsolescence by the end of the nineteenth century.

The mechanization process also made possible the production of what was essentially a new dosage form, the tablet. The Burroughs Wellcome Company in England lays claim to being the first to use the term (in 1884); it coined and registered the word "Tabloid" to exploit the form. The earliest tablets were made by a hand-operated machine invented by an English watchmaker and artist, William Brockedon, to conserve graphite otherwise wasted in the making of pencils. He soon applied his apparatus, patented in 1843, to compressing drugs. Brockedon's hand-punch machine was fol-

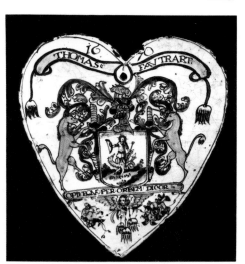

Lambeth delft pill tile decorated in polychrome
with the arms and motto of the Worshipful
Society of Apothecaries of London. English,
1670. Museum of the Royal Pharmaceutical
Society of Great Britain, London

lowed by a number of ingenious devices for compressing drugs: punch presses using a lever, screw presses, cam and flywheel presses, and others—all affecting the art of the apothecary, and all supplying medication in unprecedented quantities.

The gelatin capsule was another new dosage form developed in the nineteenth century. A soft version of the capsule was patented by two Frenchmen, F. A. B. Mothes and J. G. A. Dublanc, in 1834, and a hard version was patented in 1847 in England. The capsule did not come into general use until about 1875, when Parke, Davis undertook to have it manufactured on a large scale.

The capsule was intended to disguise the taste of medicine, make it easier to swallow, and provide a precise dose. Another and older way of accomplishing the first two of these ends was the coating of pills. Coating with gum mucilage goes back at least to Rhazes, and coating with gold or silver goes back at least to Avicenna. In the nineteenth century, coating with silver was still being practiced, and it was a most elegant art. A few drops of mucilage of acacia were placed in the palm of one hand, and pills were gently rolled in the mucilage with the forefinger of the other hand. When the pills were thoroughly coated, they were rolled around in a special box containing silver leaf until the silver leaf had adhered to the surface. The pills were then burnished by being rolled under paper on a "pill-rounder."

A simpler hand method of coating pills was to varnish them with a solution of resin. Pills were shaken in a porcelain jar with a few drops of the varnish, then put out on a greased tile to dry. Gelatin coating, first described by the French pharmacist Garot in 1838, was another technique that required hand manipulation by the pharmacist. Garot's procedure, promptly reported in the *American Journal of Pharmacy,* was to hold the pill on a pin while coating it with gelatin, filling in the pinhole later.

All these hand techniques gave way to tools and machinery. In France, in 1837, Adolphe Fortin patented a process of sugar-coating pills of cubeb and copaiba. Fortin had learned his technique from the makers of dragées, the sugarcoated nuts produced by French confectioners. Sugarcoating on a small scale was awkward, but excellent results were obtained on a large scale with the introduction of a power-driven "pan-coating" method that continued in use into the present century. Coating by machinery, under pressure, also began in the last quarter of the nineteenth century.

The coating of pills and tablets—at least forty-five different coatings were used, the so-called pearl coating, which used purified talc, being particularly popular—culminated, at the end of the century, in the development of the enteric coated pill. This advance laid the foundation for new concepts in pharmacotherapy: the importance of the form as well as the substance of a

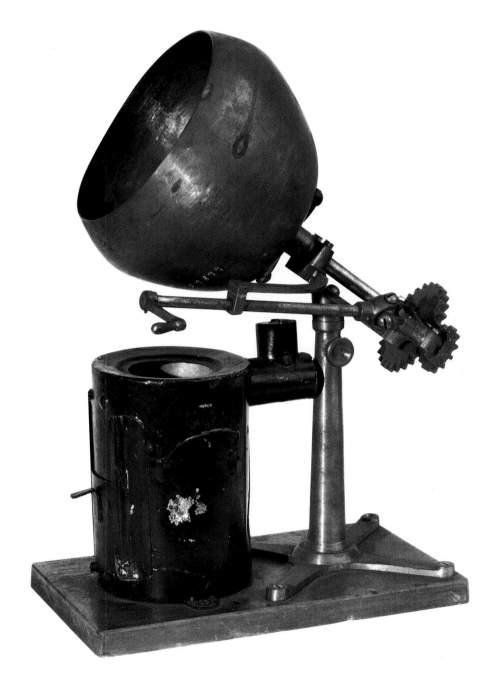

Model of an apparatus used for sugar-coating pills, submitted to the U.S. Patent Office by William Cairns. 1875. Compressed tablets and coating material were placed in the pan and then rotated. National Museum of American History, Smithsonian Institution, Washington, D.C.

medication and the control of the site and time of assimilation of medication by the body.

The idea that a medicinal preparation could be coated with a substance that was impervious to stomach fluids but could be absorbed in the small intestine was dramatically demonstrated by the dermatologist Paul G. Unna at a meeting of the Hamburg Medical Society in 1884. Unna acknowledged that there had been earlier attempts at this procedure—collodion had been suggested at least as early as 1867—but his use of what he called "keratine" really was the starting point of enteric coating.

Two other important dosage forms were introduced in the nineteenth century, the cachet and the ampoule. The cachet, or wafer capsule, was another means of overcoming the problem of unpleasant-tasting drugs. The medication was placed between two wafers, which, being made from a mixture of flour and water, were easily sealed together by a bit of moisture. The ampoule was developed to meet the needs of a new therapeutic technique that had become extremely common in the last half of the nineteenth century, intravenous injection. The glass ampoule could, together with its contents, be sterilized by heat and thus protected until the physician was ready to use it.

Both the cachet and the ampoule can be credited to an ingenious French pharmacist, Stanislas Limousin, who also developed droppers, pipettes, and an apparatus for the administration of oxygen. Limousin's ampoule kits were first produced in 1887, and although a Czech, A. V. Pel, had invented an ampoule the year before, it was Limousin's ampoule kits that were carried by physicians throughout Western Europe in the late nineteenth and well into the twentieth century.

THE PATENT
AND THE TRADEMARK

The pharmaceutical industry did not supplant the apothecary entirely on the basis of superiority of product or economy of production. Credit also goes to two legal devices that Western society developed to reward inventiveness and protect property—the patent and the trademark. The idea of the patent goes back to the feudal practice of bestowing rights of various kinds. A lord's or monarch's letter patent granted the recipient an exclusive right, usually to produce and market a product of his own invention.

The first patent given to a medicine was granted in England in 1698 to the makers of Epsom salts. Other medicines were patent-

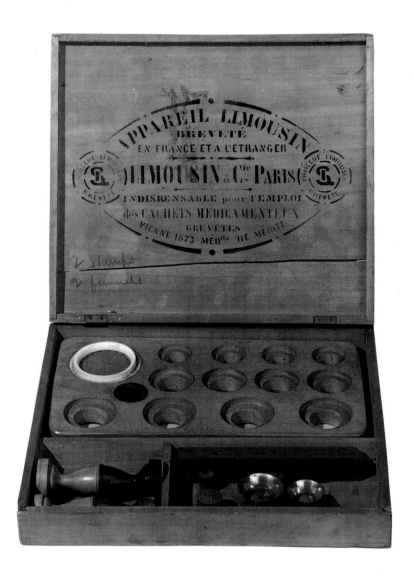

Original U.S. Patent Office model of an apparatus (Patent No. 216,197; June 3, 1879) for preparing the Limousin cachet, a dosage form in which medication was inserted between two wafers that were subsequently moistened around the edges and sealed. National Museum of American History, Smithsonian Institution, Washington, D.C.

ed in the eighteenth century, but patent laws attained their modern form only in the nineteenth century—in France in 1844, in England in 1852, in Italy in 1864, and in Germany in 1877. In 1787, the Constitution of the United States (Article I, Section 8) specifically granted Congress the power "to promote the Progress of Science and Useful Arts, by securing for limited Times to Authors and Inventors the exclusive Right to their respective writings and discoveries." The first Congress passed a patent act in 1790, but American patent law was not given its modern form until 1870. Property created by a patent was of great significance to the buregeoning industrial

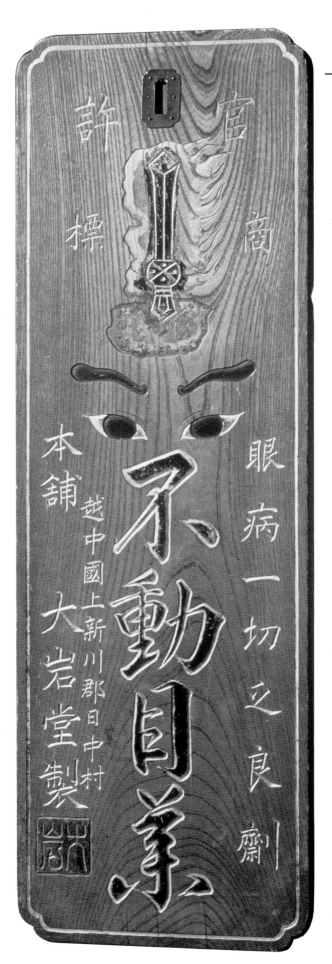

Two Japanese wooden signs (*kanban*) advertising proprietary medicines: eyedrops (left) and a medication for children (right).

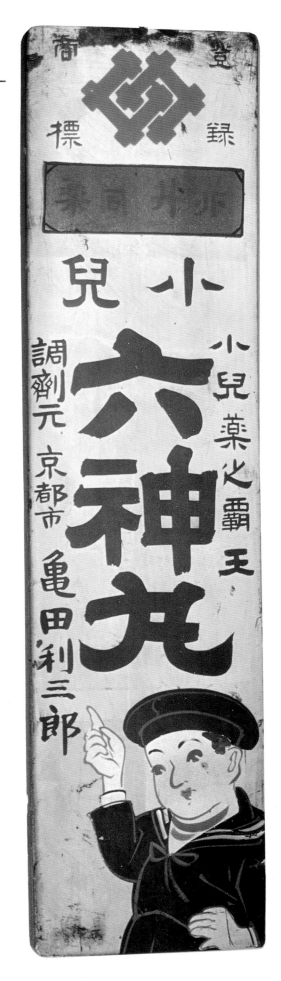

The Travelling Quack. Color lithograph by Harry Tuck. English, 1894. Itinerant medicine sellers, often illustrated in paintings and prints, continued to appear in rural areas into the 20th century.

Colored Liquids in Bottles. Chromolithograph cigarette card. English, c. 1912. On the reverse of the card (a premium with the purchase of a package of cigarettes) the question "Do you know why Chemists have large bottles of Coloured Liquid in their Windows?" was answered with the partial truth that chemists used these bottles to impress their customers.

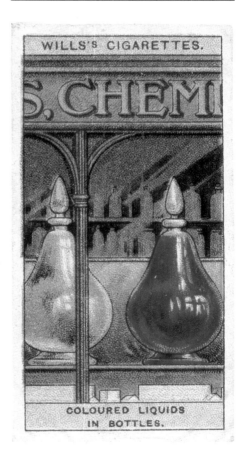

Trade card for Dr. Hand's Remedies for Children. Chromolithograph. American, c. 1885. Typically, the reverse of the card has an extensive advertisement for Dr. Hand's Colic Cure, Teething Lotion, Cough and Croup Medicine, Pleasant Physic, and other nostrums.

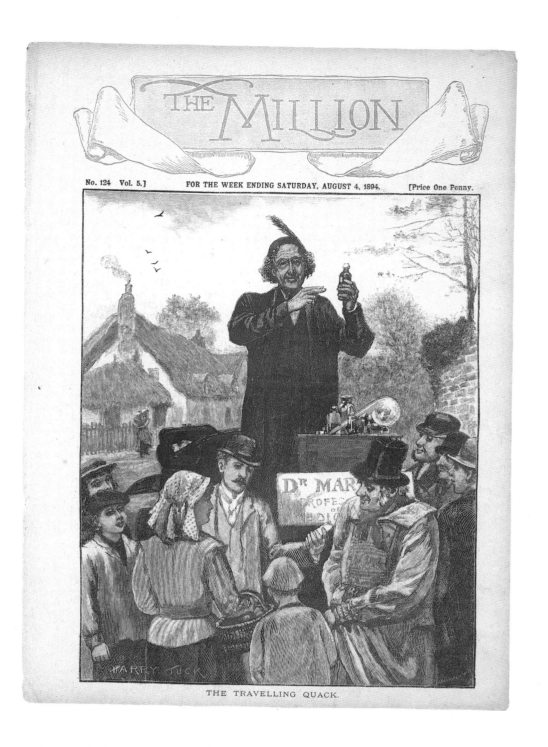

THE TRAVELLING QUACK.

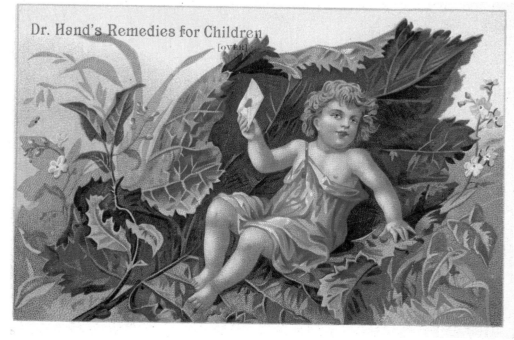

THE PHARMACEUTICAL HOUSES

The modern pharmaceutical house had its origin in the nineteenth century. The number of pharmacists who became manufacturers, mainly of their particular specialties, was legion—and some of these eventually became giants in the industry. Heinrich Emanuel Merck, for example, turned his family's pharmacy, established in 1668, into E. Merck AG of Darmstadt when he began to manufacture morphine and other alkaloids in bulk, in 1821. Nine years later John K. Smith, a Philadelphia druggist, founded what was to become Smith, Kline and French Laboratories and later SmithKline Beecham Ltd. Two pharmacists, Louis Dohme and Alpheus Phineas Sharp, established Sharp and Dohme—later (1953) merged into Merck Sharp & Dohme—in Baltimore in 1845. Ernst Schering's Grüne Apotheke in Berlin became Schering AG in 1851. The Warner-Lambert Co. was a twentieth-century combination of two houses that had been established in the preceding century, one by pharmacist William R. Warner in 1856 in Philadelphia, the other by Jordan Wheat Lambert in 1884 in St. Louis. Eli Lilly, who had been trained as a pharmacy assistant and had owned a pharmacy for a short time, founded the company that bears his name in Indianapolis in 1876. Silas M. Burroughs and Henry S. Wellcome, both graduates of the Philadelphia College of Pharmacy, founded the Burroughs Wellcome Company in London in 1880.

Important pharmaceutical houses were also established by physicians. E. R. Squibb & Sons was founded by Edward R. Squibb in Brooklyn in 1858. Dr. Squibb's enterprise flourished when he undertook to supply the Union forces with pure medicines during the Civil War. In 1885, William E. Upjohn and his brothers founded what was originally the Upjohn Pill and Granule Company in Kalamazoo, Michigan. Dr. Upjohn's company was grounded on his patent for "friable" pills; his original price list indicated that thirty of his pills were made from plant sources, twenty were chemicals, five were alkaloids, and one was a glycoside.

A number of the most important modern drug houses began, especially in Europe, as offshoots of the chemical and dye industry. Although one of the founders, Etienne Poulenc, was a pharmacist, the firm of Rhône-Poulenc began, in 1858, in a factory in Ivry-Port that manufactured fine chemicals. Farbwerke Hoechst likewise traces its origins to a chemical house, one established in 1863 in the town of Hoechst, Germany. Sandoz Chemical Works began as a dye-stuff factory in Switzerland in 1886. Charles Pfizer, a young German chemist who was a refugee from the European turmoil in 1848, established the company that bears his name in Brooklyn in 1849. Similarly, Ciba began as a small silk-dyeing plant in Basel in 1859—and became a joint stock company with a capital of 2.5 million Swiss francs by 1884. Merck & Co., the American branch of E. Merck that had become independent during World War I, began producing fine chemicals in Rahway, New Jersey, in 1899.

Pharmaceutical houses were also started by entrepreneurs who had no training as pharmacists, physicians, or chemists. J. R. Geigy AG had its origins in 1758, when the Swiss businessman Johann Rudolf Geigy founded in Basel a firm that traded in spices, coloring materials, and drugs. Similarly, F. Hoffmann-LaRoche & Co. was founded in 1896, also in Basel, by Fritz Hoffmann-LaRoche—who had once worked for a Belgian drug house but had no other background in pharmacy or chemistry.

These companies for the most part produce chemicals and ethical drugs for the pharmacist to dispense, primarily on prescription, but some also manufacture over-the-counter specialties and medical sundries. Outstanding among these manufacturers, who also emerged in the nineteenth century, were Johnson & Johnson of New Brunswick, New Jersey, founded in 1886; Boots Pure Drug Company of London, founded in 1877; and Bristol-Myers, now Bristol-Myers-Squibb, founded in Clinton, New York, in 1887.

THE DECLINING ART OF THE APOTHECARY

Industrialization had an impact on every aspect of the activity of the pharmacist. First, it led to the creation of new drugs, drugs that the individual pharmacist's own resources could not produce. Second, many drugs that the individual pharmacist was able to produce could be manufactured more economically, and in superior quality,

Engraved trade card for T. Smith, Wholesale and Retail Chemist & Druggist of Boston. English, c. 1820

by industry. Third, industry assumed responsibility—traditionally vested in the pharmacist—for the quality of the medication. Indeed, the transformation wrought by industrialization created a variety of problems. The plethora of proprietary medicines, widely and often blatantly advertised, deprived the pharmacist of a market for private specialties; it forced the pharmacist to become a vendor of questionable merchandise; it opened the way to much broader competition—from merchants, grocers, and pitchmen—than the pharmacist had previously encountered; and in several countries it opened up competition among pharmacists themselves, leading to such developments as the cut-rate drugstore and the chain store.

These problems were universal. In the United States there was friction between grocers and department stores on the one

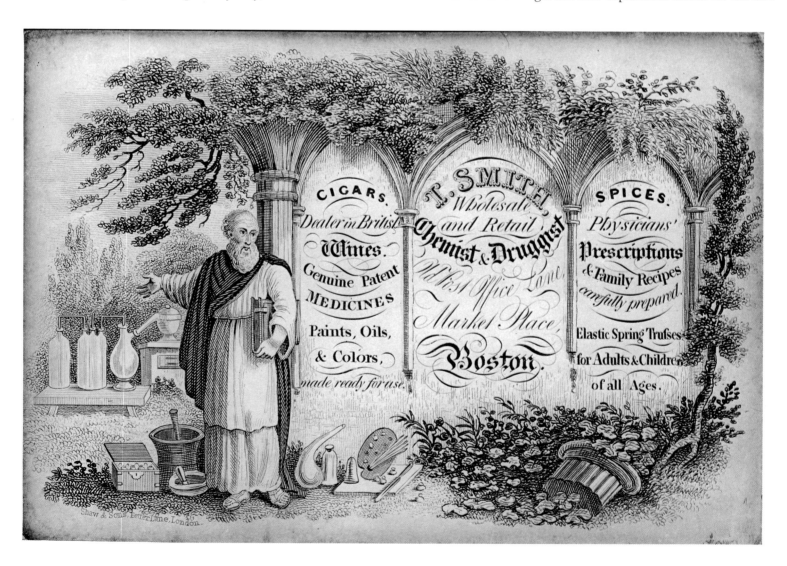

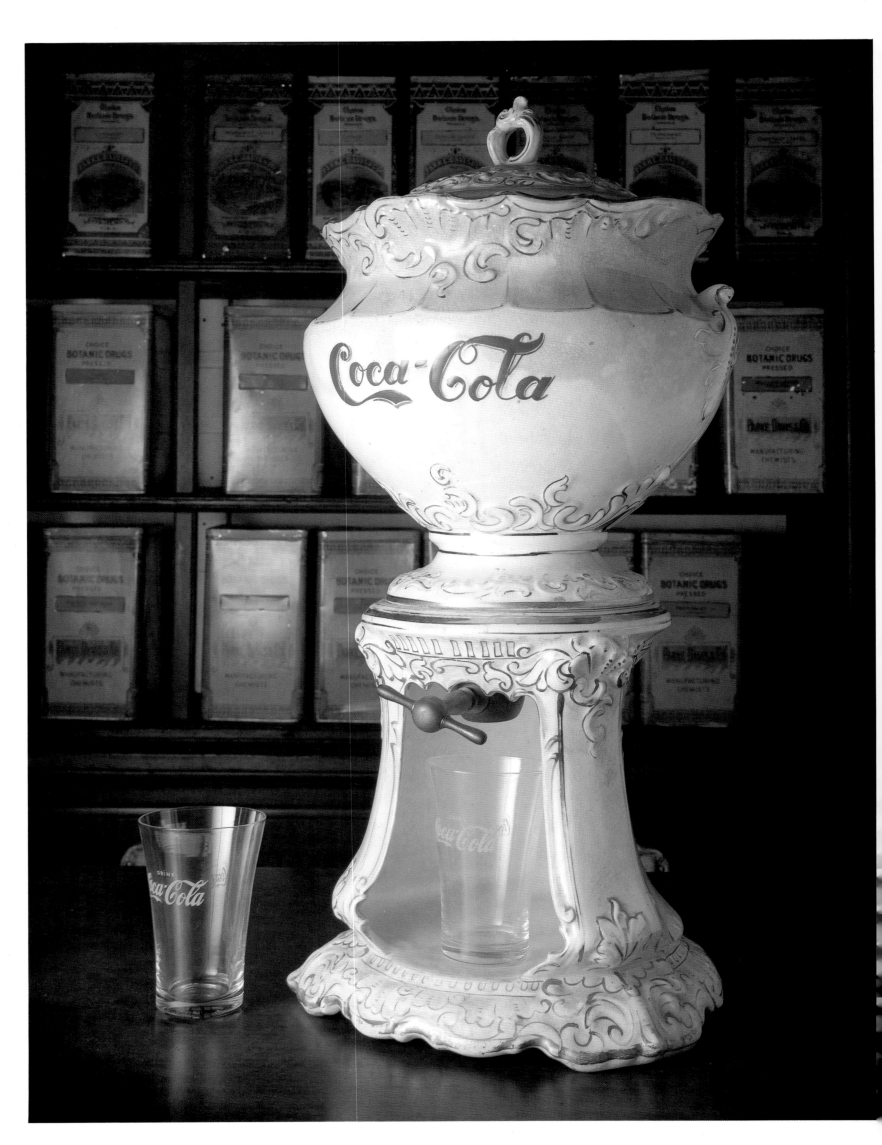

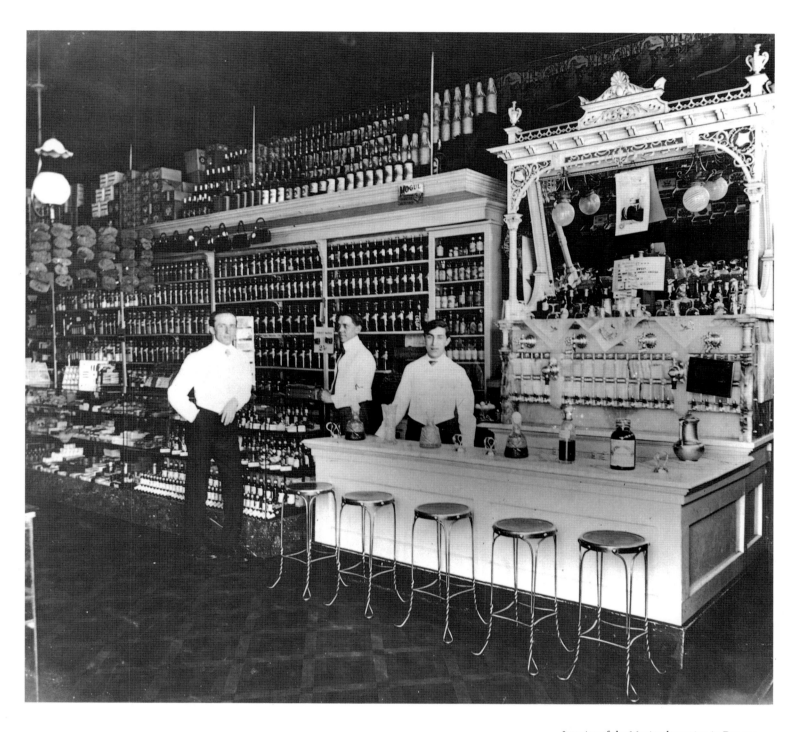

Ceramic Coca-Cola dispenser. American, c. 1900. The formula for Coca-Cola was developed in 1886 in Atlanta, Georgia, by pharmacist-physician John S. Pemberton, who, because of state prohibition laws, substituted syrup for wine as the base of his popular beverage. Originally Coca-Cola, which contained an extract from the leaves of the coca shrub (*Erythroxylon coca*), was promoted as a tonic, an aid to digestion, and a means of imparting energy to organs of respiration. National Museum of American History, Smithsonian Institution, Washington, D.C.

◄

Interior of the Moritz drugstore in Denver, Colorado, c. 1885, showing the prominent place of the soda fountain. Western History Department, Denver Public Library

Posters advertising Cachou Lajaunie. Color lithographs by Leonetto Cappiello. French, c. 1900–1920. These posters advertising a breath freshener for smokers were the work of a leading early-20th-century poster artist. *Overleaf*

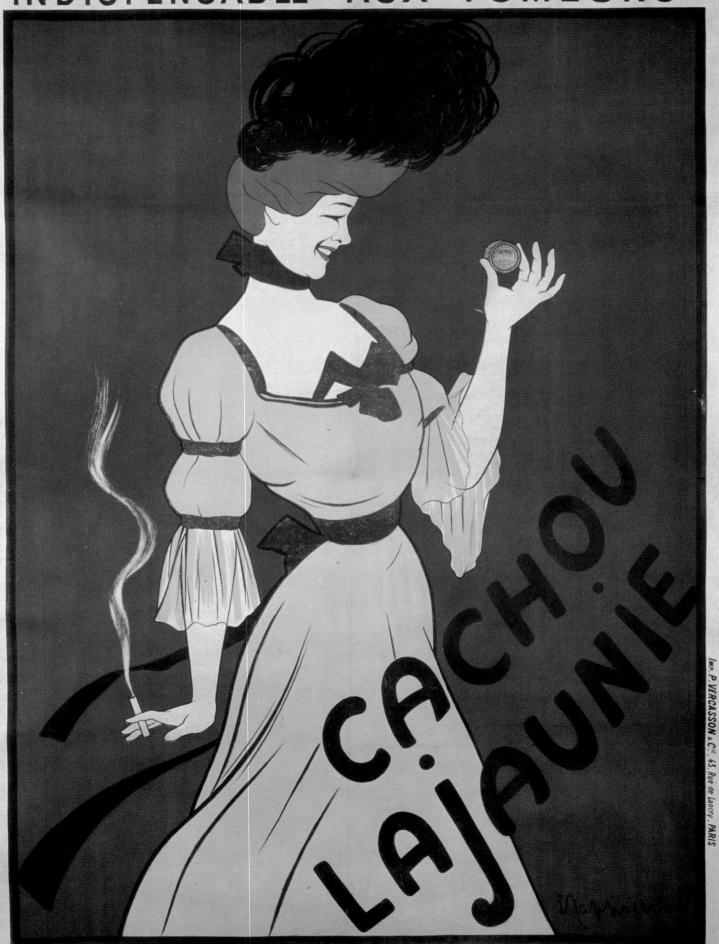

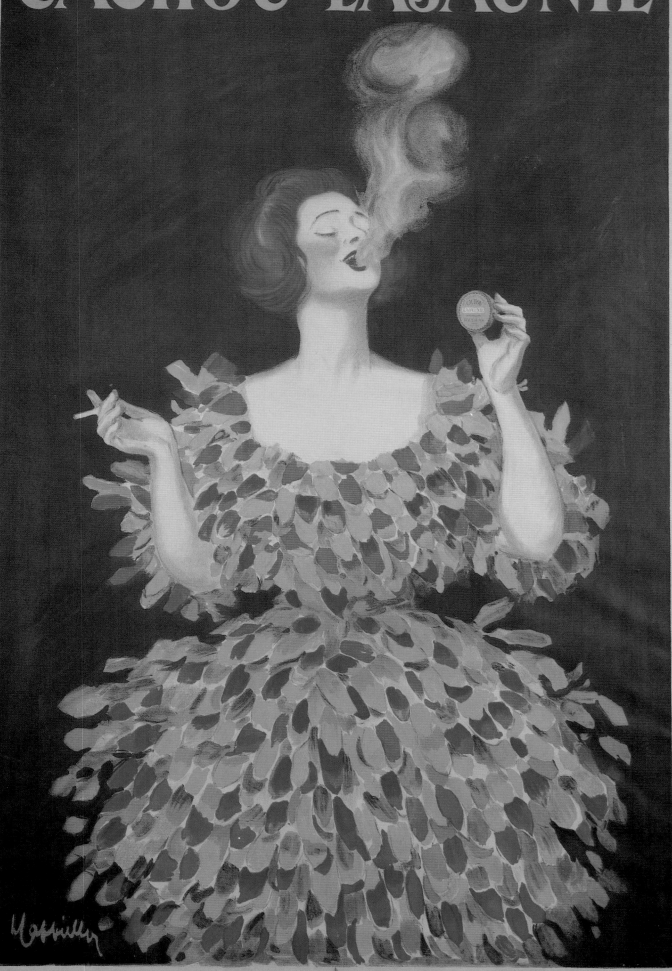

hand and pharmacists on the other; in Germany there was friction between the *Drogist* and the *Apotheker*. In France the first-class pharmacist was burdened with competition both from large numbers of second-class pharmacists and herbalists in the provinces and from the many charlatans who took advantage of legal loopholes to sell their nostrums. In the United States, Great Britain, and Holland, the pharmacist also met with competition from the dispensing physician.

The most colorful competitors of the pharmacist were the itinerant charlatans who, with little conscience and less integrity, pitched their purported panaceas across the country. These mountebanks could trace their lineage back to the *pharmakopoloi* of ancient Greece and the *pharmacopolae circumforaneae* of ancient Rome—and to the traveling medicine shows those ancients contrived, which became a feature of country life throughout medieval and Renaissance Europe. These shows offered a kind of *commedia dell'arte* and were widely depicted in prints, drawings, paintings, and caricatures of the period. They crossed the Atlantic in the eighteenth century, becoming a familiar feature of American life, and persisted into the twentieth century.

The stresses and strains that arose with the manufacture of products by the pharmaceutical and chemical industry, products intended for use by the pharmacist in compounding and dispensing, were evident early in the nineteenth century, and throughout the century pharmacists everywhere sought to stem the tide. At the outset of the century, a Prussian ordinance (1801) obligated the pharmacist to prepare every pharmaceutical and chemical preparation for which a formula was given in the pharmacopoeia. At the end of the century (1894), the *United States Pharmacopoeia* excluded products that could be made only by a patented process or that were protected by proprietary rights. The U.S.P. of 1905, although it still proscribed anything that involved secrecy and still looked askance at "unlimited" patent, or proprietary, rights, nevertheless accepted "any product of defi-

nite composition which is in common use by the medical profession." By 1905, then, the pharmacist had learned that it was economical—and also easier—to rely more and more on the pharmaceutical industry. Nonetheless, pharmacists sought to encourage the writing of prescriptions for medications that would require the exercise of the pharmaceutic art—medications "tailor-made" for the individual patient, as it was often put.

PROPRIETARY MEDICINES

Proprietary remedies, the so-called patent medicines, presented pharmacists with other problems. While they challenged the pharmacists' art, they were also a threat—an even greater one—to the pharmacists' economic well-being. And their accessibility undermined the pharmacists' function as custodians of the public health.

Many of these remedies were not new—some had existed since the Middle Ages—and they were widely used in Europe in the seventeenth and eighteenth centuries. In the eighteenth century in England the promotion of nostrums was as brazen and extravagant as it was dishonest, and in the nineteenth century, as a direct consequence of improved advertising and promotional methods, the sale of such nostrums flourished, especially in America. The proliferation of newspapers, the advent of cheap printing, the activity of itinerant pitchmen, and the improvement in mass-production techniques—not to mention the propensity for self-medication in an age when medical attention was scarce, costly, sometimes dangerous, and often given to unpleasant therapeutics—gave a tremendous impetus to the manufacture and sale of these remedies.

Proprietary medicines used in colonial America were largely imports from England. During and immediately after the Revolutionary War, substitutes and coun-

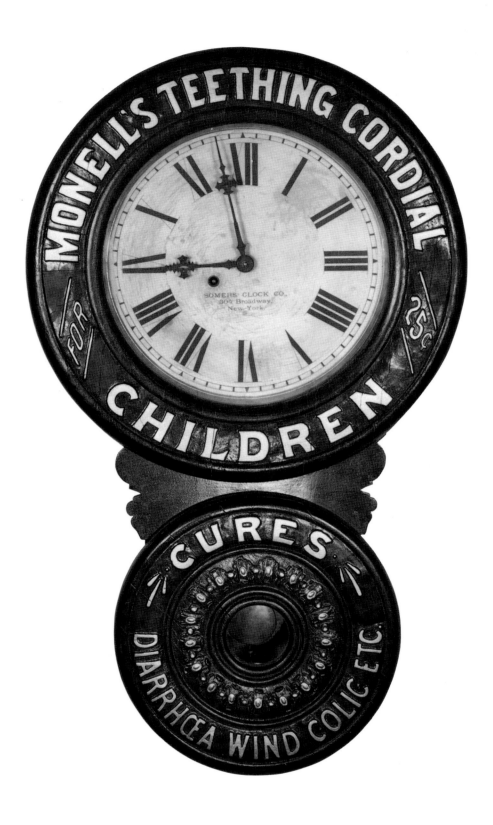

Baird Advertising Clock. American, c. 1885.
Clocks with promotional messages, made by
Baird, were given to pharmacists and merchants
who purchased a sufficient quantity of the
product advertised. National Museum of
American History, Smithsonian Institution,
Washington, D.C.

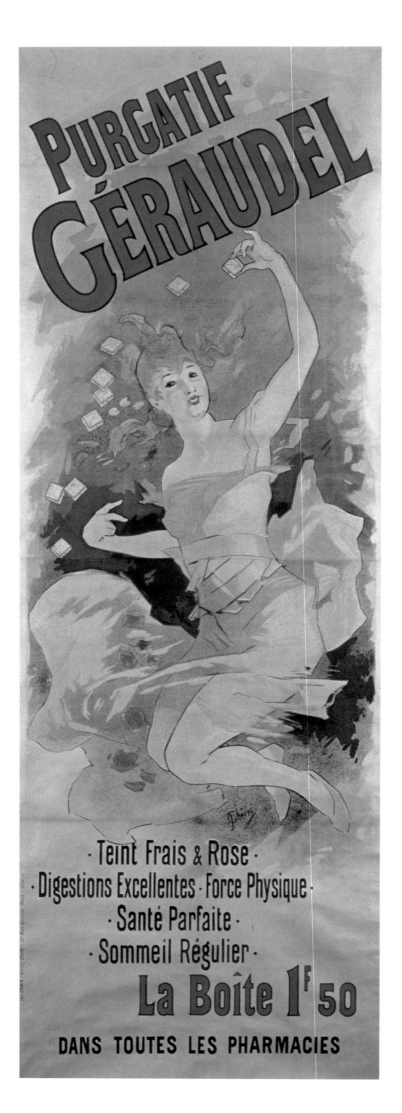

Poster for the widely advertised laxative Purgatif Géraudel. Color lithograph by Jules Chéret. French, 1891.

▶

Poster for Vin Mariani. Lithograph by Jules Chéret. French, 1894. Angelo Mariani launched his tonic at the end of the Franco-Prussian War. An advertising genius, he collected more than 1,400 testimonials from popes, kings, presidents, physicians, artists, and actors attesting to its virtues. The active ingredient in Vin Mariani was derived from the leaves of the shrub *Erythroxylon coca*, source of cocaine.

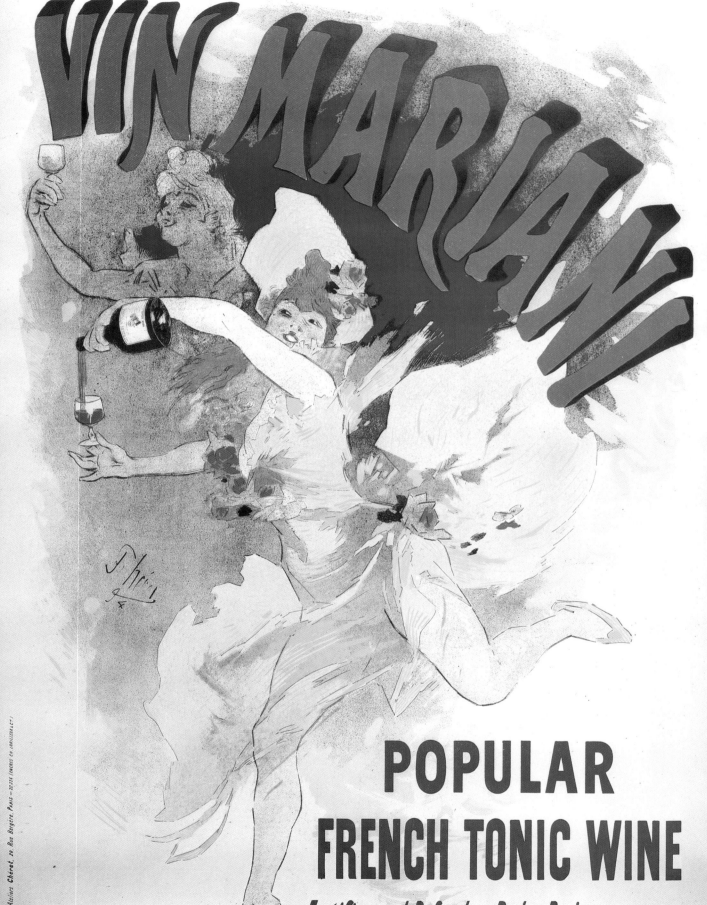

terfeits were all that were available. The first of the purely American proprietary medicines appeared in the 1790s, and the first patent for a medicine issued under the new Constitution was granted to Samuel Lee, Jr., of Windham, Connecticut, for his Bilious Pills. Others followed rapidly; by the 1840s there were more than seventy patented nostrums, and by the beginning of the Civil War catalogues of wholesale druggists carried lists of up to six hundred proprietary products. Among the best-known nostrums on these lists were Dr. Robertson's Family Medicines, prepared by a Dr. T. W. Dyott, and Swaim's Panacea, both made in Philadelphia.

In England and on the Continent there were similar developments in the 1800s. Dr. Samuel Solomon's Cordial Balm of Gilead was typical of the hundreds of products promoted in British newspapers early in the century as cures for just about everything. Beecham's Pills, Holloway's Ointment, and Eno's Fruit Salts were three of hundreds of remedies introduced later in the century. Morison's Pills, first introduced in the 1820s, claimed that humankind was subject to only one disease—impurity of the blood—and that the way to cure it was to take Morison's Number 1 and Number 2 pills. (If two pills would not accomplish the task, then four certainly would.)

The proprietary medicine business grew exponentially in the second half of the nineteenth century. Advertising, over which there were no controls, was the propelling force. In the United States, by the 1860s, partly owing to increasing levels of literacy, there were more than four thousand newspapers being published. Those in rural areas, and those devoted to special interests, especially religious or temperance groups, were principally supported by advertisements for proprietary medicines. As late as 1900 these products still led all others in outlays for national advertising.

Not surprisingly, the contribution that proprietary medicine advertising made to the success of publishing enterprises paid extra dividends, and editors were reluctant to criticize the promotional methods, often flamboyant, or the ingredients, often dangerous, in the products of nostrum promoters. Excesses were many in such advertising, for most promoters of these products were indifferent to the side effects and to the possibly addictive properties of their products. Several widely available proprietary medicines with mild-sounding names—such as Mrs. Winslow's Soothing Syrup and Kopp's Baby Friend—contained morphine sulfate as their chief ingredient. Other products, even those promoted to followers of the temperance movement, contained considerable amounts of alcohol. Hostetter's Bitters, for example, contained 39 percent alcohol, and there were competitive products whose alcohol content exceeded this proportion.

The manufacturers and promoters of proprietary medicines (aptly labeled "medical messiahs" in the title of a book published in 1967) shrewdly took advantage of the parlous state of medicine in the nineteenth century, and they often advertised that the vegetable ingredients in their nostrums were milder, more pleasant, and safer than the heroic remedies and measures employed by many physicians. Thus the promotion for Morison's Pills inveighed against the use of calomel and related products. Another stratagem was to suggest specific situations that required treatment: a prolapsed uterus could be cured by Lydia Pinkham's Vegetable Compound; catarrh could be successfully treated with Pe-ru-na.

For ailments both common and rare there was a bewildering variety of nostrums from which to choose. In France and England the cold-and-cough remedy was Geraudel's Pastilles; in Italy it was Pastiglie Paneraj; in North America it was Ayer's Cherry Pectoral. Laxatives, Indian tonics, bitters, and other liquids with high percentages of alcohol were ubiquitous. One pharmacist, complaining about the competition offered by nostrum promoters, suggested that the chief mission of some of these remedies was to open people's purses by opening their bowels.

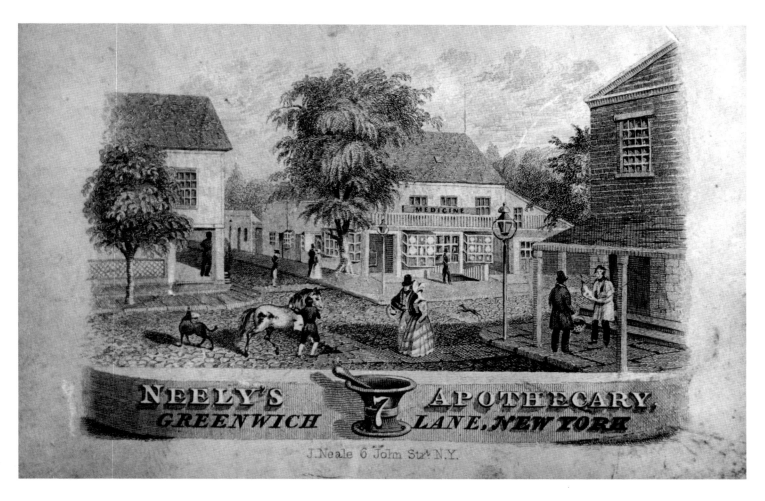

NEELY'S APOTHECARY, GREENWICH LANE, NEW YORK

J.Neale 6 John St. N.Y.

Engraved trade card for Neely's Apothecary, a New York pharmacy. c. 1835. Landauer Collection, The New-York Historical Society

Vin Mariani, a Bordeaux wine–based tonic whose active ingredient was *Erythroxylon coca*—the Peruvian source of cocaine—was a truly multinational product. First offered at the time of the Franco-Prussian War, it was widely advertised. Testimonials came from kings and queens and popes; President McKinley, Thomas Edison, and Sarah Bernhardt recommended it.

Testimonials were not an exclusive province of Vin Mariani, however. In England, advertisers favored published statements from literary men, and opium preparations received support from Coleridge, De Quincey, Shelley, Keats, Wordsworth, Byron, and Dickens, among others. Additional promotional strategies included: promises of rapid and certain relief, promises to cure all known diseases, use of distinctive symbols, claims of professional degrees or the backing of highly important institutions, claims of major scientific breakthroughs, and use of "secrets" from exotic or distant lands.

In promoting their products, vendors of proprietary medicines made use of every possible medium. Not only newspapers and magazines but billboards, booklets, broadsides, calendars, coloring books, fortune-telling books, games, jigsaw puzzles, pamphlets, paper money, playing cards, posters, riddle books, songs, therapeutic guides, toys, trade cards, and, especially, almanacs transmitted the vendors' messages. Toward the end of the nineteenth century, Ayers, Hostetters, Jaynes, and Herricks, perhaps the largest publishers of patent medicine almanacs, issued more than one million almanacs each; in its peak year, Ayers proudly boasted that it had distributed sixteen million copies of one of its issues. These were not only in English: in 1889 alone Ayers offered its almanac in twenty-one languages in addition to its nine different English-language editions, which were sent to various parts of the United States and to Australasia, South Africa, the East Indies, and Great Britain.

Eventually, promotional excesses of proprietary manufacturers became so widespread that they prompted writers and journalists, among them Edward Bok, editor of the *Ladies' Home Journal,* and Samuel Hopkins Adams, one of the early muckrakers, to expose them. Adams's series of articles, which appeared in *Collier's Weekly* under the title "The Great American Fraud," is credited with leading to the passage of the first Pure Food and Drug Act in 1906, the first restrictive legislation to curtail the freewheeling ways of nostrum producers.

The pharmacists' first reaction to the growing popularity of proprietary medicines was to imitate those that were most popular, witness the *Formulae for the Preparation of Eight Patent Medicines,* issued by the Philadelphia College of Pharmacy in 1824. Henry Beasley's popular *Druggist's General Receipt Book,* first published in London in 1850, devoted thirty-nine closely printed pages to "Patent and Proprietary Medicines, Druggists' Nostrums, etc." At least fifteen editions of Beasley's book were published in London and Philadelphia between 1850 and 1907, and many more editions of related publications by him appeared between 1841 and 1924. While some pharmacists produced their own versions of proprietaries, others went further, imitating not just the product but the bottle and the package—in short, counterfeiting the nostrum.

But as the proprietary medicine business expanded in the nineteenth century, pharmacists found themselves increasingly confronted with innumerable varieties of inferior products. Some were adulterated, others utterly worthless; some were common remedies that had been given brand names. It was disturbing to dispense such products. Worse, it hurt the pocketbook, for the sale of proprietaries entailed small profit margins. And proprietaries lent themselves to ready sale by the nonpharmacist, by chain stores, and by price-cutters. In France, a medical congress of 1872 declared, "The drug specialty constitutes for most pharmacists a kind of

vassalage. . . . The specialty is the cause of the decadence of pharmacy."

The negative attitude of the pharmacist toward the proprietary was exemplified by the exclusion of such products from convention exhibits of the New Jersey Pharmaceutical Association in the 1880s and 1890s. In the end, however, pharmacy succumbed—and by the end of the nineteenth century, in the United States at least, the proprietary had become a very significant part of the pharmacist's stock-in-trade.

THE COMMUNITY PHARMACY

The nineteenth century did not see the end of the art of compounding, but the art did give way, however grudgingly, to new technology. It has been estimated that a "broad knowledge of compounding" was still essential for 80 percent of the prescriptions dispensed in the 1920s. Although pharmacists increasingly relied on chemicals purchased from the manufacturer to make up prescriptions, there still remained much to be done *secundum artem.* They spread their own plasters, prepared pills (of aloes and myrrh or quinine and opium, for example), prepared powders of all kinds, and made up confections, conserves, medicated waters, and perfumes. They put up tinctures (of laudanum, paregoric, and colchicum) in five-gallon demijohns (which the clerk was required to agitate three times a day). And they frequently combined into a single dosage form several medicines, which today would be written and dispensed as separate prescriptions. Furthermore, they were often called upon to provide first aid and medicines for such common ailments as burns, frostbite, colic, flesh wounds, poisoning, constipation, and diarrhea.

In addition to maintaining a prescription laboratory, pharmacists usually carried the disliked but necessary patent and proprietary remedies along with herbs and locally popular nostrums of their own compounding. They also dealt in such medical accessories as leeches, trusses, and toilet articles. In the United States these sidelines included paints, dyes and glass, ink, sealing wax, and, sometimes, liquor. By and large, Continental pharmacists, protected in some areas by limitations on who might practice pharmacy, and where, were able to concern themselves with more purely pharmaceutical activities and products.

European pharmacies, in the nineteenth century, except in Great Britain, retained something of the formal appearance of their predecessors. The more elegant among them, particularly those in larger towns and cities, displayed row upon row of handsome drug jars, which no longer served their original utilitarian function but added beauty to the establishment. Bottles, scales, and boxes occupied the shelves, and the paneled interior of the shop was frequently inscribed with the names of celebrated pharmacists or important botanicals. Labeled drawers, often decorated with illustrations of the roots, herbs, or other botanicals that they contained, added to the pharmacy's mystique.

Most Continental pharmacies had a front counter, from which the pharmacist dealt with the public. This usually contained scales and other equipment, and it provided space for the performing of some professional functions. There was always a closed-off space as well, a place where the pharmacist could work out of view of the patrons. This laboratory was often rather large, for despite the inroads of the pharmaceutical industry the nineteenth-century pharmacist still had a good deal of compounding to do. There were scales, weights, mortars and pestles, and equipment such as distilling flasks, suppository molds, pill tiles and rollers, folders for powder papers, presses, cork sizers, plaster spreaders, and empty bottles and boxes to contain the prescriptions the pharmacist would prepare.

Facades of Continental pharmacies tended to blend with the surrounding architec-

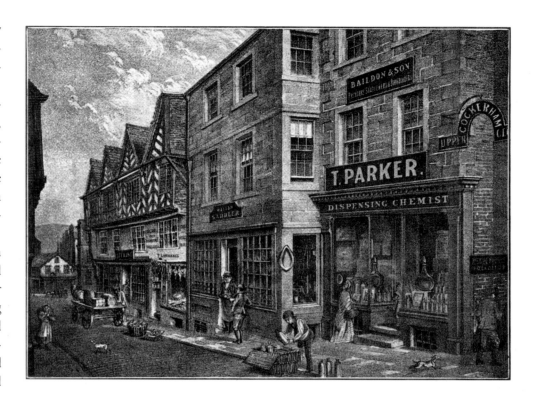

Postcard with engraved view of a street in Halifax, England, composed from photographs taken in 1861, showing the shop of dispensing chemist T. Parker. English, c. 1910

ture. Those in Germanic countries had meager window space, and displays were therefore minimal. The names of these pharmacies—the Engel-Apotheke or the Einhorn Apotheke, for example—were painted in large letters on the facade, so as to be visible from a distance. The Einhorn Apotheke displayed what was purportedly a unicorn's head and horn at the entrance. French pharmacies, in contrast, often presented a larger expanse of glass, one that made the interior more visible from the street. As a rule, faience or majolica drug jars were displayed. The name of the pharmacy was applied in porcelain or gilt to the windows, and advertisements of specialties were displayed. Sometimes elaborately patterned woodwork or ironwork enhanced the exteriors of French pharmacies, and toward the end of the century Art Nouveau exteriors began to appear, reflecting the prevailing taste.

In Great Britain, pharmacies were considerably less elegant. Shops fitted with fine cabinets and bow windows, with large specie jars and show globes containing colored liquids displayed in them, were seen only in London and a few other large cities. The coming of Jesse Boot's chain stores in the late 1870s, coupled with the tradition of offering a variety of nonpharmaceutical products, created a competitive situation in which economy was more important than style. This had its effect on the interior of the pharmacy, where space had to be provided for such products as foods, film, and hardware. It also affected the exterior appearance of the shop: the windows were filled with as many products as they would hold, and seldom presented a dignified appearance.

In the United States, only the large cities could boast of pharmacies established by trained pharmacists. The American pharmacy was either an offshoot of the general store or an appendage of a doctor's office, and it more often resembled the British druggist's shop than the Deutsche Apotheke or the Pharmacie Française. Thanks to a process that began in the nineteenth century, the modern drugstore has the ambience of a department store.

One peculiarly American development of the nineteenth century was the introduction of the soda fountain into the drugstore. This was a natural outcome of the pharmacist's knowledge of syrups and carbonation, and it transformed the "corner drugstore" into a social meeting place, in communities small and large. Elias Durand, a French-trained pharmacist who settled in Philadelphia, opened one of the first soda fountains about 1825, and from the 1860s to the 1940s the soda fountain was a fixture of the American drugstore. In the twentieth century, the pharmacy was to contribute, through the soda fountain, features that are earmarks of our society. It was in a pharmacy in Atlanta, Georgia, that Coca-Cola was first concocted, and it was in a pharmacy in New Bern, North Carolina, that Pepsi Cola originated. A much earlier contribution to social life is said to have been made in the late eighteenth century by the New Orleans pharmacist Antoine Peychard, who dispensed tonics of cognac mixed with his own Peychard bitters. This mixture—which was served in an eggcup (French *coquetier*)—was, according to one theory, the

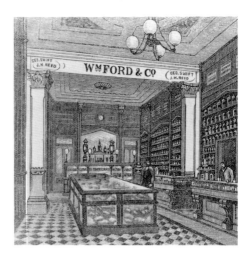

Interior views of the drugstore of Wm. Ford & Co. in Melbourne, Australia. c. 1885. National Library of Medicine, Bethesda

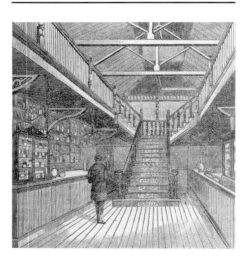

Postcard view of the interior of Murphy's Drug Store in Las Vegas, New Mexico. c. 1910

forerunner, etymologically as well as actually, of the "cocktail."

In the United States, the drugstore often had an ordinary front, distinguished only by colored show globes in the windows. The interior of the shop was usually a long rectangle, with a soda fountain behind a marble counter near the entrance. Showcases along the sides displayed tobaccos, medical accessories, toiletries, and whatever sidelines the shop might be carrying. Fixtures were ordinarily of hardwood, sometimes ornately carved. Shelves behind the counters displayed proprietaries in bottles and packages. Surrounding the prescription counter, which was typically at the far end of the store, were shelves on which medicines used in compounding were stored in matched bottles with gold or gilt-edged labels. Although hardly as impressive as the apothecary jars of the European pharmacy, these bottles, matched and orderly, did convey an impression of well-organized professionalism. Beneath the shelves would be drawers containing herbs and packaged drugs. If the shop was wide enough, there might be small tables and chairs for patrons of the soda fountain, and often there was a potbellied stove. Advertisements for various proprietaries—especially for those of the owner's own manufacture—adorned the walls, hung from the ceiling, and were displayed on the top of counters. A characteristic fragrance of herbs and volatile oils lent the shop a somewhat mysterious and exotic aura.

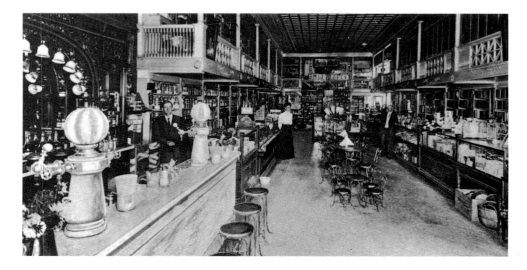

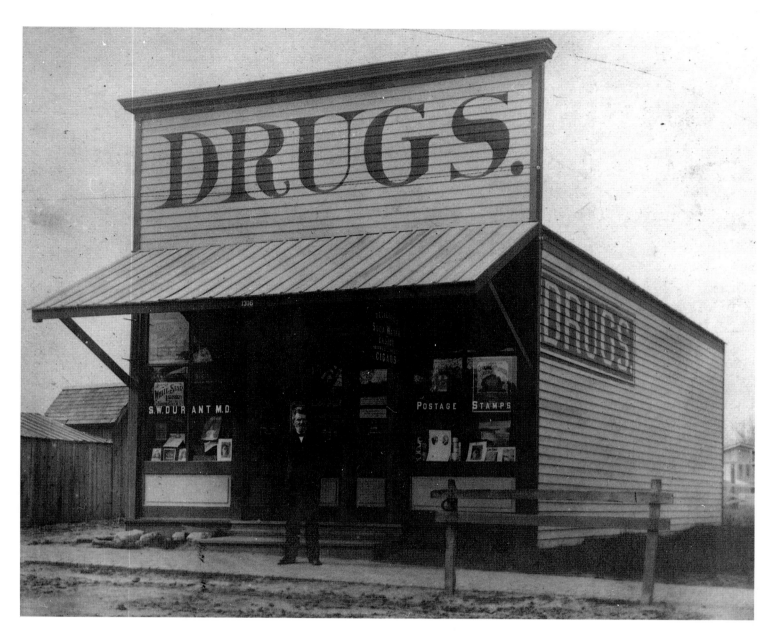

Dr. S. W. Durant standing in front of his
drugstore in Topeka, Kansas. c. 1885.
Physician-owned pharmacies in the United
States were sometimes called "doctor's shops."

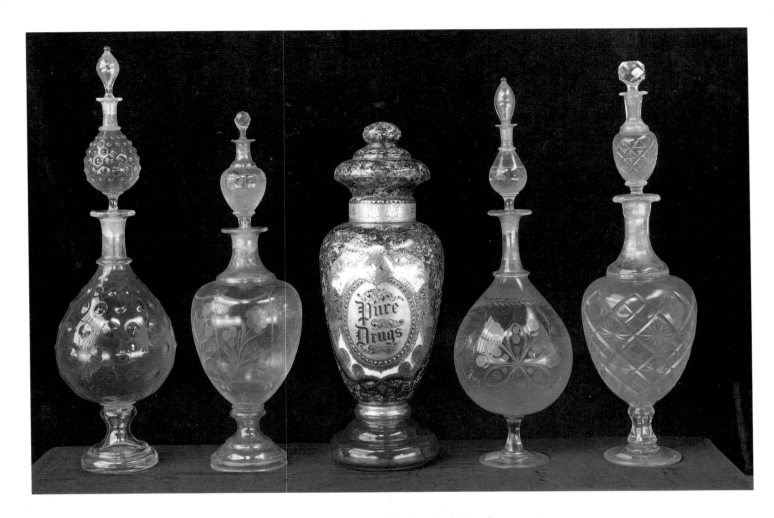

Glass show globes (display drug bottles) used
in a pharmacy in Harrisburg, Pennsylvania.
Mid-19th century. National Museum of
American History, Smithsonian Institution,
Washington, D.C.

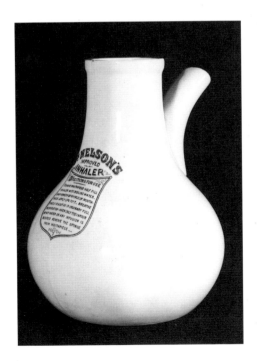

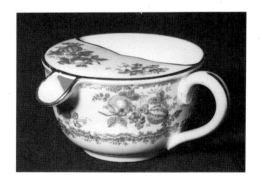

Painted porcelain invalid feeding cup.
English, 1894. Wellcome Institute Collection,
Science Museum, London

Dr. Nelson's Approved Inhaler. Ceramic.
English, c. 1875. This device provided patients
with a convenient way to inhale water vapor
impregnated with medicinal agents to relieve
coughs and colds. Wellcome Institute
Collection, Science Museum, London

THE NEW MATERIA PHARMACEUTICA

The materia pharmaceutica changed considerably by the end of the nineteenth century, when alkaloids, glycosides, and new synthetic drugs altered both the substance and the kind of medications that physicians prescribed and pharmacists dispensed.

A good deal can be learned about the medications that pharmacists were dispensing toward the end of the century from the Ebert Prescription Survey of 1885. This study covered some 15,700 prescriptions dispensed in nine Illinois pharmacies. The ingredients used most frequently—after distilled water, syrup, and glycerin—were quinine sulfate and morphine sulfate. Quinine was found 857 times per 10,000 prescriptions, morphine 519 times; next came potassium iodide (473 times), tincture of opium (463), phenol (455), and mild mercury chloride (450); ipecac was used 217 times as a syrup and 207 times as an infusion; powder of ipecac and opium, potassium bromide, tincture of camphorated opium, cinchonidine sulfate, colocynth compound, rhubarb, and ethyl nitrite were all used more than 300 times; syrup of sarsaparilla, nux vomica, potassium chlorate, hyoscyamus, saccharated pepsin, syrup of tolu, opium, and petrolatum were used 250 times or more.

The Ebert survey covered only prescribed drugs. It did not cover drugs dispensed by doctors or by nurses, in hospitals or in private practice. It did not cover drugs dispensed directly by the pharmacist, and it covered only prescriptions written in one geographic area. Nevertheless, the survey indicates both the importance of new additions to the nineteenth-century materia medica and the continued demand for traditional remedies. American pharmacists of the late 1800s were compounding or dispensing acids, cerates, decoctions, elixirs, extracts, fluid extracts, infusions, irons, liniments, mercury and its various compounds, oils, ointments, oleoresins, pills, powders, sodium compounds, solutions, spirits, syrups, tinctures, and wines. They were also dispensing many more chemicals than the above list suggests and providing customers with a variety of crude drugs.

Much of this was reminiscent of traditional pharmacy, but by the end of the century it was evident that exciting new developments were at hand. The progress of science in the nineteenth century—not simply in chemistry, physics, and botany but also in the newer sciences of physiology, biochemistry, pharmacology, microbiology, immunology, and endocrinology—had created new options in therapeutics.

Three particular innovations at the end of the nineteenth century ushered in the new age of pharmacy. Diphtheria antitoxin, developed by von Behring and Kitasato and placed in commercial manufacture in 1892, helped create a new class of therapeutic agents, the biologicals. In addition, the isolation and stabilization of adrenaline by John Jacob Abel and Jokichi Takamine at the turn of the century opened the age of hormonal therapy. And when, in 1899, the clinical value of acetylsalicylic acid, or aspirin, was demonstrated by Julius Wohlgemut and Heinrich Dreser, the most widely used drug of modern times entered the armamentarium.

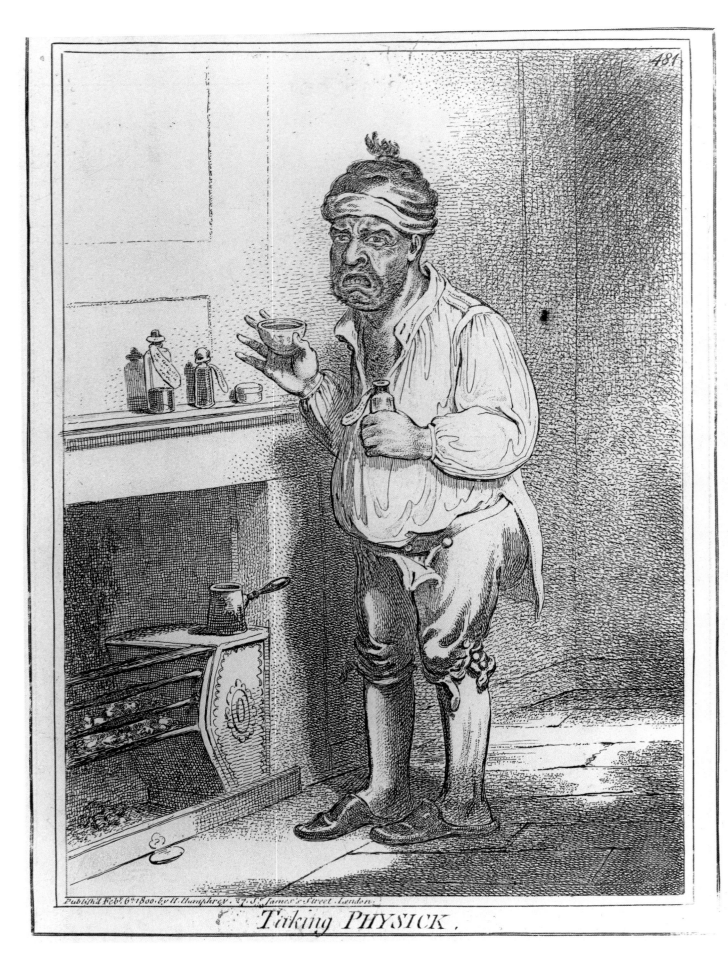

Published Feb.ᵣ 6ᵗʰ 1800 by H. Humphrey. 27 St James's Street London.

Taking PHYSICK.

Taking Physick. Color engraving by James
Gillray. English, 1800. Gillray is perhaps toying
with the notion that a medicine has to be bitter
to be effective. He conveys the patient's reaction
to the medicine's taste in a way that words
could never equal.

Chapter IX

SCIENCE, TECHNOLOGY, AND PHARMACY

T he changes in the pharmacist's traditional role that began in the nineteenth century were intensified in the twentieth. Throughout the nineteenth century, advances in science and technology whittled away at the mystique associated with the collecting, preserving, and compounding of drugs, but it was in the first third of the twentieth century that the pharmacist's role underwent radical change.

In part, this change was a result of the burgeoning of precise and efficacious pharmaco-therapeutic agents. Advances in chemistry made possible synthetic molecular alterations that provided a seemingly limitless supply of new drugs. The vast new armamentarium of chemotherapeutic agents would have been inconceivable without advances in chemistry, the discovery of antibiotic agents without advances in microbiology, the development of hormonal agents without advances in endocrinology, and the creation of new vaccines without advances in immunology. Studies in physiology and dietetics resulted in the development of a wide range of vitamins. Progress in biochemistry opened up new areas of research in pharmacology—and helped to create new pharmaceutical sciences. Nuclear physics led to nuclear medicine, radiopharmacy, and radionuclides. And biotechnology and genetic engineering opened new vistas in drug innovation.

. . . Et le mien ne drogue pas! (. . . And mine doesn't give drugs!). Color lithograph by Abel Faivre, from the French weekly *L'Assiette au Beurre,* March 22, 1902

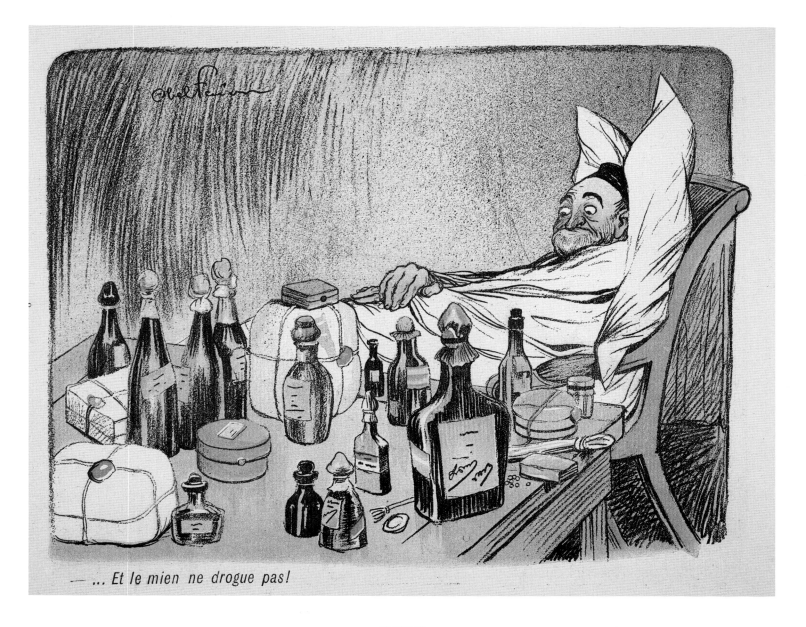

— *. . . Et le mien ne drogue pas!*

PHARMACOKINETICS AND BIOPHARMACEUTICS

An awareness of the pharmacologic effect of drugs, that is, their effect on living tissue, became essential to understanding the new sciences of pharmaceutics, biopharmaceutics, and pharmacokinetics. Pharmaceutical scientists investigated such matters as mechanisms of action, metabolism, distribution, and rates of absorption and excretion of drugs in the body. Concepts unthought of in the first half of the twentieth century became subjects of intense research in the second. These included the bioavailability of drugs, pharmacokinetic drug reactions, analytical methods of measuring concentrations of organic substances in body fluids, and the stability, shelf life, degree of ionization, solubility, particle size, and crystallization of drugs.

Pharmaceutical formulation became increasingly important as pharmacists recognized that effectiveness depended not only on the chemical entity involved but also on the correctness of the dosage and on the presentation of the drug in a form that would maximize its bioavailability. As medicines became more complex, more powerful, and more common, these considerations became more vital—and they gave pharmacotherapy a new precision and a new assurance.

The new science of pharmacokinetics drew on many disciplines. Its real beginnings date from the late 1930s, but at that time little was known about the concentration of drugs in blood or tissues. The concept of the biologic half-life of drugs (the time required for the plasma drug concentration, or the amount in the body, to decrease by half) was first demonstrated experimentally in 1953, and dissolution-rate controlled absorption was not introduced until 1959. Modern pharmacokinetic research is concerned with understanding

Microbes. Cover of a song sheet. American, 1905. In the song, one of the verses reads: "Wise men declare,/Germs throng the air,/and we'll all get our share./I wish I'd been like Adam,/And never known I had 'em." ▶

and measuring drug substances in the blood and tissues—and also with targeting the delivery of drugs in proper concentration to specific sites. The development of time-related medications, transdermal pumps, intranasal and bronchopulmonary administration techniques, and microcapsule implants, all mark advances in the technology of drug delivery.

NEW SCIENCE, NEW DRUGS

The ongoing search for new drugs to combat disease, provide comfort, and prolong life has been given special impetus in the twentieth century by economic motivation. The health of the worker is a primary concern in an industrialized society; illness is costly. Industry was quick to realize that there were economic advantages to more effective drugs.

Serum Therapy and Vaccines

The battle against microbes set in motion by the scientific verification of the germ theory of disease led to the use of aseptic and antiseptic procedures in surgery; in therapeutics and preventive medicine it was to lead to a new array of agents that were of concern to the pharmacist and the pharmaceutical industry, namely, serums and vaccines.

Therapeutic serums, or antitoxins, contained the antibodies developed in the blood of animals, mainly horses, in response to the injection of toxins. The first of these, diphtheria antitoxin, proved its value almost immediately after it was developed, in 1890. It was in commercial production by 1892. In New York, the Board of Health, which was producing its own diphtheria antitoxin in 1895, established—mainly in pharmacies—"culture stations" where the antitoxin was sold and where physicians were supplied with diagnostic kits.

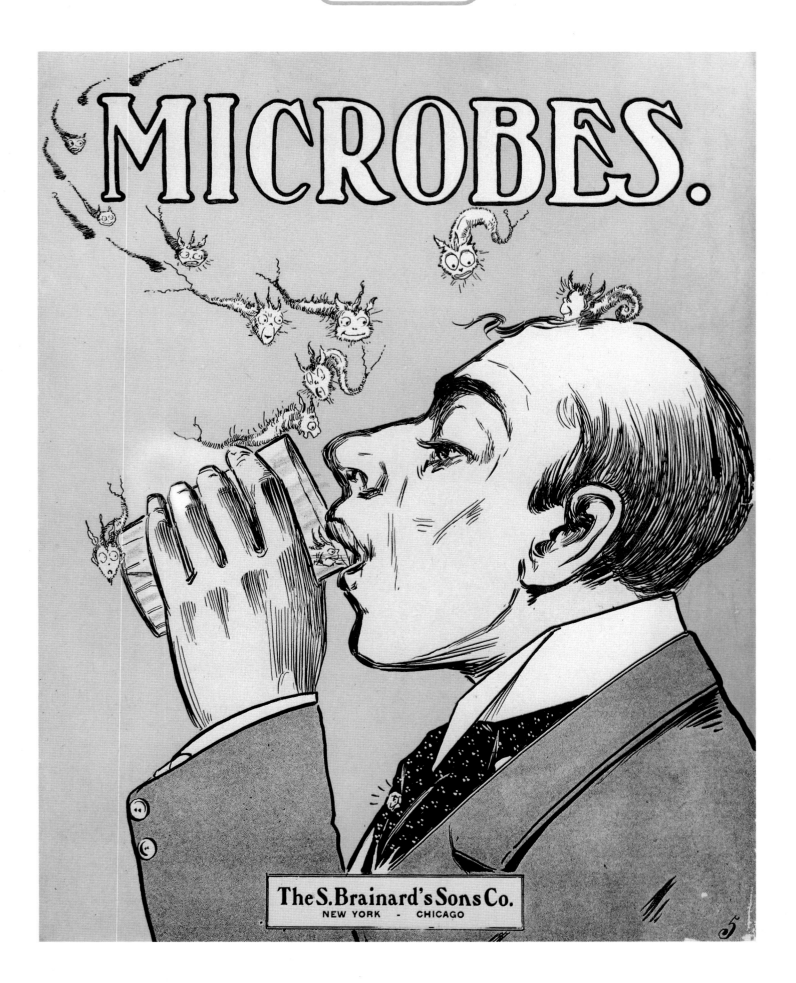

Serums for pneumococcal pneumonia and meningococcal meningitis, derived from injecting animals with whole bacteria, soon followed. Serum therapy was the only means of combating certain infections until chemotherapeutic agents became available in the late 1930s.

Vaccination against specific diseases, that is, providing immunity against diseases, had its modern development with the introduction of a vaccine for rabies by Louis Pasteur in 1885. The early twentieth century saw the development of vaccines, or toxoids, produced by killing or treating the microorganism or its toxins with heat or chemicals so that their toxicity was eliminated but their antigenic properties were retained. Starting in the 1930s, increased knowledge and improved techniques made development of new vaccines possible. A vaccine against typhus was dramatically successful: among thousands of American troops immunized during World War II, only sixty-four came down with typhus—and all of those had mild cases and recovered. The effort to develop a vaccine against influenza ran into complications because of the variety of new strains that were repeatedly encountered; this made it necessary to create a new vaccine as each variant strain was isolated.

The most spectacular developments in the field of vaccines involved those against poliomyelitis. The popularity of President Franklin D. Roosevelt, who had been a victim of poliomyelitis, gave impetus to the creation of the National Foundation for Infantile Paralysis, which raised huge sums from the American people to support research. Eventually two vaccines were developed, an injectable vaccine, by Jonas E. Salk (1955), and an oral vaccine, by Albert B. Sabin (1961). Widespread use of these vaccines has practically eliminated polio in developed countries.

Important, if less dramatic, are the vaccines that have been developed against such common childhood diseases as whooping cough, measles, rubella, and mumps. Current therapy makes use of multiple vac-

cines: DPT (diphtheria, pertussis, tetantus); DPT-Polio; and MMR (measles, mumps, rubella). Vaccines have been developed against hepatitis B: the first one, derived from plasma, was introduced by Merck Sharp & Dohme in 1982; a newer one was genetically engineered from yeast in 1987 by the Chiron Corporation and marketed by Merck Sharp & Dohme.

Vaccines and serums were not without their problems—occasionally devastating problems. Public and professional demands for the setting of standards of strength and purity led to legislation controlling the manufacture of these "biologicals," as they were called. As early as 1896, laws regulating the manufacture, sale, and distribution of biologicals had been enacted in France, Germany, Italy, and Russia. In the United States, the Biologics Control Act of 1902—passed four years before the Pure Food and Drug Act—provided for the inspection and licensing of establishments producing biologicals.

Hormones

The basis of the science of endocrinology had been laid in the middle of the nineteenth century, when the English physician Thomas Addison identified the disease of the suprarenal capsules that bears his name. By the end of the century, rapid advances in biochemistry and endocrinology led to new knowledge of glands and internal secretions. Several of these secretions were produced synthetically, among them epinephrine, which had been isolated by John Jacob Abel in 1897, adrenaline, isolated by Jokichi Takamine in 1900, and thyroxine, isolated by Edward C. Kendall in 1916. The isolation of insulin, in 1922—one of the twentieth century's major medical breakthroughs—was accomplished by the Canadian scientists Frederick G. Banting, Charles H. Best, John J. R. Macleod, and James B. Collip.

A search that ensued for biologically active substances in the adrenal cortex produced no fewer than twenty-eight steroids,

Poster advertising Bayer's Aspirin to the Netherlands market. Color lithograph by Jan Lavies. Dutch, c. 1910 ▶

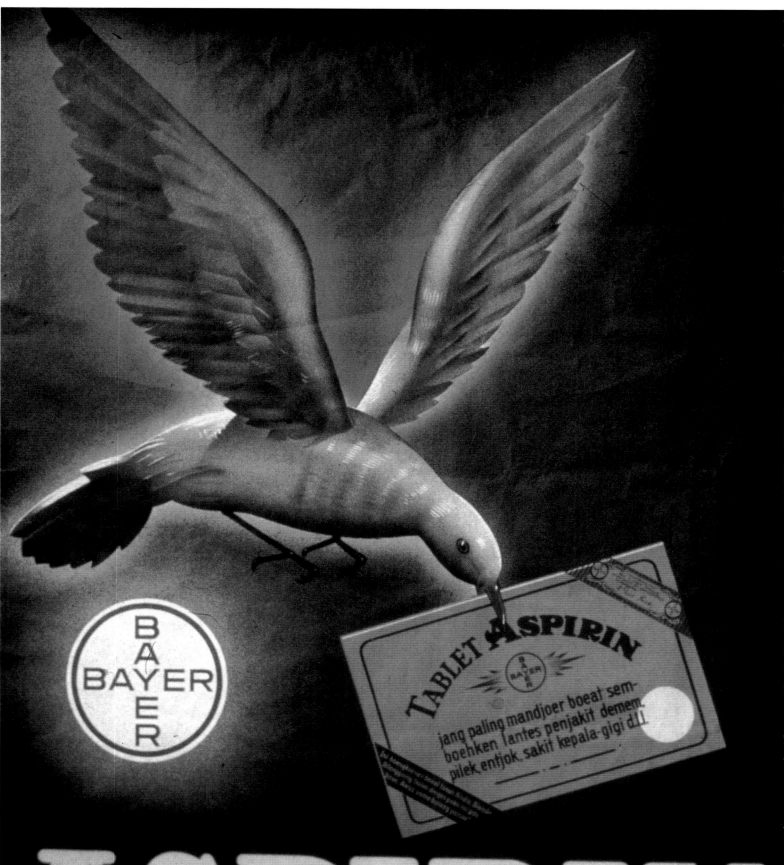

previously unknown crystalline compounds. The most important of these, cortisone, was extracted by three researchers independently in the late 1930s, and synthesized in 1946 by Lewis H. Sarett of Merck Sharp & Dohme. It was found effective against Addison's disease by Edward Kendall and against arthritis by Philip S. Hench. Of the ninety chemical entities made from these and related hormones that were introduced by the American pharmaceutical industry from 1940 to 1984, cortisone and adrenocorticotropin (ACTH) have proved particularly valuable. Indeed, cortisone and related products have become something of a twentieth-century panacea; a recent compilation describes hydrocortisone as indicated in endocrine, rheumatic, and hematological disorders, in collagen, dermatological, ophthalmic, respiratory, and gastrointestinal diseases, and in other conditions.

Interest in sex hormones led to the isolation of estrone in 1929 and to its synthesis by 1948. In 1934 and 1935, respectively, the hormones progesterone and testosterone were isolated. The first oral hormone product that was inexpensive to manufacture was diethylstilbestrol (DES), synthesized by Charles Dodds in England in 1938. Prescribed to prevent miscarriages, it found a ready reception in many parts of the world. Unfortunately, DES was to demonstrate the long-term, unsuspected, and unpredictable perils in the introduction of drugs: diethylstilbestrol was to prove particularly dangerous to the daughters of women who had undergone DES therapy. Although the risk was low, "DES daughters," especially between the ages of fifteen and twenty-two, could develop clear-cell cancer of the vagina and cervix and other vaginal and cervical problems. Moreover, the mothers themselves, after a considerable time lag, showed a noticeable increase in the incidence of certain types of cancer. Even "DES sons" were not immune to problems involving the reproductive organs.

Hormone therapy was to give medicine its first real weapons against infertility, menstrual and menopausal complications, and sexual dysfunction. Most dramatic was the development of oral contraceptives. In 1951, the first oral progestin, norethindrone (Norinyl™), was developed by Carl Djerassi of the Syntex Corporation. The possibilities attracted a great deal of research, and in 1960 in the United States a combination product of progestin and estrogen—which has come to be known as "the Pill"—was approved by the Food and Drug Administration. Six years later, it was estimated that one of every six women under thirty using any method of contraception was using this one. No other single drug has had the tremendous social impact of the Pill; marriage, the family, birth rates, patterns of human sexuality, the role of women, all have been affected by this single product of pharmaceutical research.

It was to be expected that hormonal contraceptive drug therapy would be followed by abortifacient drug therapy. Mifepristone (RU 486), developed largely through the work of Etienne-Emile Baulieu, a French endocrinologist, and introduced by Roussel in France, was first reported in 1982. It proved to be an effective oral means of terminating early pregnancies. (It is usually administered along with prostaglandin.) RU 486 offers decided advantages over surgical abortion: ease, privacy, safety, and economy. The implications for society are far-reaching—both the social impact of the contraceptive pill and the mainly religious objections to it were given a new dimension by the abortion pill. Two countries, France and China, promptly approved its use; in France, Roussel was forced at first to take it off the market by antiabortionist pressure but was required to return it to the market by government order.

Vitamins

In 1796, the British navy was finally convinced, on the basis of the experiments of the Scottish physician James Lind—experiments that went back to 1757—that lemons cured scurvy and that eating fresh vegetables prevented it. This was a purely empirical discovery: it was not until the last decades of the nineteenth century that definitive studies of various food elements were carried out on the basis of physiological chemistry.

The realization that certain elements in food were necessary for the maintenance of health came in the late nineteenth century. Considerable research—first on animals, then on humans—demonstrated that some diseases were caused by diets deficient in certain substances and that such deficiency diseases (among them beriberi and pellagra) could be prevented and cured by proper diet. A search to find the responsible substances began. In 1910–12, Frederick Gowland Hopkins of Cambridge University definitely established the existence of vitamins, but it was Casimir Funk, a Polish-born American chemist who did his research in France, Germany, England, and the United States as well as his homeland, who gave them their name. In the belief that these vital substances were amines, he originally called them "vitamines"; the final e was later dropped.

In the United States, vitamin A and vitamin B (later shown to be a complex of vitamins) were isolated in 1914–15, vitamin E in 1922, and nicotinic acid, or niacin, the factor whose absence caused pellagra, in 1937. More specific isolations and syntheses followed: vitamin B6 in 1930, pantothenic acid in 1940, biotin in 1943, vitamin B12 in 1948.

Advances in vitamin research were not limited to the United States. In 1928, Albert von Szent-Györgyi, at the Biochemical Laboratory of Cambridge University, isolated what he named "hexuronic acid," later to be renamed ascorbic acid—vitamin C. American researchers affirmed its antiscorbutic activity, and in 1933 British and Swiss chemists succeeded in synthesizing it. Dutch, British, German, and American scientists contributed to the identification, isolation, and synthesis of vitamin B1, or thiamine.

Chemotherapeutic Agents

Vaccination and serum therapy won the first battles in the war against infectious diseases, but after these victories the conflict was far from over. The weapon that won the next battle was chemotherapy, first wielded by the physician-physiologist-chemist Paul Ehrlich, who shared a Nobel Prize in 1908 for his work in immunology. Ehrlich's quest for a chemical agent that would kill or limit the growth of infectious organisms in the body without destroying the host cells epitomized the interdisciplinary demands of pharmaceutical research. It was Ehrlich who introduced the term "chemotherapy." His "magic bullet," arsphenamine, was the first synthetic chemotherapeutic agent. (Previously, only quinine could combat infection without injuring the host cells; vaccines and antitoxins operated on an immunological basis.) Arsphenamine, an effective antisyphilitic, was patented in 1907, although its effectiveness was not demonstrated until two years later. It was the 606th chemical combination that Ehrlich and his coworker Sahachiro Hata tested, and the process of its discovery illustrates the complex and toilsome nature of the work of the modern researcher.

A quarter of a century was to elapse before another chemotherapeutic agent was discovered. In 1932, Gerhard Domagk, a physician who was the director of research in experimental pathology and bacteriology for I.G. Farben Industrie in Elberfeld, Germany, observed that prontosil, a dye synthesized by the firm's chemists, cured mice infected by deadly doses of hemolytic streptococci. Domagk's finding was not announced until 1935. In the same year, Drs. Jacques Tréfouël, Theresa Tréfouël, Frédérico Nitti, and Daniel Bovet, at the Pasteur Institute in Paris, announced that they had broken prontosil down in the way it was broken down in the body and had isolated the active portion, later to be called sulfanilamide. A new era, the era of "sulfa" drugs had begun. Arsphenamine had proven effective against only one type of microorganism, the trypanosomes; the sulfas were to prove effective against a wide range of microorganisms.

To the medical professions and to the public the sulfonamides produced a series of what seemed like miracles. The success of sulfanilamide unleashed an almost frantic search for analogues, resulting in the finding of several useful agents, including sulfapyridine, sulfadiazine, and sulfisoxazole. Not only did the sulfonamides prove effective in combating infectious diseases; they also provided an effective means of prophylaxis. For the first time in history, drugs could effectively intervene in streptococcal infections, puerperal fever, erysipelas, meningococcal meningitis, shigella dysentery, gonorrhea, and other diseases. In the treatment of pneumonia the sulfa drugs soon eliminated the need for pneumonia typing and replaced serum therapy. They did not cure all infections, but in many cases they shortened the duration, lessened the incidence of complications, and lowered the fatality rate.

Antibiotics

Within a decade of the introduction of sulfanilamide, humankind was to receive a still greater boon in the form of penicillin, the first of an entirely new class of drugs, the antibiotics—drugs that are derived from living organisms and are capable of inhibiting or destroying other living organisms. Like the chemotherapeutic agents, penicillin and the wide range of antibiotics that followed had the ability to attack infecting organisms without doing harm to the host.

The antibiotic effect of a substance produced by the mold *Penicillium notatum* was first noted in 1928 by Alexander Fleming, a Scottish physician and bacteriologist at St. Mary's Hospital in London whose trained eye recognized this effect in a culture plate that had been left unattended and exposed to air. Fleming, who named the substance

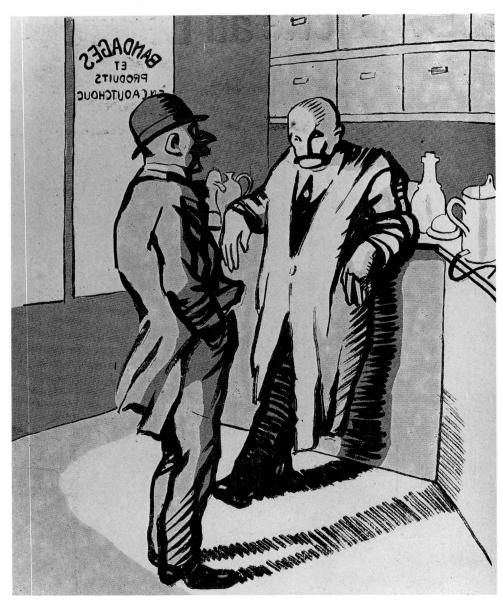

Les Victimes de la science. Lithograph by Juan Gris in *L'Assiette au Beurre,* October 8, 1910. The entire issue of the satiric weekly of this date was devoted to cartoons on 606 (arsphenamine). Here the pharmacist is commenting that 606 has killed his sales of prophylactics.

penicillin, did not—although its medical potential did occur to him—pursue his interest further when his chemist colleagues proved unable to purify it.

The actual introduction of penicillin into medicine was the work of a group of researchers at Oxford University, led by the Australian physician and pathologist Howard Florey. The exceptional team of scientists that Florey gathered around him included the biochemist Ernst Boris Chain, a refugee from Hitler's Germany, and the British biochemist Norman Heatley. Attracted to Fleming's account of penicillin, Florey's team succeeded in obtaining enough pure penicillin for experimental use on laboratory animals. In May 1940 they injected eight mice with streptococci: four were untreated and died; four were injected with penicillin and lived.

During 1940, the Oxford team conducted a number of clinical tests of penicillin, but they were handicapped by the low productivity of their laboratory, and not until August of 1941 were they able to publish a report. The results in the ten cases reported on were so favorable as to make large-scale production imperative; the potential value of penicillin in wartime was obvious. Florey sought to involve the British pharmaceutical industry, but since it was beset by wartime problems and could offer only a minimum of help, Florey turned to the United States and its pharmaceutical industry. The Northern Regional Research Laboratories of the United States Department of Agriculture at Peoria, Illinois, contributed significantly to penicillin culture, and the American pharmaceutical industry made heroic strides in penicillin production. In 1942, only enough penicillin to treat one hundred patients was produced, but by the time of the Allied invasion of Europe, in 1944, there was sufficient penicillin, from British as well as American sources, to treat all severe battle casualties in the American and British forces.

Just as the sulfonamides had replaced antipneumococcal serum, so penicillin replaced the sulfonamides in the treatment of pneumonia. Penicillin also offered superior results in the treatment of meningitis, endocarditis, staphylococcic infections, streptococcic infections, and gonorrhea. In 1943 it was shown that penicillin could cure syphilis, and the subsequent decline in the prevalence of that disease was spectacular. Spectacular, too, was the recovery rate of British soldiers wounded in World War II who were treated with penicillin—it was 95 percent.

The next antibiotic to be found was streptomycin, a drug derived not from fungi or bacteria but from an intermediate form of life, the actinomycetes. The discovery of streptomycin, in 1944, was the culmination of a long and persistent exploration of soil microbiology by Selman

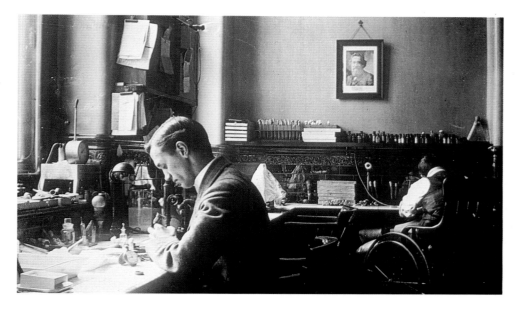

Sir Alexander Fleming (1881–1955), Scottish bacteriologist and discoverer of penicillin, in his laboratory at St. Mary's Hospital Medical School, London. c. 1935.
St. Mary's Hospital Medical School Library

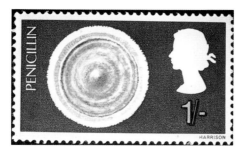

British postage stamp honoring the discovery of penicillin. 1967. Collection Dr. Albert Lyons, New York

Waksman and his associates at the Agricultural College of Rutgers University. Streptomycin was the first drug to prove effective against pathogenic tubercle bacilli. It and a later discovery, isoniazid, made great strides toward the conquest of "the great white plague."

As the quest continued, scientists in both institutional and industrial laboratories took up the search for more aminoglycosides, the class of antibiotics of which streptomycin was the prototype. Neomycin, kanamycin, gentamycin, tobramycin,

The Man who doubted if HOWARDS' ASPIRIN was the BEST. Color lithograph by H. M. Bateman. English, c. 1925

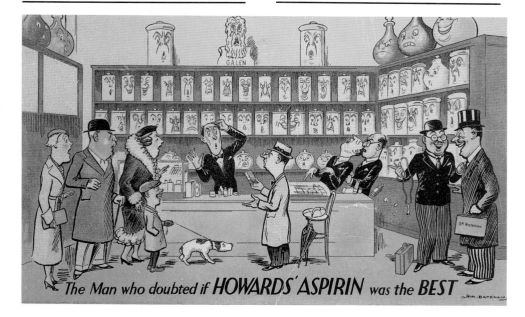

sisomycin, amikacin, and others were developed. These are broad-spectrum antibiotics—effective against a variety of bacteria—but like all antibiotics they are subject to problems: bacteria develop resistance to them, and they frequently have side effects.

At Yale University, in 1947, Paul Burkholder, searching through soil microorganisms, came upon what was to be called *Streptomyces venezuelae*, after an organism found in the soil of Venezuela. From it, scientists at Parke, Davis extracted a substance that proved effective against rickettsias, the extremely small bacteria responsible for such diseases as typhus, Rocky Mountain spotted fever, and Q fever. The cures that antibiotics could achieve were dramatically illustrated when this new substance, chloramphenicol, was given to twenty-two of the sickest patients during a 1947 typhus epidemic in Bolivia. All were thought to be dying (for one the death certificate had already been prepared). All twenty-two recovered. The new antibiotic proved effective against typhoid fever as well. Chloramphenicol (Chloromycetin™) was the first of the broad-spectrum antibiotics to be used clinically, but an alarming number of reports linking it with blood dyscrasias led to a decline in its use. However, the drug continues to be valuable for several severe infections, particularly typhoid fever, that cannot be managed with other agents.

Similar researches, mainly in industrial laboratories, introduced other broad-spectrum drugs, the tetracyclines. These included chlortetracycline (Aureomycin™) and oxytetracycline (Terramycin™). In addition, another group of antibiotics was derived from actinomycetes, the cephamycins. Like penicillin, the cephamycins are B-lactam antibiotics, that is, they contain a B-lactam ring. The effectiveness of the cephamycins, especially cefoxitin (Mefoxin™), against gram-positive cocci is comparable to that of other antibiotics, and they show greater activity against a variety of gram-negative rods and anaerobic microbes.

The sulfonamides, penicillin, and the

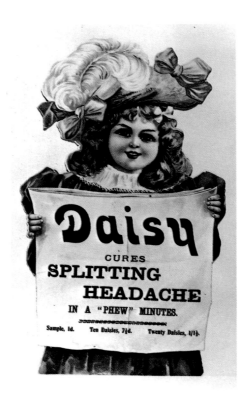

Advertisement for an analgesic. English, c. 1900

actinomycetes-derived antibiotics by no means conquered infection. They did not always work effectively: there were organisms that did not respond; there were problems of distribution and concentration of these drugs in the body; there was the development of tolerance in the patient and of the spontaneous development of resistant strains of microorganisms.

Resistance to penicillin, the "wonder drug," aggravated by its promiscuous use in over-the-counter products such as salves, throat lozenges, and nasal sprays, became particularly troublesome. By 1955, the government agencies responsible for public health in most countries restricted the dispensing of penicillin in order to mitigate the development of resistance.

The tedious process of screening bacteria and fungi for antibiotic potential was paralleled by attempts to synthesize and modify the penicillin molecule. Particularly active were John C. Sheehan of the Massachusetts Institute of Technology and scientists of the Beecham Research Laboratories in England. The latter spent two years determining that the nucleus of the penicillin module was 6-aminopenicillanic acid, and they studied 1,241 configurations of that molecule to arrive, in 1960, at the "semisynthetic" penicillin named methicillin, an antibiotic effective against penicillin-resistant organisms. This was followed by a spate of semisynthetic penicillins that proved effective against certain gram-negative bacteria while retaining their action against gram-positive bacteria. The first of these, a Beecham product, was ampicillin (Penbritin™), announced in 1961.

Before these developments took place, scientists began to derive antibiotics from a new source, the mold *Cephalosporium acremonium*, first recognized by Giuseppe Brotzu in 1948. The former rector of the University of Cagliari in Sardinia found the mold at a sewer outlet off the coast of that island. His laboratory work and clinical tests—with an admittedly impure filtrate—led him to send a culture to Florey at Oxford. There a team that included Heatley,

Edward P. Abraham, G. G. F. Newton, and Henry S. Burton succeeded in identifying three antibiotics, two of which—cephaloporin N and cephalosporin C—were active against both gram-positive and gram-negative microbes. There followed many new derivatives: cephalothin and cephaloridine in the 1960s, cephapirin and cefazolin in the 1970s, and cefuroxime in the 1980s.

This account hardly exhausts the subject of antibiotics. There are a host of miscellaneous antibiotics that are all of some value and importance, among them macrolides, polypeptides, and antifungus and antitumor agents. The impact of immunization and antibiotic therapy on human life is evident in mortality statistics. In the United States, between 1935 and 1970, mortality rates for influenza and pneumonia dropped from 103.9 to 30.9 per 100,000; for tuberculosis, from 55.1 to 2.6; for gastroenteritis, from 14.1 to 1.3; for syphilis, from 19 to 2. By 1970, deaths from diphtheria, typhoid, dysentery, whooping cough, scarlet fever, and meningococcal infections had fallen almost to zero. The incidence of poliomyelitis fell from 37 per 100,000 in 1952 to near zero in 1970.

It would be a mistake to attribute these benefits entirely to antibiotic drugs, however. Where infectious diseases are concerned, the long-term mortality trend had been in steady decline before the advent of antibiotics. Improvements in sanitation, living conditions, personal hygiene, diet, and medical and nursing care were undoubtedly prime contributors to this trend. It is also likely, although difficult to prove, that some of the pathogenic organisms were losing their virulence—or that the human system was making successful new adjustments to host-parasite relationships with certain microbes. Nor must it be forgotten that immunization and serum therapy had combated disease with considerable effect even before the introduction of chemotherapeutic and antibiotic agents, and that public health agencies, with their programs of mass inoculation, played a highly significant role in the process.

Chemical Therapeutics

Immunization, serum therapy, hormones, vitamins, chemotherapy, and antibiotics all led, in one way or another, to isolation, extraction, and synthesis of active agents. In the process, there developed what has been called "chemical therapeutics," that is, the use of pharmaceuticals, largely from synthetic chemical sources, not only to combat infections, endocrine imbalance, and deficiency disease, but also to correct or ameliorate every known human dysfunction—neurological, metabolic, cardiac, vascular, and allergic among others (see table, p. 206).

Chemical therapeutics began early in the twentieth century with the barbiturates, a class of "sedative-hypnotic" drugs that derived from barbituric acid. In 1903, Emil Fischer and Joseph von Mering introduced barbital, which was followed by phenobarbital, developed in 1912. In the following years more than 2,500 barbiturates were synthesized, and about 50 of them found clinical use. Most notable of these were phentobarbital and secobarbital, introduced in 1941 and 1945, respectively.

Although the barbiturates are still valued as central nervous system depressants, they came, with the introduction of the tranquilizing agents, to play a lesser role in sedation. The first of these agents was reserpine, a drug discovered in the old-fashioned way—by laboriously extracting the alkaloid from a plant, in this case *Rauwolfia serpentina,* long known and used in India. This extraction was accomplished at the Ciba Research Laboratories in Switzerland, and the alkaloid was first marketed in 1953. There followed a galaxy of psychopharmacological drugs—developed after it was noticed that certain antihistaminic substances were useful in treating psychoses. The first to be obtained by chemical synthesis, chlorpromazine, was developed in France by Rhône-Poulenc and made available in 1954. Roughly fifty more products of this class appeared in the next two decades; the most important among them were meprobamate (Miltown™), marketed in 1955, prochlorperazine (Compazine™) in 1956, chlordiazepoxide hydrochloride (Librium™) in 1960, and diazepam (Valium™) in 1963. That tranquilizers became popular as soon as they were put on the market is perhaps an indication of the frenetic pace of modern life. For a decade and more, central nervous system drugs have been the leading class of drugs sold domestically by American manufacturers, usually accounting for about one-fourth of all sales. They have also been the second-largest class of drugs (second to anti-infective drugs) sold abroad by American firms, accounting for over 14 percent of such sales in 1976, for example.

With the advent of these drugs, the treatment of the mentally disturbed entered a new age. The spectacular improvement of mental patients to whom certain of these drugs had been administered led to a rapid—even precipitous—reduction in the number of patients in mental hospitals. After 1955, drug therapy largely supplanted convulsive therapy and surgery in the

AIDS—Don't Pass It On. American poster, c. 1985. Many infectious diseases have been controlled by therapeutic advances, but others, most notably AIDS, are the targets of large-scale biological and pharmacological research activities. ▶

Technicians using computers to control major steps in the synthesis of an angiotensin-converting enzyme at a Merck chemical plant in Ireland. 1988

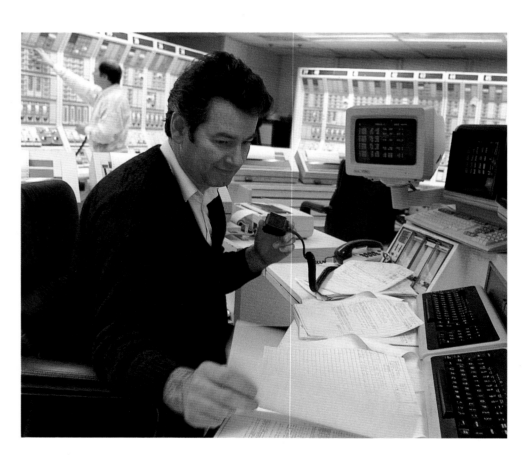

treatment of psychoses: chlorpromazine calmed the manic agitated patient, chlordiazepoxide soothed the highly anxious patient, and imipramine (Tofānil™), first reported by Geigy in 1957, aroused withdrawn patients sufficiently to enable them to communicate with a therapist.

Cardiac drugs, usually among the three leading classes of drugs sold by American companies, accounted for 17 percent of all sales in 1983. In 1987, this was the class of drugs most often dispensed in community and chain-store pharmacies. Before the present century the most commonly used drugs for the heart were digitalis, quinidine, and nitroglycerine. All continue in regular use; nitroglycerine is now available in the form of pads applied to the skin for transdermal assimilation, as well as in sublingual tablets.

Based on new understanding of physiological processes, such as the recognition of both alpha and beta nerve receptors in the adrenergic portion of the nervous system, rapid advances were made in the 1950s in the development of drugs to deal with cardiovascular problems. By the 1960s, the physician had a choice of a large array of antihypertensives, antiarrhythmics, antianginals, vasodilators, hypolipedmics (cholesterol-reducing), and other drugs. To point up a few: the antihypertensives methyldopa (Aldonet™) and clonidine hydrochloride (Catapres™) were made available by Merck Sharp & Dohme in 1962 and Boehringer Ingelheim in 1969, respectively; the beta-blocker propranolol hydrochloride (Inderal™) was synthesized by Imperial Chemical Industries of Great Britain in 1964; the vasodilator isoxuprine hydrochloride (Vasodilan™) was introduced by Mead Johnson in 1959. The hypolipedmic clofibrate (Atromid-S™) was introduced by Imperial Chemical Industries in 1963, to be followed by related drugs, of which fenofibrate (Lipanthyl™), introduced by Fournier of France in 1975, gained wide acceptance in Europe. Other agents directed toward the reduction of cholesterol in the bloodstream included

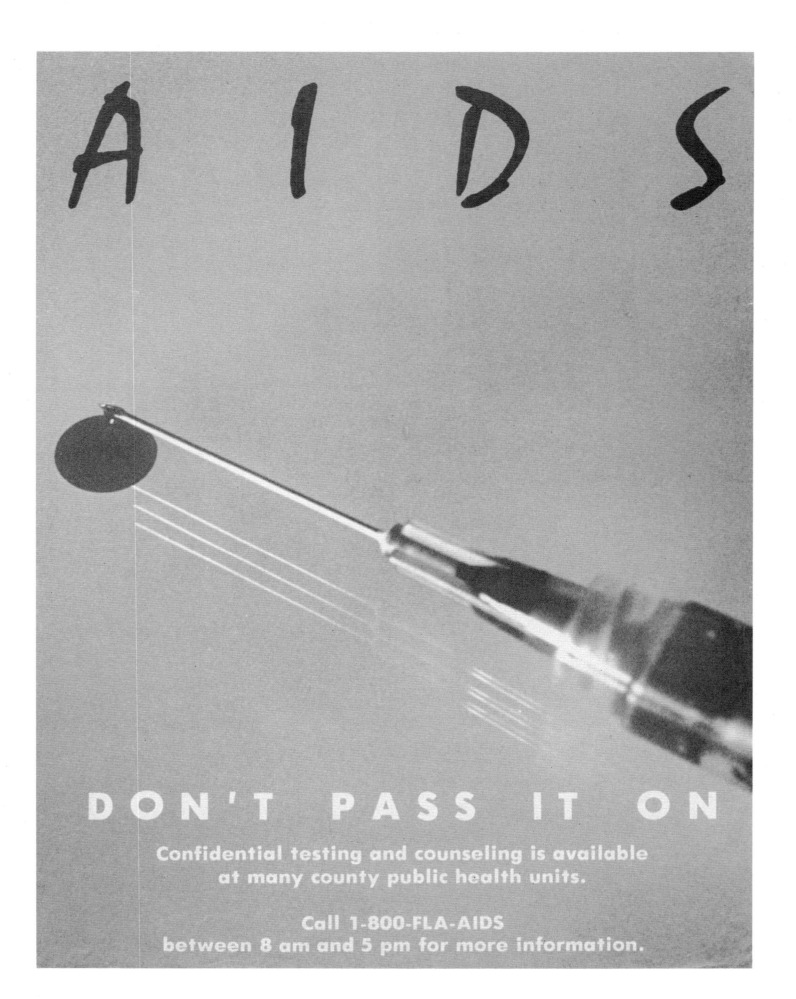

cholestyramine resin (Questran™), introduced by Merck Sharp & Dohme in 1968, colestipol hydrochloride (Colestid™), introduced by Upjohn in 1978, and lovastatin (Mevacor™), introduced by Merck Sharp & Dohme in 1988. In addition, new approaches involving inhibition of the angiotensin-converting enzymes have been introduced by Squibb and by Merck Sharp & Dohme. In the United States, in the two decades from 1960 to 1981, deaths from hypertensive heart disease declined by 71 percent, those from hypertension by 53 percent, those from cerebrovascular disease by 34 percent, and those from atherosclerosis by 39 percent.

Undoubtedly changed habits of eating and exercising, the decrease in smoking, and new surgical procedures played a part in the decline in deaths from cardiac and vascular diseases, but there can be little doubt of the impact of the new chemical agents.

The chemical therapeutic agents that twentieth-century research has made available for the physician to prescribe and the pharmacist to dispense are legion, and their number is constantly increasing. Among these weapons in the war against illness and infirmity are analgesics, anaesthetics, diuretics, antispasmodics, muscle relaxants, and anti-inflammatory agents (see table). Similarly, the expansion of the concept of chemotherapeutics to include anticancer agents and antiviral agents has added substantially to the materia pharmaceutica. The development of antiviral agents took on particular urgency with the challenge of the scourge of the late twentieth century, the human immunodeficiency virus (HIV) responsible for AIDS. A number of such agents were explored, and in 1984 azidothymadine (AZT), first synthesized in 1964, was shown by scientists of the National Institutes of Health and Duke University to be useful. Its production and marketing (as Retrovir™) were undertaken by Burroughs Wellcome. The great advances in drug therapy that the twentieth century has witnessed seem but a prelude to greater things to come.

NEW SINGLE CHEMICAL ENTITIES INTRODUCED IN THE UNITED STATES MARKET, BY THERAPEUTIC CLASS, 1940–1988

Anaesthetics	28
Analeptics	3
Analgesics	36
Antagonists and antidotes	21
Anthelmintics	13
Antiarthritics (nonhormonal)	13
Anticoagulants	12
Anticonvulsants	16
Antihistamines	37
Anti-infectives	227
Anti-inflammatory agents (nonhormonal)	15
Antinauseants	12
Anti-obesity preparations	17
Antivirals	5
Ataraxics	58
Bronchodilators	16
Cancer chemotherapy	39
Immunosuppressants	2
Cardiovascular preparations	102
Cholesterol-affecting agents	14
Coagulants	5
Convulsants	1
Cough and cold preparations	24
Dermatologic preparations	58
Diabetic therapy	12
Diuretics	38
Enzymes	10
Eye preparations	19
Fertility agents (nonhormonal)	1
Gastrointestinal preparations	76
Hematinics	15
Hemostatics	2
Hormones	91
Hospital solutions	8
Muscle relaxants	38
Oxytocics	5
Parasympathomimetics	7
Psychostimulants	23
Sedatives and hypnotics	23
Thyroid therapy	9
Vitamins and nutrients	16
Unclassified	50
Total	1,217

Source: PMA Statistical Fact Book, 1986. Table 2–9 (PMA Analysis of Paul de Haen data)

Chapter X

THE ROLE OF THE INDUSTRY

The economic realities of the marketplace—which include the continuing competition among pharmaceutical companies in Europe, Japan, and America and the ever-increasing costs of research—have led to a spate of mergers and acquisitions. One of the earliest mergers was the union, in 1953, of Merck & Company, a chemical firm supplying products to the pharmaceutical industry, and Sharp & Dohme, Inc., a major pharmaceutical company. In 1970, the Warner-Lambert Pharmaceutical Company, itself the result of a 1955 merger, acquired Parke, Davis & Company. Their merged assets amounted to over $1 billion, and the company boasted of installations in forty-seven countries and of twelve major research centers in five countries.

In another 1970 merger, two Swiss pharmaceutical giants, Ciba Ltd. and J. R. Geigy joined forces to form Ciba-Geigy Ltd. In 1974, Hoechst AG of Germany purchased a majority interest in the French drug company Roussel Uclaf S.A., thereby creating Hoechst-Roussel Pharmaceuticals, one of the largest of the international titans. In the years that ensued, other transactions followed the pattern: the E. I. Du Pont de Nemours Company acquired Endo Laboratories; Dow Pharmaceuticals acquired Merrell-National Laboratories and then Marion Laboratories; William H. Rorer, Inc., acquired the pharmaceutical division of Revlon, Inc., and was later acquired in turn by Rhône Poulenc; Smith-Kline Beckman Corporation merged with the British Beecham Group PLC to form SmithKline Beecham Ltd.; the Squibb Corporation merged with the Bristol-Myers Company to form Bristol-Myers Squibb.

This concentration has created ever larger companies with ever larger levels of capitalization, sales, and profit. It has made efficient manufacturing and marketing operations essential. By the 1960s, the pharmaceutical industry had become an important segment of international trade and international finance. The industry thrived not only because it met vital needs of society but also because the uniqueness of its product gave it an advantageous position in the marketplace. The producer had the benefits of a patent for a number of years, and although the situation might change after a patent had run out and a generic drug entered the market, the peculiar physician-patient-pharmacist relationship still operated to lift the pharmaceutical product out of the ordinary competition of the marketplace.

The pharmaceutical industry's economic success is apparent from the statistics. The total world sales of pharmaceuticals for the twelve months ending in June 1989 were estimated at $103.5 billion. In 1989, the members of the (American) Pharmaceutical Manufacturers Association alone projected worldwide sales of $51.5 billion.

These large sums represent but a small fraction of the overall health-care expenditures in the United States and other developed countries. In the United States, in 1987 the amount spent on health ($500.3 billion) amounted to only 11.1 percent of the gross national product, and less than 7 percent of that ($34 billion) was spent on "drugs and medical sundries." The largest expenses for health care, by far, are hospital costs and physicians' fees.

THE INDUSTRY AND PHARMACEUTICAL RESEARCH

The growth of the pharmaceutical industry entailed the establishment of research laboratories designed not only for the development of new drugs but also for the development of analogues of drugs introduced by competing companies. The reliance on science, and the creation of laboratories by pharmaceutical houses to put science to use, had started in the nineteenth century. In Germany, Hoechst organized its

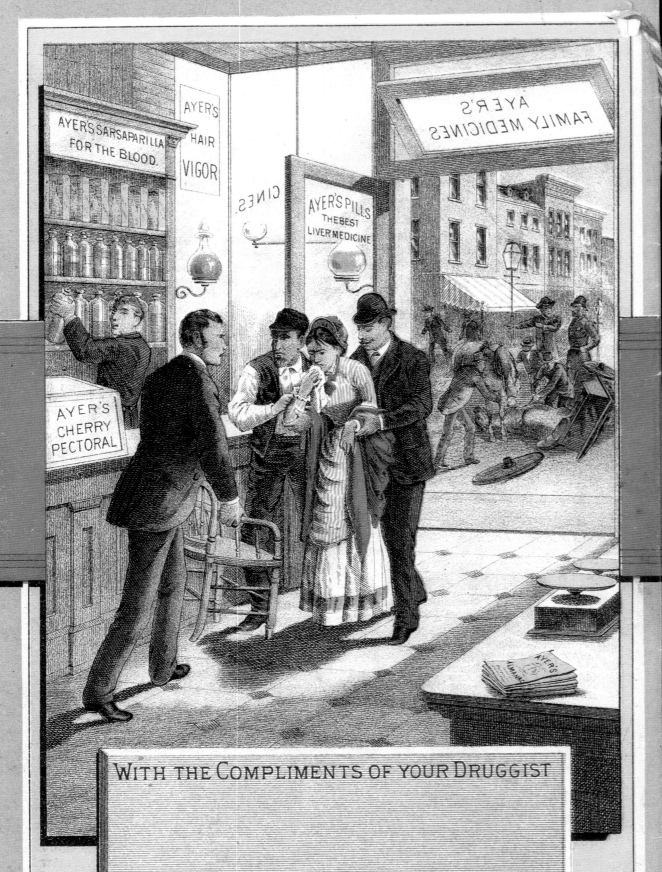

WITH THE COMPLIMENTS OF YOUR DRUGGIST

The pharmacy as first-aid station. Back cover of *Ayer's Book of Emergencies,* published by J.C. ◄ Ayer & Co., Lowell, Massachusetts, 1888

Postcard view of tablet manufacture in Vichy, France. c. 1905. The equipment punched one tablet at a time. State-of-the-art rotary presses are capable of punching 350,000 to 400,000 tablets per hour on the highest-speed machines.

Labeling and packaging ampoules at Parke, Davis & Co. in Detroit in 1930. The labor-intensive methods then required to ensure the safety of injectable products have been superseded by advances in automation.

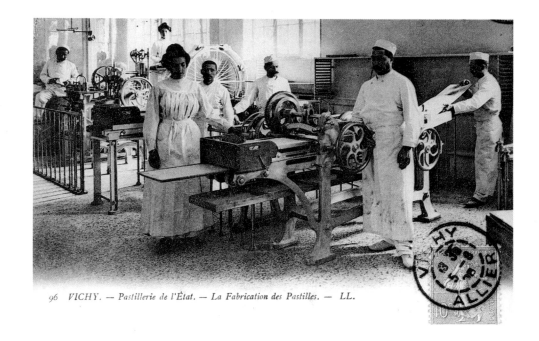

96 VICHY. — Pastillerie de l'État. — La Fabrication des Pastilles. — LL.

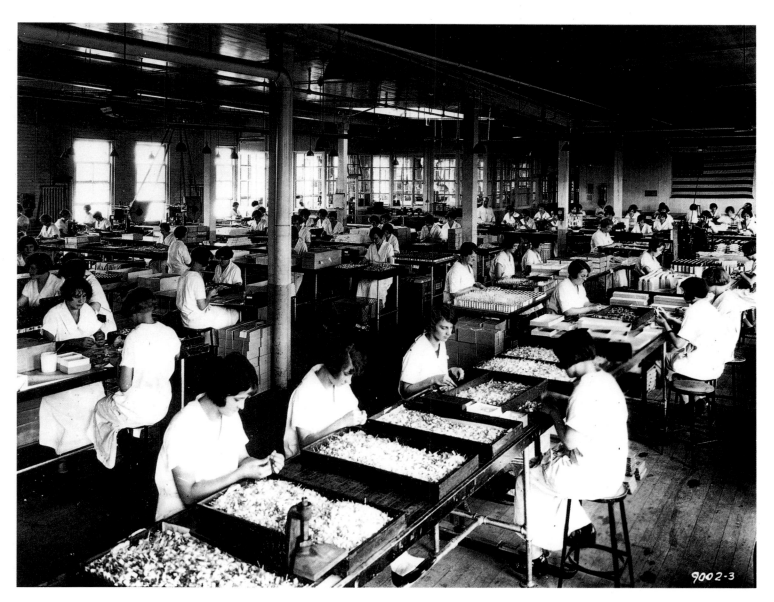

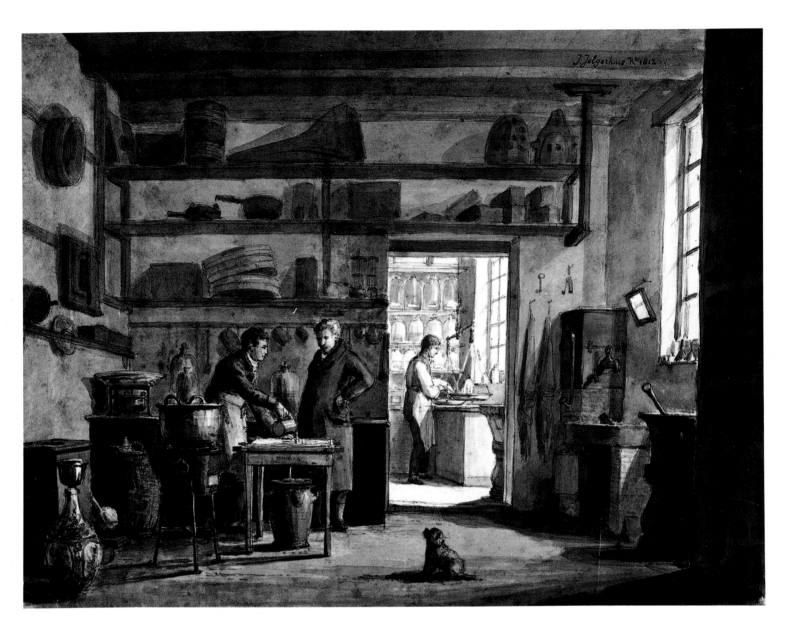

The laboratory of the pharmacy of A. d'Ailly. Painting by Johannes Jelgerhuis. Dutch, 1818. Amsterdams Historisch Museum

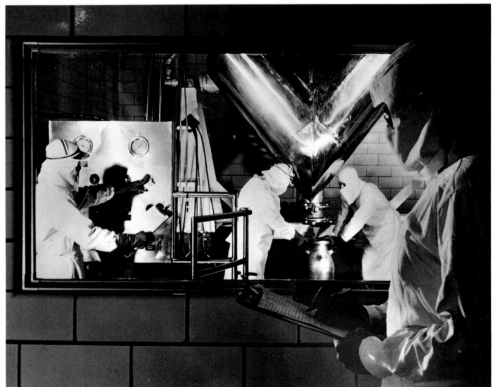

Antibiotic compounding operation at Squibb's New Brunswick, New Jersey, plant. 1959. Working in areas controlled by exacting sterile technique, technicians are filling cylinders with an antibiotic that has just been mixed by revolving the large triangular metal container.

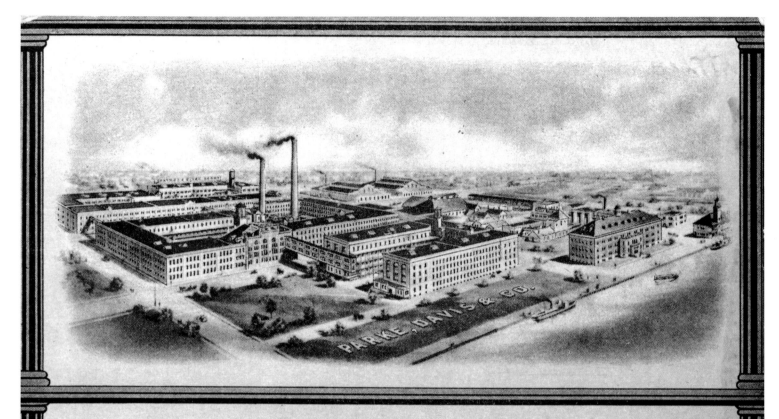

PARKE, DAVIS & CO., INC., LABORATORIES AND MAIN OFFICES, DETROIT, MICH.

The plant is located on the Detroit River, at the foot of McDougall and Joseph Campau Avenues. It occupies 16 acres of ground, and the floor-space of the buildings amounts to 836,418 square feet, or about 19 acres.

Postcard view of the Parke, Davis & Co. manufacturing plant in Detroit. c. 1910. Parke, Davis and the H. K. Mulford Company of Philadelphia pioneered in the pharmaceutical industry's development of research laboratories.

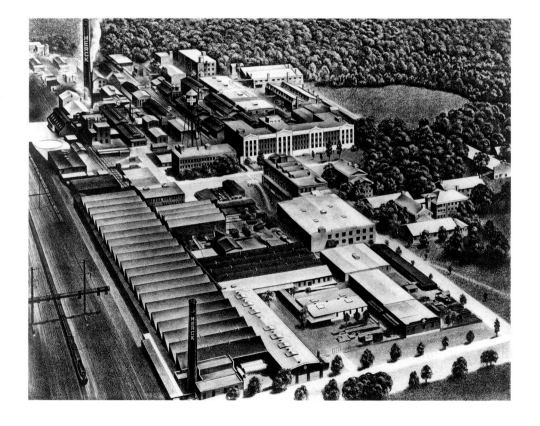

Merck. Lithograph by Louis Lozowick after an aerial photograph. American, 1942. In this rendering of the Merck plant and offices in Rahway, New Jersey, the artist has omitted the smoke coming from the chimneys, added a train moving in the direction of Philadelphia on the tracks of the Pennsylvania Railroad, and beautified the area at the upper right. Ars Medica Collection, Philadelphia Museum of Art

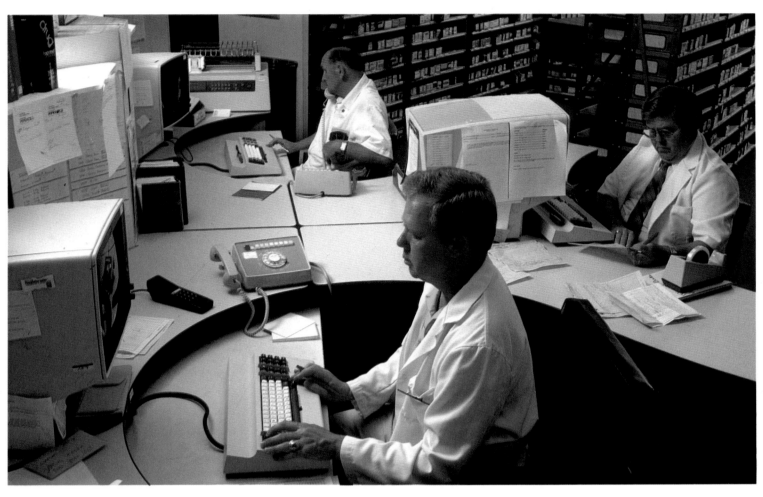

Pharmacists filling prescriptions by computer, University Hospital, Augusta, Georgia. 1987

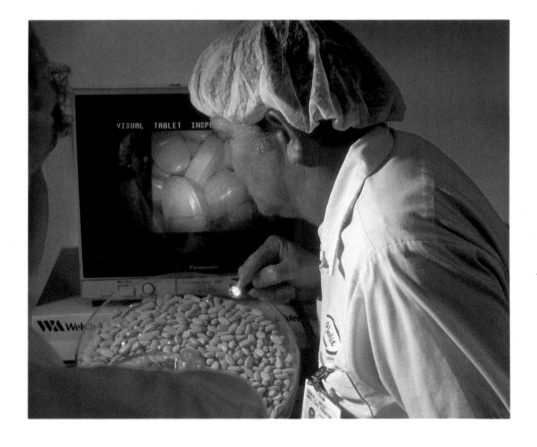

Inspecting finished tablets with the aid of a fiber-optic probe. c. 1985. Technological advances have not eliminated the need for trained personnel to locate and remove imperfect (broken or discolored) tablets.

Workers in the granulating area of a pharmaceutical manufacturing plant wearing suits for protection against toxic fumes. c. 1985. Such suits are also essential to keep the environment free of foreign particles. ▶

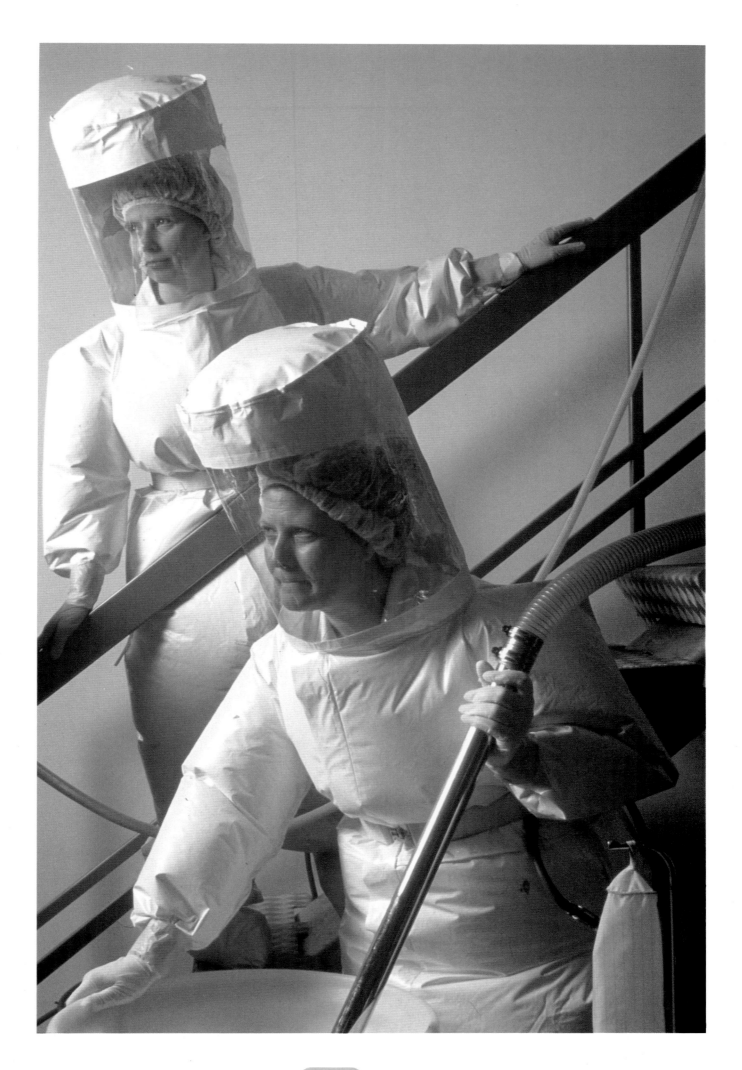

research activities and directed its attention to synthetic medicines in the 1880s. Parke, Davis boasted of a scientific staff in the 1890s, and Smith, Kline and French had an "analytical laboratory" by 1893. In Great Britain, Burroughs Wellcome established its physiological laboratory in 1894.

The laboratories that were established in the first decades of the twentieth century were essentially "service" laboratories, concerned with testing raw materials and standardizing finished products. After World War I, research of a broader, more fundamental nature was undertaken, but modern research in the pharmaceutical industry in the United States did not begin until the 1930s. The Merck Research Laboratories were founded in 1933; the Squibb Institute for Medical Research was established in 1938. These developments in the United States were paralleled in Germany, Great Britain, France, Switzerland, and, somewhat later, Japan.

The result was the creation of superb research laboratories for the isolation, preparation, synthesis, physical production, quality evaluation, and clinical testing of drugs. Vast resources—financial, scientific, and engineering—have been brought into play. The pharmaceutical industry has integrated the work of scientists in a host of disciplines: chemists, chemical engineers, biochemists, biochemical engineers, virologists, biophysicists, immunologists, microbiologists, statisticians, epidemiologists, mycologists, geneticists, pharmacologists, pharmacognosists, toxicologists, biologists, physicians, pharmacists, and clinicians. To this long list should be added workers in some of the newer disciplines: enzymologists, immunotherapeutists, peptide chemists, and pharmacogeneticists.

The financing, management, and integration of even a part of this enterprise would probably be beyond the capacity of universities or private institutions; only government would have the resources. It is estimated that from the 1940s to 1984 the American pharmaceutical industry expended over $30 billion on research and devel-

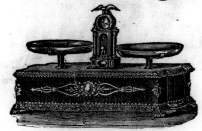

Broadside advertising the Henry Troemner company and featuring the Hoffman balance (patented in 1866). Philadelphia, c. 1885. National Library of Medicine, Bethesda

opment. That the pace has accelerated markedly is evidenced by the fact that for 1989 alone the member companies of the (American) Pharmaceutical Manufacturers Association estimated an expenditure of $7.3 billion on research and development.

Modern pharmaceutical research has kept pace with scientific advances. It was based, after its 1930s beginnings, largely on chemistry and pharmacology. Standard approaches have been the alteration of molecular structure, chemical synthesis, large-scale screening of potential drug sources, and new chemical combinations. Experimentation with the arrangement of molecules could have beneficial results, as in the development of hydrocortisone, which was free of some of cortisone's side effects. But this approach also resulted in the production of "me too" drugs, that is, slightly different drugs performing the same function as those of a competitor. Synthesis could mean tremendous economies and the supplying of quantities not otherwise attainable.

In the period between 1930 and 1960, pharmaceutical research was mainly empirical and serendipitous. The observation by an outside researcher, in 1949, of the increased excretion of sodium in sulfanilamide therapy was taken note of by the research program, already in existence for six years, at the Merck Sharp & Dohme laboratories, and after six more years of research this observation led to the development of chlorothiazide and a new diuretic therapy. Similarly, the observed relaxing effects of rauwolfia led to the development of reserpine and a whole new group of tranquilizing and antihypertensive drugs.

The 1960s brought radical change: pharmaceutical research moved from an empirical, intuitive approach to a rational and targeted one. This came about as a consequence of the explosion of scientific knowledge, particularly in the area of biochemistry. The starting point of research began to be analysis of a disease or condition and identification of the physiological processes involved. Currently, with the aid of an awesome array of new procedures and equipment, the biochemistry of these processes is studied and key chemical actions are selected for pharmacological intervention. One approach is to identify the enzymes involved in the biochemistry of a disease and to find drugs to inhibit them. Another is to analyze cellular receptor sites and find blocking agents. Opportunities for a "rational pharmacology" are obvious: it has become possible to design an ideal drug for a particular need through the use of the computer and for the computer to offer alternatives with which the chemist can work.

GOVERNMENT AND PRIVATE RESEARCH

The many new drugs developed in the twentieth century (see table, page 206) point up the enormous contribution to human health and well-being that has come from the concentration of scientific and technical knowledge available in the laboratories of the pharmaceutical industry. But the discoveries, all based on years of study and research in the basic sciences, have not come from the industry alone, as we have seen. Insulin was the discovery of Banting, Macleod, Best, and Collip, working at the University of Toronto. Penicillin was discovered by Fleming at St. Mary's Hospital in London, and its therapeutic value was recognized and production begun by the Florey group at Oxford University. Streptomycin was discovered by Waksman and associates at Rutgers University, and its antituberculosis potential was recognized by William H. Feldman and H. Corwin Hinshaw at the Mayo Clinic. At the Mayo Clinic, too, thyroxine was isolated, by Edward C. Kendall, and the corticosteroids were derived through the work of Kendall and Philip S. Hench. Chloramphenicol resulted from the research of Paul Burkholder at Yale University. Heparin, the blood-thinning drug, was a 1959 contribution of Jay

McLean at the Johns Hopkins University. Polio vaccines were the work of Jonas E. Salk at the University of Pittsburgh and of Albert B. Sabin at the University of Cincinnati.

Government agencies and government aid have also played a fundamental role in drug research and production. Agencies such as the National Institutes of Health in the United States and the Medical Research Council in Great Britain have not only become heavily involved in research; they have also provided financial support for university and institute laboratories and investigators. The role of private philanthropic organizations such as the Rockefeller Foundation has also been significant.

In the United States, the assumption of responsibility by the federal government for the quality of drugs began in 1902 with the Biologics Control Act of that year. Under this act, the Public Health and Marine Hospital Service was granted the power of inspection and licensing of plants manufacturing vaccines, serums, and related products. The Hygienic Laboratory of the service, which was charged with testing the purity and strength of such products, became the National Institute of Health in 1930. The scope of activity of these governmental agencies expanded, and they are credited with the elimination of tetanus as a complication of smallpox vaccination, with the development of vaccines against Rocky Mountain spotted fever and typhus, with the improvement of the antityphoid vaccine, and with the production of all the tetanus vaccine available in the United States at the time of World War I. The National Institute of Health developed into the National Institutes of Health, whose extensive internal research activities are exemplified by the development of AZT and whose sponsorship and financing of external research programs have been noted. In addition, the N.I.H. provides essential coordination of the work of universities, industrial laboratories, and research institutes.

Such governmental and institutional involvement in pharmaceutical research in no

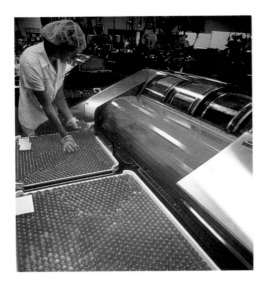

Inspecting empty capsules to ensure quality control. c. 1980

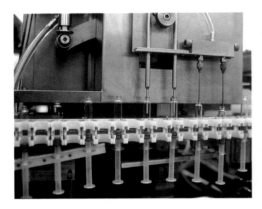

Packaging line for filling syringes, Parkedale Pharmaceutical Complex, Rochester, New York. 1982.

Drying coated tablets. 1975. After the tablets leave the coating pan they are shaken and tossed, to speed their drying, as they move across a screen.

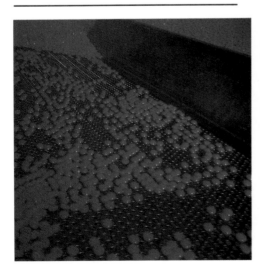

Monitoring bottles on a pharmaceutical packaging line. 1985 ▶

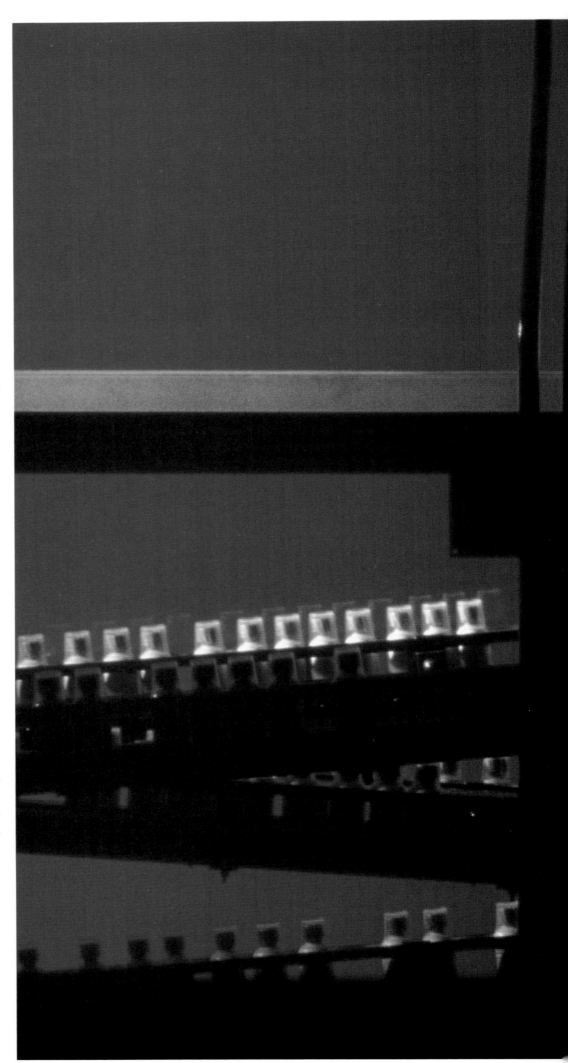

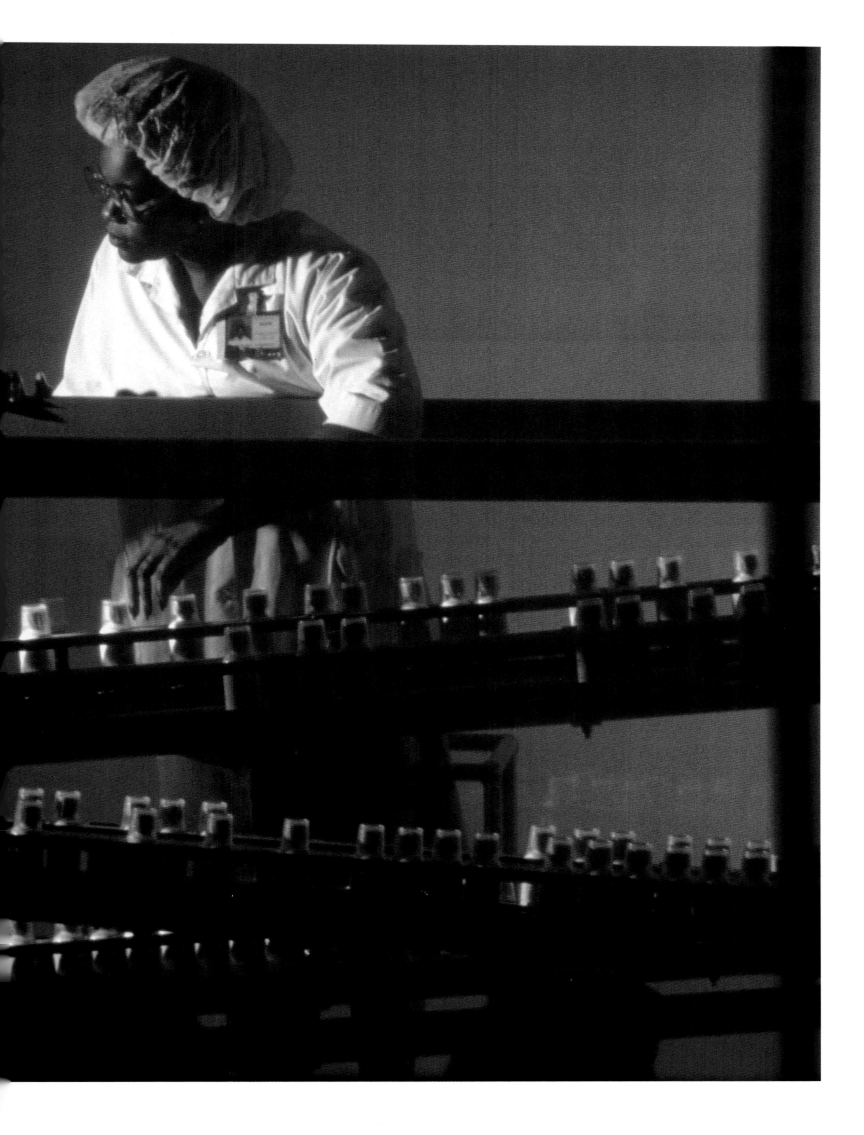

way diminishes the accomplishments of industry, the source of many breakthroughs. To cite a few examples, aspirin originated with Bayer, the sulfonamides with I.G. Farben, chlorpromazine with Rhône-Poulenc, vitamin B12 with Merck & Company, the thiazides with Merck Sharp & Dohme, reserpine with Ciba in Switzerland, and the semisynthetic penicillins with Beecham Industries. Most antibiotics and almost all the new chemical therapeutic agents introduced since 1960 can be credited to industry laboratories.

The introduction of new entities is not the only major contribution that industry has made. It has contributed on two other fronts. One is the giving of financial support to research done by private investigators. The other, which is more significant, is the processing, producing, and distributing of new medicinal agents of the highest quality. If it had not been for the work of Merck Sharp & Dohme in developing production techniques, streptomycin and related antibiotics might have remained mere bibliographic curiosities. The same might be said about insulin, which became widely available after Eli Lilly developed a means of mass-producing it. Similarly, Hoffmann-LaRoche began to manufacture vitamin C in quantity after it had developed a process for the bulk production of synthetic vitamins.

INDUSTRIAL RESPONSIBILITY

Modern scientific quality-control techniques began to make an impact on the industry in the 1920s, and by the 1950s "total quality control" had taken hold. Given the critical nature of its products, it was imperative for the industry to use exacting

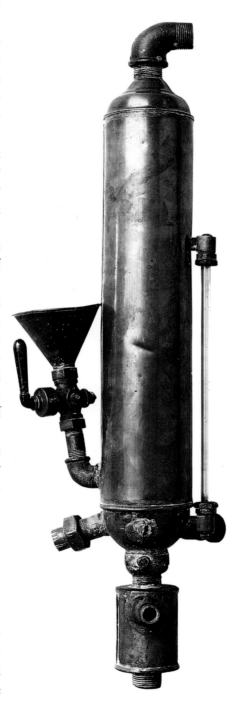

A still used in the preparation of fluid extracts. Cincinnati, c. 1880. National Museum of American History, Smithsonian Institution, Washington, D.C.

quality-control procedures. These were concerned not only with the therapeutic integrity of the final product but with characteristics demanded by the new sciences of pharmaceutics: particle size, stability, dissolution rate, hydrating or dehydrating capacities, and viscosity.

The pharmaceutical industry's capacity to provide society with means of combating disease, ameliorating discomfort, and prolonging life places upon it a tremendous social obligation. As in every industry that has developed in a capitalist society, there is a tension between the demands of society and the demands of the profit motive. The industry has been given wide latitude to carry on research, and to develop and produce as it pleases, but in the main its efforts have been directed at serious public health problems, and there have been notable successes, especially in treating infections and cardiovascular, rheumatic, and mental problems. Yet critics have pointed out that the industry has also been responsible for a proliferation of drugs that offer no new therapeutic advantage, that it makes use of high-powered marketing techniques to increase profits rather than to meet medical needs, and that in the process it contributes to unnecessary increases in the use and cost of drugs.

The Kefauver Hearings, held in the United States Senate in 1959–60, and the Sainsbury Report, issued in Great Britain in 1967, were particularly critical of the industry on such scores. Governments, especially those with social security systems that provide health care, have imposed certain restrictions on the industry. As one method of controlling costs, Spain, Italy, the Netherlands, Belgium, and France require drug manufacturers to establish the prices of their products in consultation with a government agency.

Chapter XI

THE TWENTIETH-CENTURY PHARMACIST

The most notable change in pharmacy in modern times has been the virtual disappearance of the preparation and compounding of medicines. Whereas in the 1920s, 80 percent of the prescriptions filled in American pharmacies required a knowledge of compounding, by the 1940s the number of prescriptions requiring compounding had declined to 26 percent. As far back as 1971, only 1 percent, or less, of all prescriptions combined two or more active ingredients. Moreover, the pharmacist's commitment to maintaining the quality of the drugs dispensed has been reduced to knowing such facts as the length of shelf life and the effect of exposure to light—and judging the reliability and reputation of the manufacturer.

All this meant that the pharmacist's education and activities had to undergo change. At the same time that the scientific education of pharmacists was steadily becoming more demanding, their role in the provision of health care was becoming more and more circumscribed. Moreover, they were increasingly subject to government and institutional requirements that diminished the importance of the patient-pharmacist relation. And, especially in the United States and Great Britain, competition from prescription departments in chain and department stores tended to demean both the role and the dignity of the pharmacist as a health-care professional. The urban blight that attacked neighborhoods was inevitably a threat to the friendly neighborhood pharmacist.

The reaction to these conditions was apparent in the drop in the proportion of graduates of American schools of pharmacy who were planning to go into the field of community pharmacy. In 1947, about 90 percent of graduates planned to go into some aspect of community pharmacy; in 1973, that figure had dropped to 76.6 percent; in 1988, it stood at 57.1 percent. Whereas only 3 percent of graduates planned to go into hospital pharmacy in 1947, 14.4 percent did so in 1973 and 25.1 percent in 1988. A questionnaire responded to by 770 pharmacists in actual practice in 1982 indicated that almost 30 percent were in hospital practice.

HOSPITAL PHARMACY

As a professional activity, hospital pharmacy goes back to the Arab world and to medieval times, but it was not until the nineteenth century that modern hospital pharmacy had its real beginnings. In large measure this was a French contribution—an outgrowth of military pharmacy, which was highly developed in France. In 1814, a system of pharmacy internships in the great Parisian hospitals was inaugurated; later, appointments to the post of hospital pharmacist, or apothecary, went only to those who had served an internship and had passed a competitive examination. The internship program was important not only in the recruitment of hospital pharmacists but also in stimulating young pharmacists to become scientists. In the 1800s, French hospital pharmacists made original contributions to leading journals, became members of learned societies, and were appointed to professorships on various faculties. Hospital pharmacists in France had two fundamental prerogatives as health-care professionals; first, they were in charge of a pharmacy on the premises, where they compounded and prepared the remedies used in the hospital; second, they were not required to perform any but pharmaceutical functions. In Austria and the German states, in contrast, medications were frequently provided by local apothecaries, and the operation of the hospital pharmacy was under the domination of the chief medical officer. In England and in Italy, the hospital apothecary was involved in medical care that not only required accompanying the physician on rounds but also being clinically responsible for patients when the physician was not in attendance.

Postcard view of the Pharmacie Limousin.
French, c. 1910
Overleaf

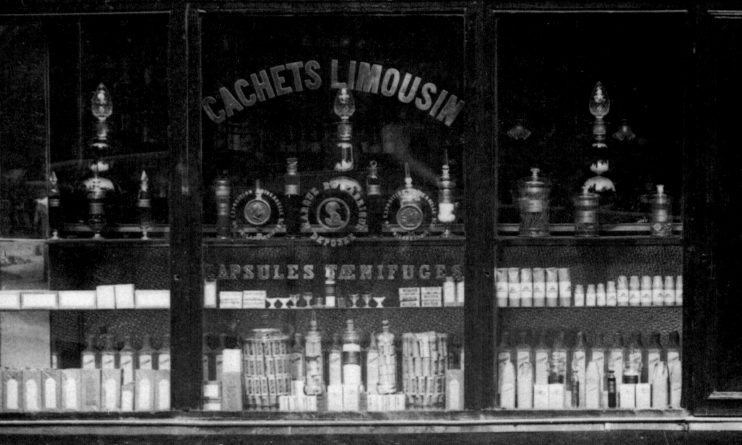

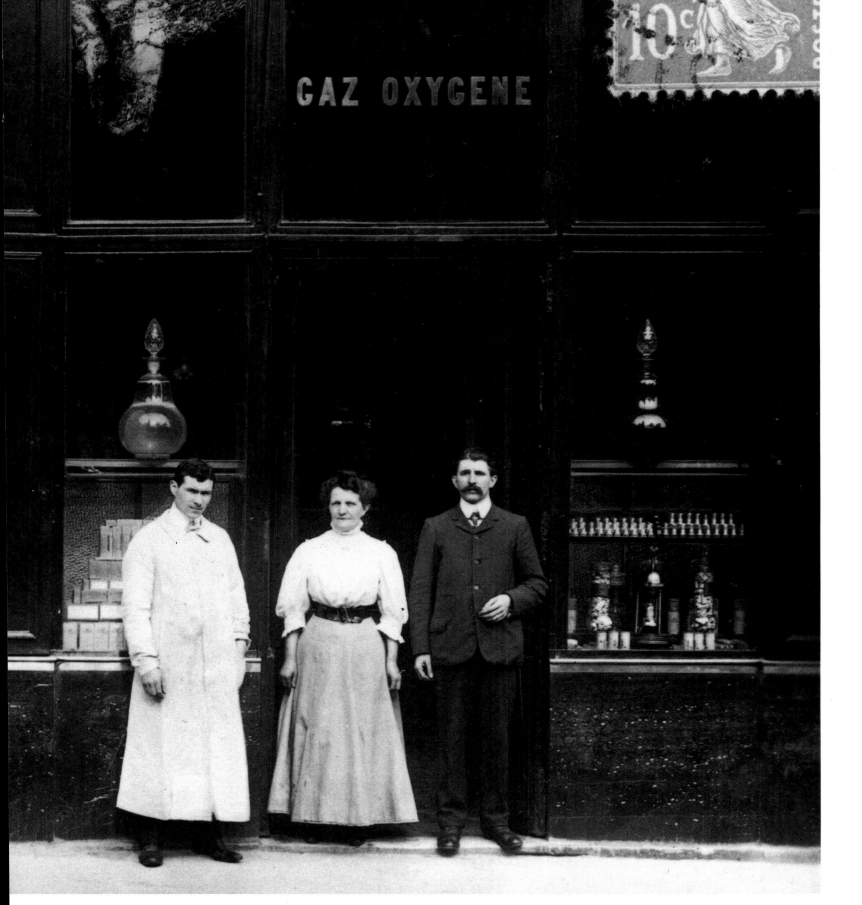

The importance of hospital pharmacy was evident as hospitals were established in French and British North America. In the seventeenth century, in Sillery, near Quebec, and in Montreal the sisters of the Hôtels-Dieu were trained and required to provide pharmaceutical services, and they continued to do so in the eighteenth century. In the 1730s and 1740s, two Jesuits trained as apothecaries served at the Hôtel-Dieu in Quebec, but the first appointment of a hospital pharmacist was in 1725, at the Royal Hospital in New Orleans. There the apothecary was provided with a laboratory—and personal perquisites to make the post attractive—and was required to provide medicines for the hospital and the garrisons. In British America, a hospital pharmacy was included in the first general hospital, the Pennsylvania Hospital, in Philadelphia, established in 1751. An apothecary, charged with making up medicines daily, was appointed in 1752. At the New York Hospital, the apothecary appointed in 1790 was given clinical responsibilities as well, following the British pattern, but after 1811 the duties of the position became entirely pharmaceutical.

The hospital reform movement that began in the last quarter of the nineteenth century had, by 1920, led, in the United States, to improved service to patients and more efficient organization. This trend increased the need for pharmacists, offered them new opportunities, and gave them a highly professional alternative to community practice. The progress of hospital pharmacy is evident: by 1936 a Subsection on Hospital Pharmacy was established under the Section on Practical Pharmacy and Dispensing of the American Pharmaceutical Association; by 1942 the American Society of Hospital Pharmacy had established its independent existence, and throughout the 1980s it maintained a membership of some 21,000 pharmacists.

Hospitals had begun as charitable institutions designed to provide care for the poor. The early hospital pharmacy could not afford to stock all the medicines that the

Interior of a German pharmacy. Engraving by Daniel Nicolaus Chodowiecki. German, 1783. Typically, an animal—here a narwhal—is suspended over the counter.

public pharmacy was required to keep on hand, and it became customary for a hospital to compile its own minimum list of drugs, or formulary. One of the most widely known of these hospital formularies, or "pharmacopoeias for the poor," was the *Pharmacopoeia pauperum* issued by the Royal Infirmary of Edinburgh in 1752. A compilation covering a group of hospitals appeared in London in 1773: *The Practice of*

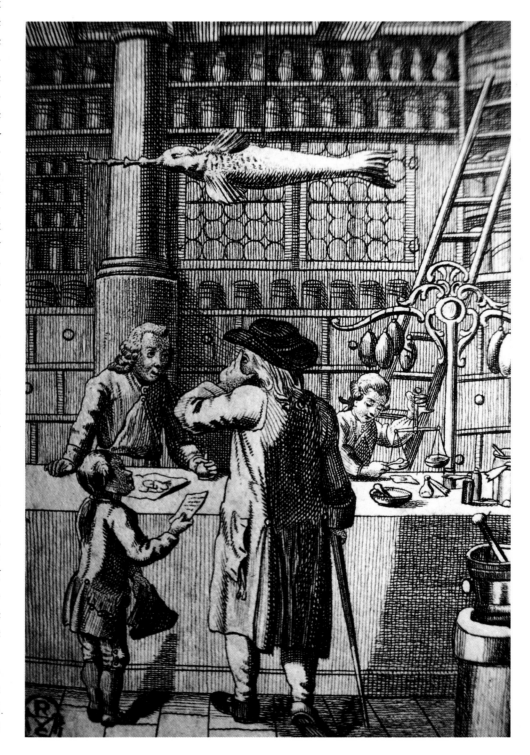

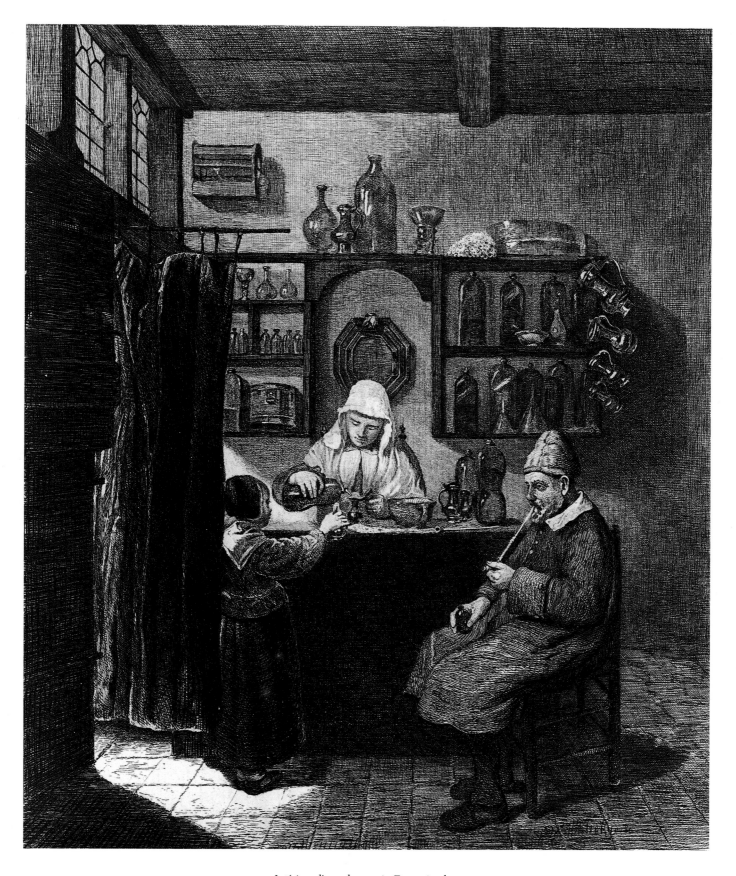

Intérieur d'une pharmacie. Engraving by
Gustave-Marie Greux after Quiringh van
Brekelenkam. French, c. 1875. This scene of a
19th-century Dutch pharmacy gives a rare
glimpse of a woman pharmacist at work. The
many women pharmacists of modern times had
relatively few precursors in earlier centuries.

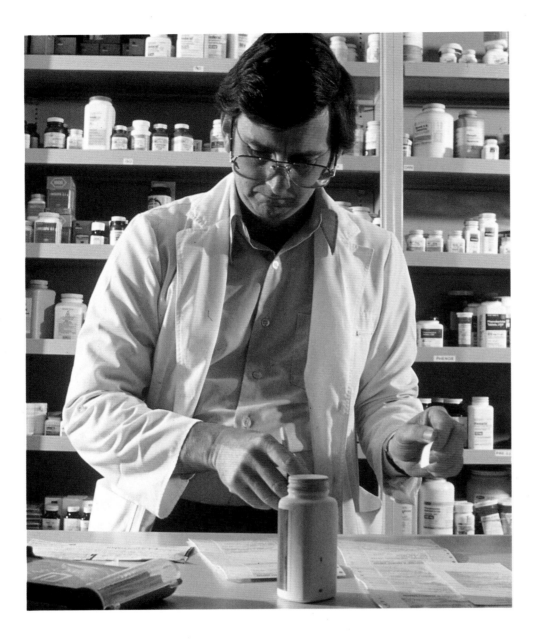

Hospital pharmacist dispensing medicine, Stanford University, Palo Alto, California. c. 1986

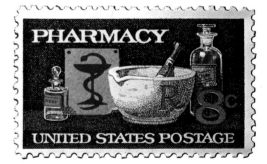

United States postage stamp, issued in 1972, honoring the profession of pharmacy—in the words of the United States Postal Service, "the friendly and dedicated men and women" who "stand with the medical profession as partners in health." Collection David L. Cowen, Rossmoor, New Jersey

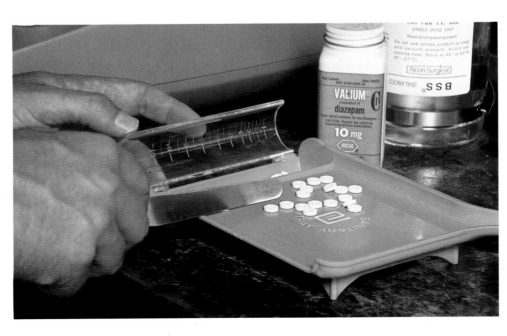

Pharmacist counting out tablets to fill a prescription

the British and French Hospitals, viz. the Edinburgh, Military and Naval Hospitals, L'Hôtel Dieu, La Charité and Les Invalides included formulas in use at all these institutions. A historic example of the hospital pharmacy formulary is one first issued in America during the Revolution—the Lititz Pharmacopoeia, so named after a Pennsylvania town that was the site of an army hospital. Compiled in wartime (1788) "for use of the military hospital belonging to the army of the Federated States of America," it was of necessity a belt-tightening formulary.

The practice of preparing hospital formularies continued throughout the nineteenth century and into the twentieth. The modern hospital formulary is a compilation of the drugs that are available in the hospital pharmacy. Except in special circumstances, the staff doctors are expected to select from it the medications they prescribe. A "pharmacy committee," made up of staff physicians and the hospital pharmacist (who is usually the permanent secretary of the committee), evaluates and selects the pharmaceuticals to be listed in the formulary. Often the staff physicians give the hospital pharmacist their prior consent to the choice of the brand of the drug (or the generic form) to be dispensed, within the guidelines of the formulary. The process of evaluating the drugs to be included in the formulary provides a basis for the selection of the drugs that are of greatest value in patient care; the prior consent given to the pharmacist, especially with the increase in generic products, makes possible economies in the cost of medication.

CLINICAL PHARMACY

Clinical pharmacy is a concept that arose in the United States in the 1940s and became nationally prominent in the 1960s. Essentially an offshoot of hospital pharmacy, it derived from the pharmacist's desire to have a more direct role in providing health care to the patient—to shift the focus

Mixing the Last Dose. Cartoon by Herbert Johnson in the *Evening Times,* Trenton, New Jersey, December 4, 1908. President Theodore Roosevelt, preparing his forthcoming message to Congress, is the pharmacist. The metaphor has been found apt by numerous political cartoonists, and other presidents, statesmen, and politicians, including Andrew Jackson, Abraham Lincoln, Ronald Reagan, Benjamin Disraeli, and William Gladstone, have been shown in similar settings.

of the pharmacist's activity from the product to the patient. The underlying assumption of clinical pharmacy is that the services of pharmacy must center on the safe use of drugs by the public. The mainstream function of pharmacy is clinical in nature; it revolves around supervision of drug use. Clinical pharmacists participate in the distribution of drugs in a clinical situation: their work takes them out of the pharmacy and onto the hospital floor. They interpret orders for medication on patients' charts, prepare medication for dispensing by the nursing staff, and, in consultation, provide drug information as required. Clinical pharmacists bring to patient care the knowledge, judgment, skills, and ethical grounding acquired in the course of their special training.

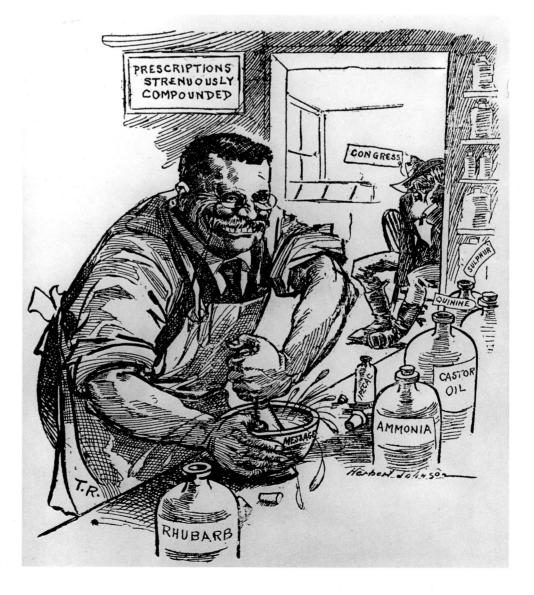

It would be a mistake to believe that all this is new. The clinical pharmacist has been reverting, perhaps unknowingly, to the involvement in clinical practice that characterized hospital apothecaries in eighteenth-century Britain and Italy. Like their earlier colleagues, modern clinical pharmacists accompany physicians on their rounds and consult with them as appropriate; unlike their predecessors, they neither examine nor prescribe. In modern practice the emphasis on clinical pharmacy reflects both the profession's ambition for greater recognition as a major force in the delivery of health care and its aim of making use of a highly scientific training and body of knowledge. In this connection there has also been a movement to involve the hospital pharmacist in the prevention of infection through improved hospital hygiene.

THE COMMUNITY PHARMACIST

The community pharmacist, probably from the time of the first pharmacy shop in the Middle Ages, advised patients, giving instructions, warnings, and recommendations and consulting with physicians about drugs. The development of clinical pharmacy in a hospital environment has carried over into the community pharmacy, where the pharmacist has assumed greater responsibility in patient monitoring and consultation. The 1969 code of ethics of the American Pharmaceutical Association, while emphasizing the pharmacist's role as "an essential health practitioner," departed from traditional practice by approving the pharmacist's disclosure of confidential information "when the best interest of the patient demanded it." The pharmacist was thus freed from the rigidity of the confidentiality requirement and could interact with the physician more directly in the care of the patient. Even more significant was the omission from the 1969 code of the age-old

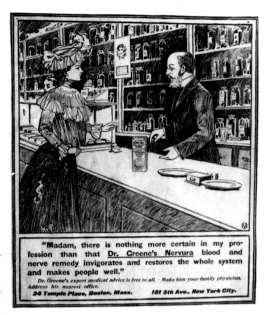

Advertisement for Dr. Greene's Nervura, a proprietary medicine, in *Popular Magazine*. American, 1902. The pharmacist prescribing remedies, as here, and the physician dispensing medications have sometimes caused problems by confusing the roles of the two professions.

Weighing Out Medicines in a Chinese Drug Store, San Francisco. Illustration by W. A. Rogers in *Harper's Weekly,* December 9, 1899. These pharmacists are carrying out very old, traditional Chinese pharmaceutical practices.

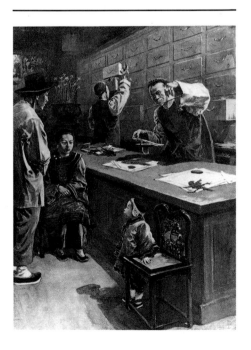

Two views of Laney's Red Lion Pharmacy in Cumberland, Maryland. c. 1890 ▶

---

provisions, explicitly stated in earlier codes, that required strict adherence to the physician's prescriptions and denied the pharmacist the right to discuss drug action with the patient.

There is a growing appreciation of the role of the pharmacist in the delivery of primary health care, powered partly by the widespread concern about misuse, side effects, and other perplexities surrounding modern medicines. A study conducted for the American Pharmaceutical Association in 1987 indicated that 87 percent of the 266 pharmacist respondents were "involved in some type of patient counseling." In California, the pharmacist is permitted to prescribe drugs in an institutional setting; in the state of Washington, pharmacists may develop protocols with physicians under which the pharmacist may prescribe for the physician's patients; and in Florida a 1985 law provides for the establishment of a state formulary from which the community pharmacist may prescribe for a patient. The modern pharmacist, trained in all aspects of pharmacy and pharmaceutics, has increasingly moved into the role of consultant—not only to the patient but also to the physician, to the hospital and other health-care facilities, to the insurance company, and to the government.

THE REGULATION OF DISPENSING

In the nineteenth century, control over the purity of food and drugs was largely left to the individual states. The century saw a frightening level of drug addiction, to a great extent iatrogenic, since opium and its derivatives were among the most frequently prescribed drugs. There was also a tremendous growth in the consumption of proprietary medicines, many of them addictive. Yet well into the century the pharmacist's freedom to dispense drugs had been limited only by professional ethics (filling a prescription required dispensing precisely

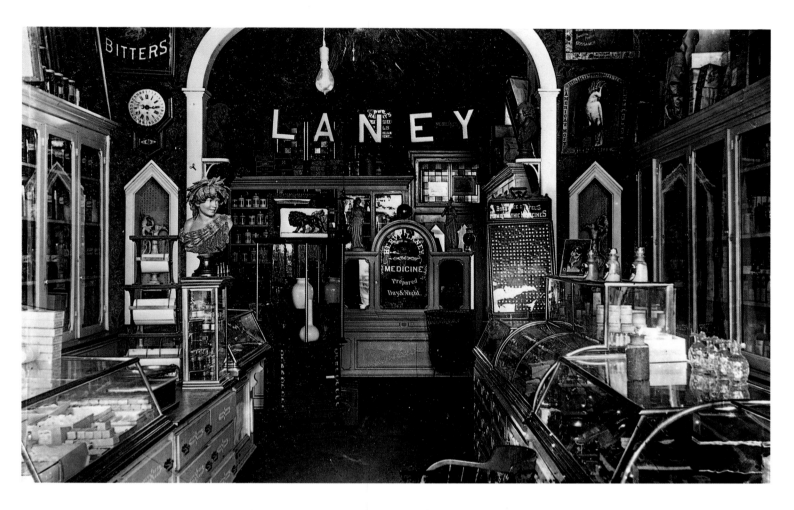

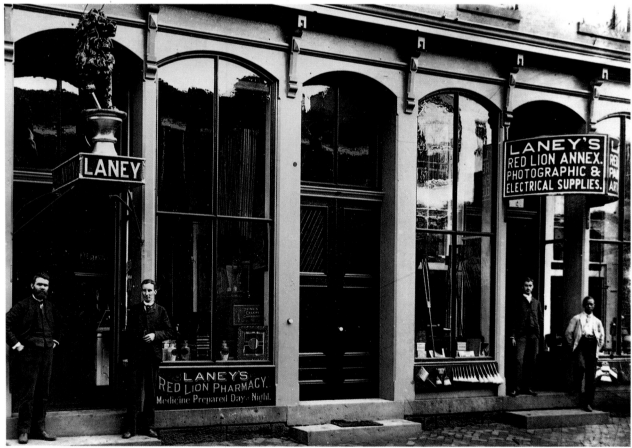

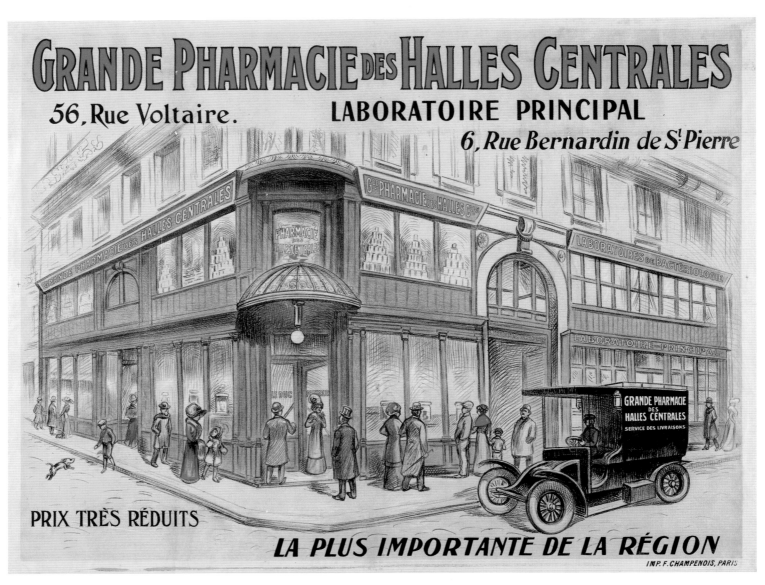

Poster for the Grande Pharmacie des Halles Centrales in Le Havre. Color lithograph. French, c. 1905. The pharmacy's delivery vehicle has a prominent place in this promotion piece. Ars Medica Collection, Philadelphia Museum of Art

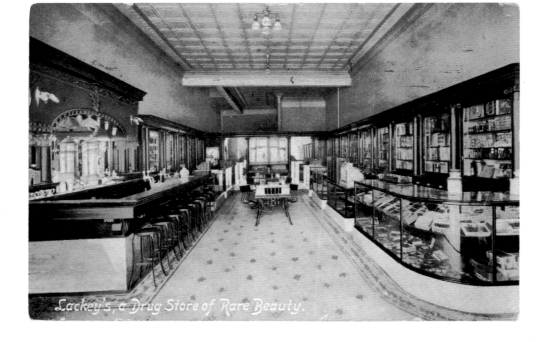

Postcard view of the interior of Lackey's pharmacy, "a Drug Store of Rare Beauty," in Fort Worth, Texas. 1908

Poster for Pharmacie Canonne, "La Pharmacie des Gens Economes," Paris. Color lithograph by Bellenger. French, 1944 ▶

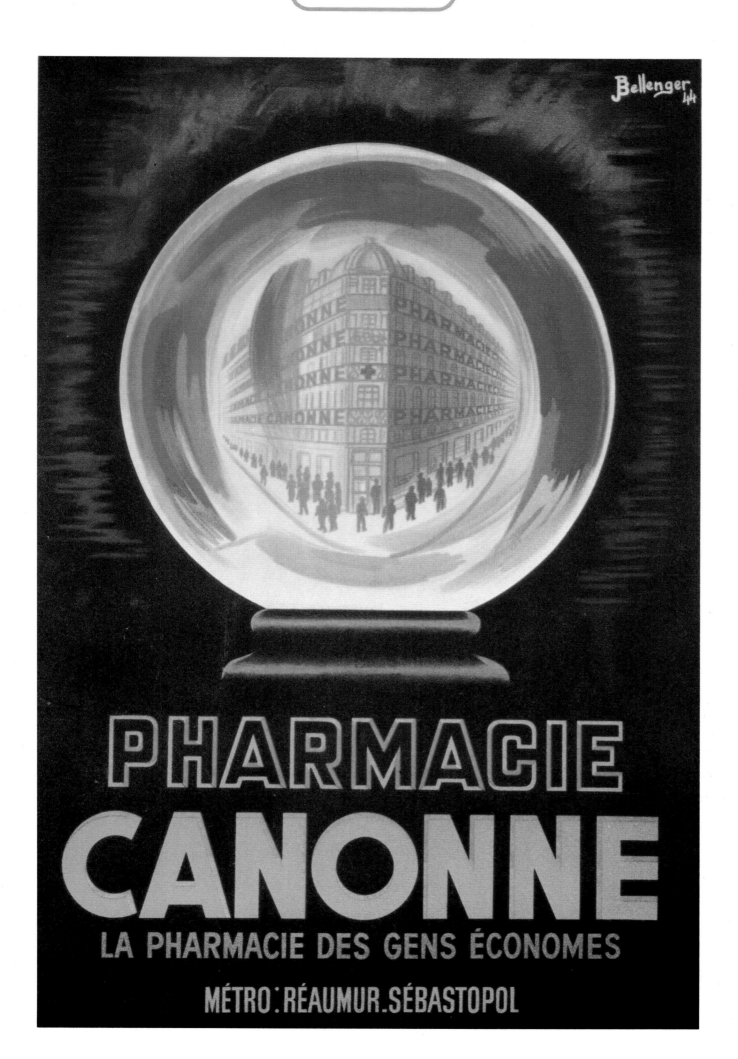

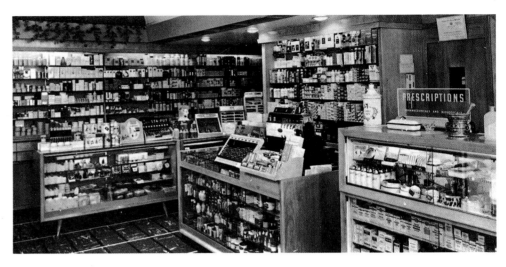

what the physician prescribed) and by the fact that the drugs dispensed were subject to inspection by professional or quasi-public pharmaceutical boards. The pharmacist could in fact dispense drugs without a prescription; opium could be obtained over the counter.

The twentieth century added to the pharmaceutical armamentarium a vast range of new chemical drugs—effective, powerful, and often potentially dangerous. Under these circumstances, such considerations as the purity, efficacy, and safety of drugs became matters of public concern, and the freedom of the pharmacist and the pharmaceutical industry to create and market new products—and the right of the physician to prescribe these products—were radically curtailed.

In the United States, regulation on the national level began with the Pure Food and Drug Act of 1906. The act sought to correct abuses in the proprietary medicine industry by requiring, among other things, listing on the label the presence and the amount of certain dangerous drugs—alcohol, the opiates, chloral hydrate, acetanilide—and by proscribing "false and misleading" statements on the label. The effectiveness of the act was limited by court decisions that narrowly defined "false and misleading" and by the absence of any provision for the control of advertising.

The inadequate 1906 law was superseded in 1938 by the Food, Drug, and Cosmetic Act, which covered ethical as well as proprietary drugs. Its most significant provision pertaining to drugs was the requirement that a new drug had to have the approval of the Food and Drug Administration, predicated on the demonstrated safety of the drug. The legislative demand for this more rigorous regulation had been spurred by the public furor over 107 deaths reported in 1937 from an "elixir" of sulfanilamide in which diethylene glycol was used as the solvent. In 1962, the Kefauver-Harris Amendments added the significant requirement of proof of efficacy for F.D.A. approval. The passage of these amendments was

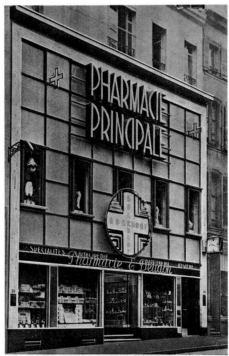

E. DELIDON, 20, Rue Saint-Dizier, NANCY
TÉLÉPHONE 68.57   Compte Chèques Postaux Nancy N° 248

Postcard views of pharmacies in New York, Philadelphia, and Nancy, France, of the period 1930–1959

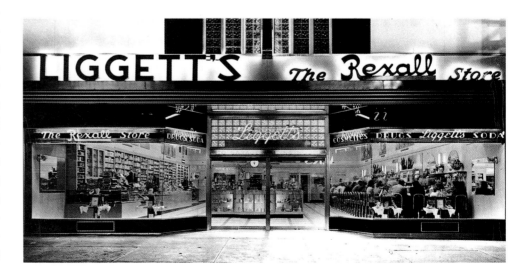

sparked by another tragic finding—that thalidomide, a sleeping pill developed in Europe, but never marketed in the United States, caused birth deformities.

With the new requirement of proof of efficacy added to the requirement of proof of safety, putting a new drug on the market became a detailed, lengthy, and time-consuming process, both in the preparation and in the approval routine. Requirements in the United States are among the most stringent in the world, and it may take from seven to ten years from the time a chemical substance becomes an active product candidate to the time when it receives final approval. Legislation passed in 1984 restored some of the effective patent life lost during the F.D.A. approval process.

The problem of narcotic addiction that had plagued the nineteenth century continued into the twentieth. In the United States the only measure taken to deal with the narcotics problem was the provision in the Pure Food and Drug Act of 1906 requiring that the label of a proprietary medicine containing a narcotic drug name the drug. The international scope of the narcotics problem led to an international conference at The Hague, which produced, in 1912, the Hague Opium Convention. This treaty obligated its signatories to place controls over opium and coca traffic; the United States set the pattern for such regulation in the Harrison Narcotic Act of 1914. Under that law, the pharmacist could dispense addictive substances only on prescription, and only physicians having a special federal license could prescribe or dispense such substances. It was with the Harrison Act that the United States began its ongoing campaign to curtail the illicit drug trade and to curb addiction through law enforcement agencies. This policy is in contrast with that of Great Britain, which has adopted an approach that treats addiction as an illness requiring medical attention.

Even before the Harrison Act, state legislatures in the United States had passed laws prohibiting the dispensing of narcotic substances except by prescription. Such legis-

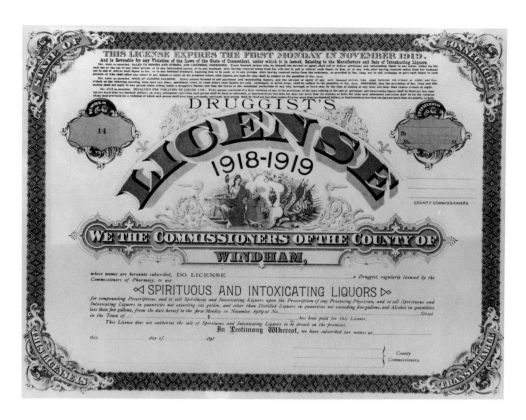

Druggist's license, dated 1918–1919, issued in Windham County, Connecticut, authorizing the holder "to use Spiritous and Intoxicating Liquors for compounding prescriptions upon the Prescription of any Practicing Physician, and to sell Spiritous and Intoxicating Liquors upon the Prescription of any Practicing Physician...."

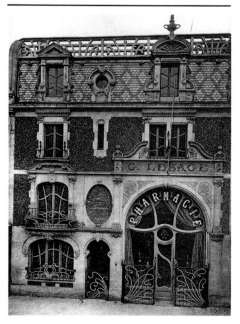

Postcard view of the pharmacy of G. Lesage, La Délivrande, with a fine Art Nouveau facade. French, c. 1910

lation had been met with some ambivalence by pharmacists, who recognized the need but anticipated a loss of business. However, by 1915 most states had passed laws modeled after the Harrison Act, sometimes on the initiative or with the approval of pharmaceutical associations. Indeed, the record of pharmacy, where abuses could readily have occurred, was praiseworthy. Pharmacists have long been numbered among the forces arrayed against the social degradation and the serious social and political problems of contemporary society created by the use of and traffic in illicit drugs. In 1962, the United States Commissioner of Narcotics stated that there was no evidence pointing to "pharmacists as being in any way responsible for one case among 46,000 nonmedical addicts known to the authorities." Pharmacists, he continued "accounted for uncovering more forged prescriptions than federal, state, and city authorities combined."

The control of narcotic substances set the precedent for the control of the plethora of powerful medicinal agents that became available in the latter half of the twentieth century. In the United States, "controlled

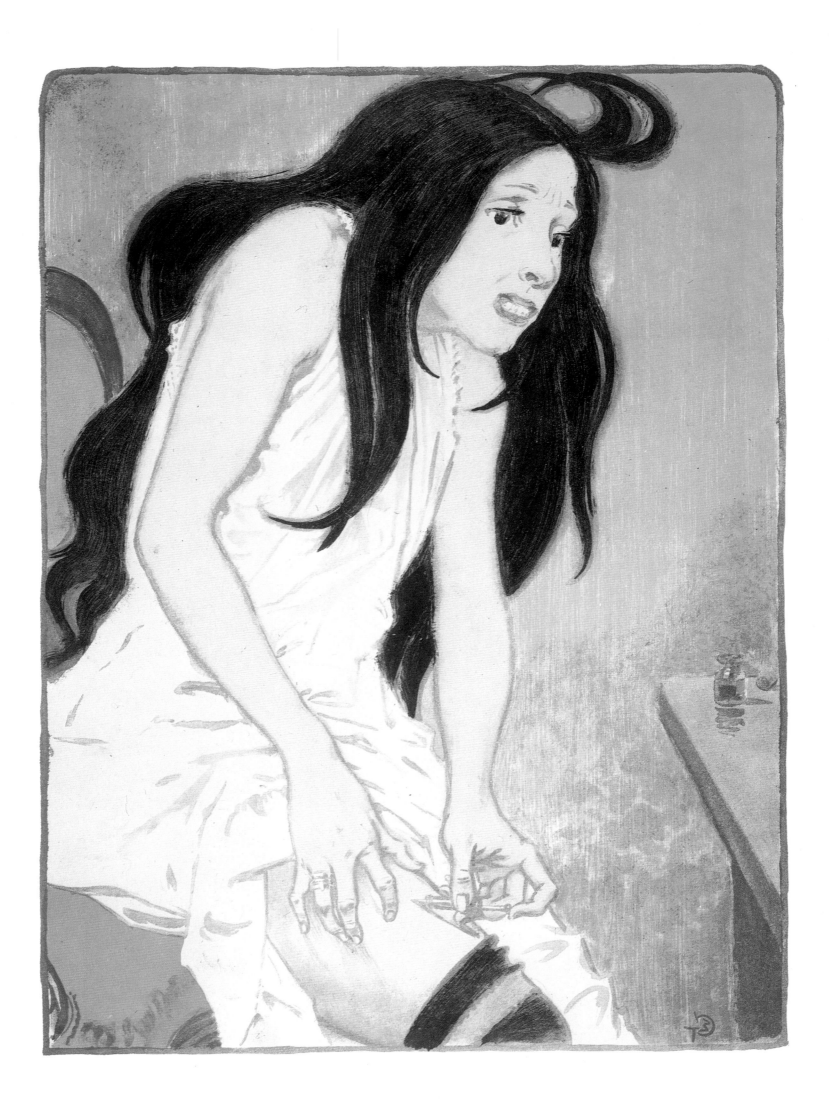

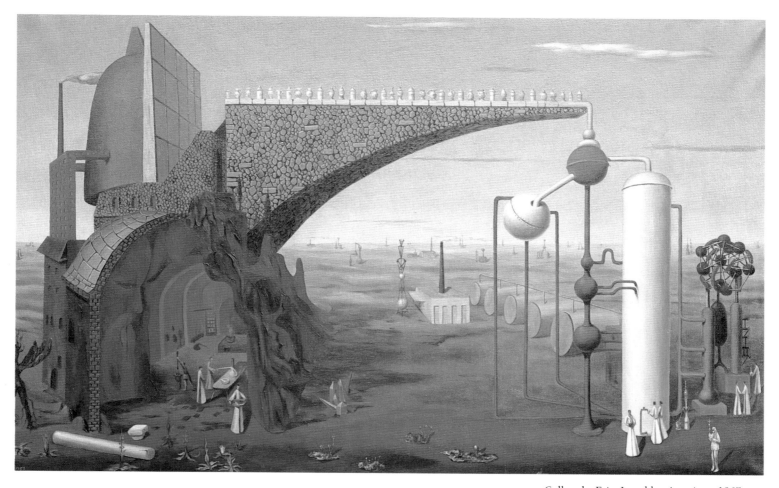

Morphinomanie. Color lithograph by Eugène-Samuel Grasset. French, 1897. A striking image of the intensity and horror of drug addiction. Ars Medica Collection, Philadelphia Museum of Art

◄

The Citadel of Drugs. Painting by Franco Assetto. Italian, 1955. A surrealist view of the progress of pharmacy. Associazione Titolari di Farmacia della Provincia di Torino, Turin

Collage by Fritz Janschka. American, 1967. Pharmaceutical advertisements, trade cards, homeopathic pills, and pages from proprietary medicine booklets are combined in this inventive work. Collection Philadelphia College of Pharmacy and Science

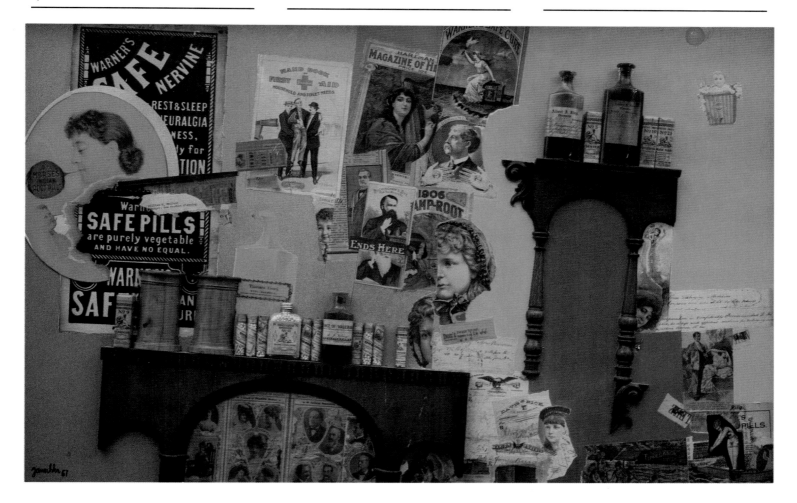

substances"—narcotic, tranquilizing and psychoactive drugs—can be dispensed only under a complex and strict set of conditions laid down by federal laws. Federal law established another class of drugs, "legend drugs" (controlled substances and legend drugs are not mutually exclusive classes), which are restricted to sale and use under medical supervision and bear the legend "Federal law prohibits dispensing without a prescription."

PHARMACY AND SOCIAL CONTROLS

Pharmacy in the twentieth century functions in a socioeconomic framework that owes much to the program of social insurance inaugurated by Bismarck in Germany. In 1883, the Iron Chancellor, seeking to head off the mounting socialist furor and the growing strength of labor, established a system of national health insurance. A network of local health insurance bodies was created. It was financed by employer and worker contributions, but in some instances the government paid the worker's share. These local bodies exerted considerable control over both physician and pharmacist, and numerous restrictions were placed on the pharmacist in the dispensing of medicines. Most important, pharmacists operated within a closely regulated system, and their incomes were based on government price lists.

By the 1950s, social security systems were worldwide and most of them covered pharmacy. In countries where private enterprise predominated, pharmacists continued to be entrepreneurs, though their activity and their income were circumscribed.

In Great Britain, national health insurance was first provided in 1911, but it covered only about one-third of the population. The National Health Services Act, which went into effect in 1948, provided health insurance for everyone. Since Na-

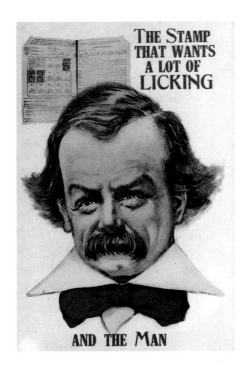

The Stamp That Wants a Lot of Licking—and the Man. Postcard. English, 1912. The government in which David Lloyd George was chancellor of the exchequer brought national health insurance to Great Britain in 1911. To finance it, employers paid the tax by purchasing stamps at the post office and affixing them to employees' records.

tional Health provides complete medical, surgical, dental, hospital, and pharmaceutical care, the British chemist-and-druggist runs a private enterprise in which it is mainly the government, not the patient, that pays the costs of medication.

In France, as in Germany, pharmacy continued to be a private enterprise. The Code de la Santé Publique restricted ownership of pharmacies to pharmacists and prohibited pharmacists from owning more than one pharmacy. The prices charged by the pharmacist for official preparations are based on a governmental *tarif pharmaceutique* and are arrived at with agreement of the manufacturer. For "reimbursed specialties"—that is, ethical drugs with brand names—the patient pays the pharmacist directly and usually receives a refund for part of the cost from the insurance fund. The amount refunded varies with the nature of the drug prescribed.

Socialized medicine made little headway in the United States. The medical establishment, sometimes joined by organized pharmacy, opposed any suggestion of compulsory health insurance, considering it not in keeping with the American way. Indeed, the medical establishment opposed as unethical medical contracts under which voluntary health insurance programs operated. In time, however, the medical establishment was forced to become involved in, and even initiate, such programs. By the 1940s, large groups of people were covered by one type of voluntary insurance program or another. But compared with programs in other countries, benefits were limited in scope. In the 1950s, expanded coverage of voluntary health insurance began to include pharmaceutical services, and insurance programs covering prepaid prescriptions developed.

Except for relief and welfare programs during the Depression, and except for provisions of the Social Security Act that covered the disabled, the aged, and the sick poor, the United States government did not become involved in official health insurance coverage until the 1960s. It was not

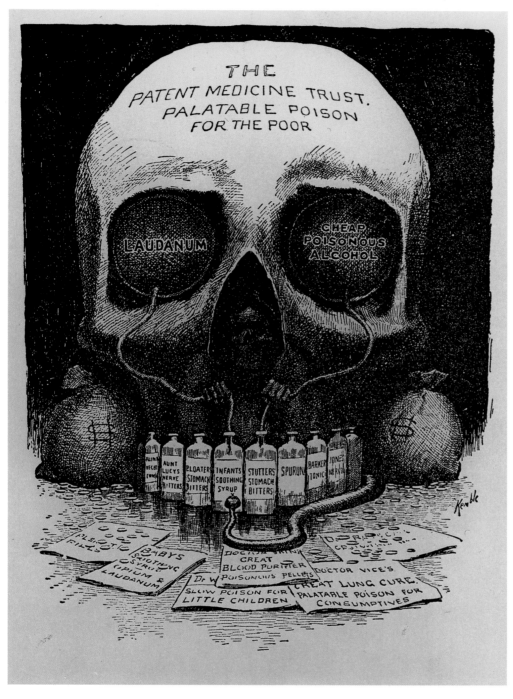

until 1965 that the federal Medicare and Medicaid programs were established. The former is an insurance program paid for by contributions from both individuals and their employers; it covers portions of most aspects of medical and surgical care. Pharmaceuticals are not included, except as part of hospital care. Medicaid is not an insurance program but a system of federal and state allowances for medical care for the medically indigent. Under Medicaid, states can provide for prescription service.

Cartoon by Edward W. Kemble in *Collier's Weekly,* June 3, 1905, illustrating Samuel Hopkins Adams's series of articles on proprietary medicines, entitled "The Great American Fraud." This exposé contributed to the passage of the Pure Food and Drug Act of 1906.

Increasingly, the pharmacist receives governmental and private third-party payment of fees. These arrangements may not be entirely to pharmacists' liking, for they now find themselves involved in bureaucratic procedures, their independence as practitioners impinged upon, and the value of their services determined by others. These are the adjustments the pharmacist must make in a complex society that attempts to provide health care for all.

WOMEN IN PHARMACY

A concomitant of the twentieth-century reform of hospitals and the rise of hospital pharmacy was the opportunity it provided, especially in the United States, for women to find a vocation in pharmacy. It had not been easy for women to enter the profession in the nineteenth century. The history of pharmacy, like that of other professions, is one of the virtual exclusion of women on the basis of the familiar clichés about women's intellectual inadequacies, biological handicaps, and unsuitability for work outside the home—clichés that began to be challenged by proponents of the women's movement from the mid-nineteenth century onward. The first female to receive a degree in pharmacy in the United States was Mary C. Putnam (1842–1906), who graduated from the New York College of Pharmacy in 1863. However, she did not practice pharmacy but became a physician, like her husband, Abraham Jacobi, a noted pediatrician. Other, less noted young women became pharmacists, but it was not until the American Conference of Pharmaceutical Faculties stated, in 1879, that women should be admitted to schools of pharmacy, that explicit invitations to women were included in school announcements. Yet during the academic year 1889–90 there were only 60 female, as compared with 2,811 male, students enrolled in schools of pharmacy in the United States; women did not compose even 5 percent of the total number of students enrolled in pharmacy programs at the end of the century. An unusual venture, the Louisville School of Pharmacy for Women, in Kentucky, had functioned for only nine years, from 1883 to 1892.

In the twentieth century, under the impact of the "second wave" of the women's movement in our time, the barriers to women's entry into pharmacy, as well as other professions, began to come down. It is perhaps no coincidence that this change came at about the same time that hospital pharmacy was beginning to flourish. In the United States in 1954, fewer than 10 percent of undergraduate pharmacy degrees went to women; by 1971 this had reached 20 percent and by 1976, 30 percent. In 1988, it was estimated that about 60 percent of students in American colleges of pharmacy were women. In 1985, for the first time, pharmacy degrees awarded to women in the United States outnumbered those awarded to men, 3,092 to 2,643. At the Faculty of Pharmacy of the University of Toronto, female students constituted over two-thirds of the student body in the decade 1975–85.

The reasons for the preponderance of women currently entering the field of pharmacy in the United States and Canada are not hard to find. Pharmacy offers an opportunity to attain professional status and carries with it a considerable degree of independence. And the new institutional patterns provide opportunities exceeding those of the community pharmacy.

In Europe, a similar pattern of discrimination against women in pharmacy prevailed until late in the nineteenth century. The Pharmaceutical Society's School in London did not officially admit women as students until 1872, and it was not until 1879 that the Society admitted a woman to membership. In Germany, where women were not admitted to universities until the end of the nineteenth century, they were denied access to the study of sciences altogether until 1908. Women were allowed to work in pharmacies, however, from 1898.

Perhaps the most typical illustration of discrimination against women is to be found in Poland, although that country has the distinction of being the first to give degrees in pharmacy to women. In 1824, master of pharmacy degrees were conferred by the Jagiellonian University on two Sisters of Charity, Filipa and Konstancja Studzinska, who had been obliged to study privately with the Associate Professor of Pharmacy because, as was stated in their diplomas, "decency did not allow them to take advantage of the lectures in a public place." However, the examinations that they passed were given before the Dean and Senate of the University.

The profession of pharmacy was clearly opening up to women in Europe in the late nineteenth century. Between 1863 and 1872 the universities of Paris, Zurich, Lausanne, Bern, and Geneva, in that order, began to permit women to study pharmacy. In the Netherlands, a woman was admitted to the practice of pharmacy in 1872, and pharmaceutical diplomas were conferred upon fifteen women in the next twenty years. In Belgium, seventeen women qualified as pharmacists between 1881 and 1891, and in Sweden discrimination against women in the study and practice of pharmacy ended in 1891. The tremendous change that has taken place is illustrated by the fact that in 1985 women constituted 57.5 percent of the pharmacists on the lists of the French Ordre des Pharmaciens.

It should be noted that women did have an association with pharmacy in premodern times. Widows of pharmacists were usually permitted to continue to operate their husbands' shops, and although they were generally required to hire a pharmacist "provisor," they sometimes simply assumed the role and title of pharmacist without being licensed. The involvement of nuns in monastic pharmaceutical activities, going back at least to the Renaissance, has already been cited. The major role played by women in pharmacy before the days of equality of the sexes, however, was as pharmacy assistants. In Europe, this reflected not only the prevailing patronizing attitude toward women but also the limited opportunities available to men, given the limitations on the number of pharmacies and the difficulty in breaking into a system of concessions and privileges. It is still common in Europe to find women as pharmacists serving patrons under the supervision of the shop owner. But with the breakdown of the limitations on ownership, number, and location of pharmacies, ownership of pharmacies by qualified women has become somewhat more common.

EDUCATING THE NEW PHARMACIST

Pharmaceutical education had to make rapid adaptations to several forces that came together in the twentieth century: the decline in compounding, the vast array of new drugs requiring knowledge of medicinal chemistry, the advances in pharmacology, the development of new sciences of pharmaceutics, and the rise of hospital and clinical pharmacy were some of the forces at work.

The most obvious impact of these forces on pharmaceutical education was the lengthening of the time required to obtain a pharmaceutical degree. A survey made in 1954 showed that of the forty-seven countries for which there was information, thirty-one required four or more years of education. A survey made in 1980 showed that in the eleven states of the European Economic Community (Common Market) and the seven states of the Council for Mutual Economic Assistance (COMECON) only two, Great Britain and West Germany, had arrangements that still made possible qualification with fewer than four years of education. The practical requirement of clerkship or internship in a pharmacy, harking back to apprenticeship days, remained in force, with the length of time required varying from country to country.

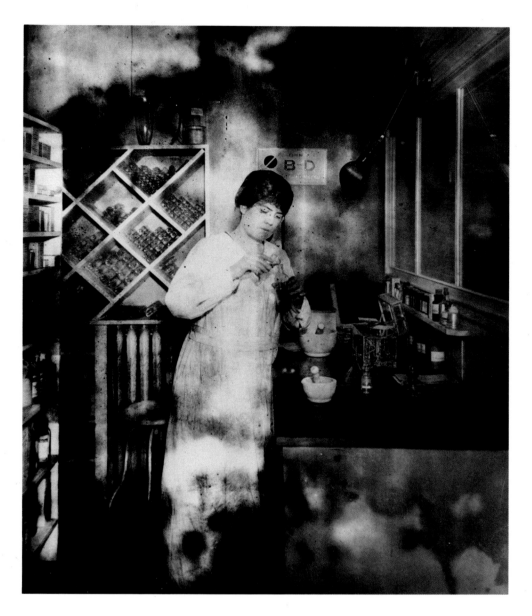

Pharmacist preparing a prescription in Denver, Colorado. c. 1910

West Germany, for example, required only three years of pharmaceutical study in 1954, but they had to be preceded by two years and followed by one year of practical work in a pharmacy.

In the United States, a two-year program leading to the graduate in pharmacy degree was superseded by a three-year program leading to that degree; in 1925, a three-year program of study was made a requirement for accreditation of schools of pharmacy. In 1932, a four-year program leading to a bachelor of pharmacy or bachelor of science in pharmacy degree was made mandatory. But four years proved insufficient to prepare pharmacists for the new roles they were beginning to assume—to produce broadly educated pharmacists versed in the new scientific advances. Consequently, a five-year program, also leading to the bachelor's degree, went into effect in 1960. By 1986, twenty-eight schools offered, in addition to the five-year program, a six-year program leading to the doctor of pharmacy degree, and six schools offered only the six-year program. In the academic year 1987–88 American schools of pharmacy conferred 5,376 baccalaureate degrees and 972 doctor of pharmacy degrees.

The new doctorate in pharmacy did not supplant the ongoing graduate work in the pharmaceutical sciences. The first doctor of philosophy degree in pharmaceutical sciences in the United States was granted by the University of Wisconsin in 1902; by 1927, at least nine schools were offering master's degrees and four were offering the Ph.D. In 1987–88, records show that 264 doctor of philosophy degrees were awarded by 46 American schools of pharmacy, and 353 master of science degrees were awarded by 51 schools. European universities offered similar doctoral programs in the pharmaceutical sciences.

INTERNATIONAL PHARMACY

In 1865, on the joint invitation of the pharmaceutical associations of north and south Germany, an International Congress of Pharmacy was held in Brunswick. This was the first of a series of such congresses held at irregular intervals until 1935. After 1935, the congresses continued to meet, but usually in connection with meetings of the Fédération Internationale Pharmaceutique. The impetus for the initial congress was the distress of pharmacists over the impact of proprietary medicines on the profession and their determination to develop international standards for drugs. The congresses proved valuable as a forum for the discussion of scientific advances and common problems.

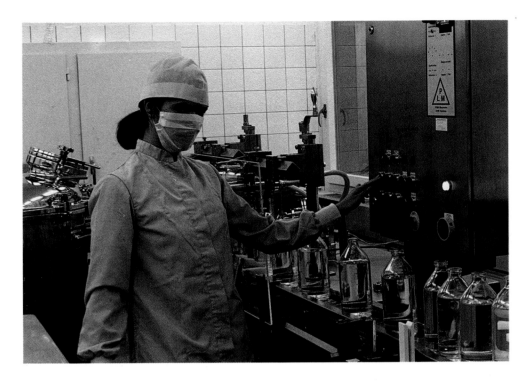

Large-scale production of intravenous parenterals in the Stadtspital Waid, Zurich. 1980s

Loosely organized, these congresses had neither permanent staff nor permanent membership. The Dutch Pharmaceutical Association therefore proposed the creation of a permanent body, and in 1911 the Fédération Internationale Pharmaceutique (F.I.P.) came into existence, with headquarters and a secretariat at The Hague. The first general assembly of the F.I.P. was held at The Hague in 1912, and, except when prevented by the exigencies of war, the organization has continued to meet annually. Originally a federation of national pharmaceutical associations, the F.I.P. opened its membership to other interested organizations and to individuals, and in 1988 eighty countries were represented in its membership.

There have been some tangible accomplishments in which the F.I.P. has played a significant role. An International Agreement for the Unification of the Formulae of Potent Drugs, which had resulted from a conference called by Belgium in 1902 and been ratified by eighteen states in 1906, was revised and enlarged by a committee of the F.I.P. The revision, which set standards for twenty-seven potent drugs, regulating method of preparation, nomenclature, and maximum doses, was accepted by the second intergovernmental convention on the subject in 1925, with twenty-six governments signing the final protocol. The agreement was ratified in 1929.

In 1937 the League of Nations set up a Technical Commission of Pharmacopoeial Experts to establish an international pharmacopoeia. After World War II, the World Health Organization established the W.H.O. Expert Committee on the Unification of Pharmacopoeias. An active committee, it produced the two-volume *Pharmacopoea Internationalis,* published by W.H.O. in 1951 and 1955. It appeared in English, French, and Spanish, and later in German and Japanese translations. A second edition appeared in 1967; the last segment of its third edition was published in 1988. The *Pharmacopoea Internationalis,* which never attained legal status, serves, as intended, as a reference and guide for national pharmacopoeias.

Success came to two other international efforts. The *Pharmacopoea Nordica* gained recognition as the national pharmacopoeia in Norway, Sweden, Denmark, Iceland, and Finland in the 1960s. In 1963, a European Pharmacopoeia Convention signed under the auspices of the Council of Europe provided for the compilation of a *European Pharmacopoeia*. Intended to provide "uniform control methods and standards of quality for medicines," it was published in two volumes in 1969 and 1971 and updated thereafter. By 1989, nineteen countries, including all the countries of the European Economic Community except Spain, had given official status to the *European Pharmacopoeia*.

A new dimension was added to the practice and regulation of pharmacy by post–World War II international developments: the World Health Organization issued a series of guidelines known as "Good Practices in the Manufacture and Quality Control of Drugs," and the European Community has become active in establishing standards for the quality control of drugs, standards for the education of the pharmacist, and arrangements for the reciprocal recognition of pharmaceutical qualifications within the member states.

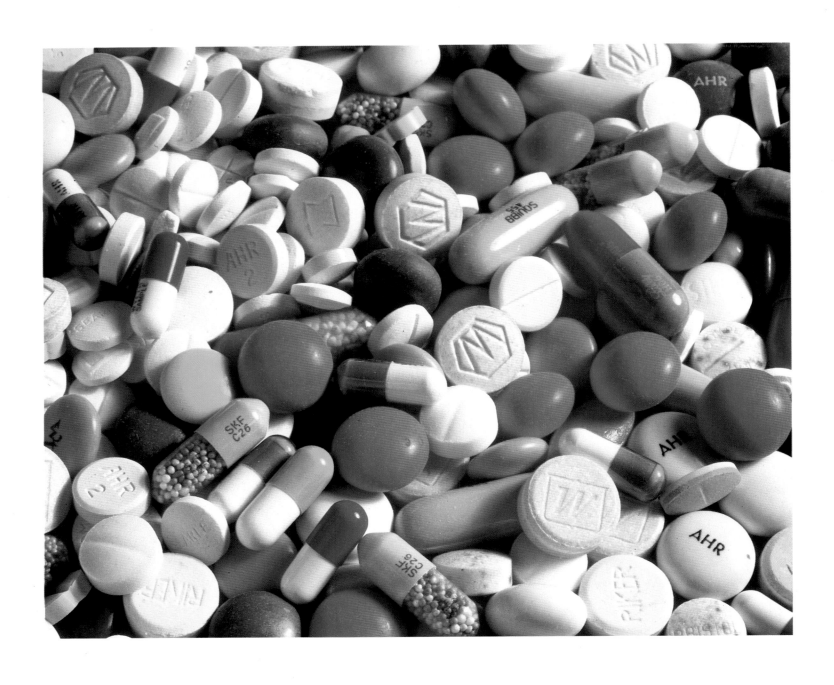

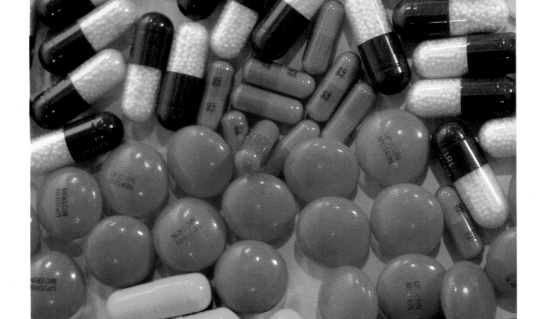

Coated tablets and sustained-action capsules.
c. 1980. Modern oral dosage forms are designed
in a variety of shapes and colors, in part to
provide accurate identification.

The practice of pharmacy has always had to reconcile the conflicting demands of commercial and professional aspirations. It is no accident that there exists, in the United States, both an American Pharmaceutical Association and a National Association of Retail Druggists. The contemporary movement toward hospital, institutional, and consulting pharmacy will undoubtedly continue, and in such settings the pharmacist will take on an increasingly important role in the delivery of health care. The future of the community pharmacy is less certain: these pharmacists have found it difficult to make full use of their expertise from behind the modern prescription counter. In some countries this is because of the availability of technical assistants who can perform the essential services of the pharmacy shop. In other countries, primarily the United States, it is because physicians have continued to dispense pharmaceutical products to their patients.

Contemporary pharmacists are faced with social changes that have made them part of a bureaucratic system, governmental or private, of drug delivery. Already aware that much of the advice they are capable of giving has been programmed into computers and will automatically appear on the prescription label, they face the specter of the complete automation of dispensing. Such considerations undoubtedly mean great changes in the pharmacy shop, the practice of pharmacy, and pharmaceutical education.

Regardless of the direction pharmacy takes, the search for effective pharmaceuticals will remain a challenge that must be met. It has been a long road from the local guilds of medieval towns to the Fédération Internationale Pharmaceutique. The overwhelming changes in the materia pharmaceutica—from crude natural products of the vegetable, animal, and mineral kingdoms to highly complex chemical substances—are symbols of our ascent from magic, tradition, and trial-and-error empiricism to science and technology.

Moreover, there is a dynamism in the approach modern civilization takes to pharmacotherapy. The history of pharmacy has been punctuated by revolutionary changes, and a new and even more exciting revolution is just beginning. Biotechnology, genetic engineering, and space exploration suggest that the golden age of pharmacotherapy is still to come. The use of recombinant DNA, for example, has made it possible to obtain large quantities of complex human proteins; insulin, interferon, and growth hormones have already been obtained by this process.

The pharmaceutical industry in the United States and other countries has sensed the potential of this new research and has become heavily involved in it. Research conducted in space can provide attributes not available on earth, such as microgravity and lack of atmospheric attenuation, and pharmaceutical researchers are anticipating a variety of new pharmaceutical products created "out of this world." A new era of pharmaceutical discovery is at hand. Thanks to it, humanity can look forward to further prolongation of life, amelioration of pain and discomfort, and improvement in the quality of life.

SOURCES

The following references are sources used by the authors, not a complete bibliography of the areas covered. Works named in the text are not listed here unless they served as specific sources. An asterisk (*) denotes a reference also used in a subsequent chapter or chapters.

GENERAL

Bouvet, M. *Histoire de la pharmacie en France des origines à nos jours.* Paris, Editoriale Occitania, 1937.

Burns, E. M., and Ralph, P. L. *World Civilization from Ancient to Contemporary.* 3d ed. New York, Norton, 1964.

Cowen, D. L. "Pharmacy and Civilization," *American Journal of Pharmaceutical Education,* 22, 1958, pp. 70–76.

[Cowen, D. L., ed.] *Medallic History of Pharmacy.* Chicago, Medical Heritage Society, 1972.

Dann, G. E. *Einführung in die Geschichte der Pharmazie.* Stuttgart, Wissenschaftliche Verlagsgesellschaft, 1975.

Flückiger, F. A., and Hanbury, D. *Pharmacographia: A History of the Principal Drugs of Vegetable Origin.* London, Macmillan, 1874.

Matthews, L. G. *History of Pharmacy in Britain.* Edinburgh, Livingstone, 1962.

Schelenz, H. *Geschichte der Pharmazie.* Berlin, Springer Verlag, 1904.

Schmitz, R. *Mörser, Kolben und Phiolen aus der Welt der Pharmazie.* Stuttgart, Franckh'sche Verlagshandlung, 1966.

Shryock, R. H. *The Development of Modern Medicine.* New York, Knopf, 1947.

Sonnedecker, G. *Kremers and Urdang's History of Pharmacy.* 4th ed. Philadelphia, Lippincott, 1976.

Wittop Koning, D. A. *Art and Pharmacy.* Vols. 1–5. Deventer, Ysel, 1957–80.

Wooton, A. C. *Chronicles of Pharmacy.* London, Macmillan, 1910.

CHAPTER I. ANCIENT ANTECEDENTS

Anati, E. *Palestine Before the Hebrews.* New York, Knopf, 1963.

Basham, A. L., ed. *A Cultural History of India.* Oxford, Clarendon Press, 1975.

Breasted, C. *The Edwin Smith Surgical Papyrus.* Chicago, University of Chicago Press, 1930.

————. *A History of Egypt.* New York, Scribner's, 1946.

Bryan, C. P. *The Papyrus Ebers.* London, Bles, 1930.

*Buess, H. "Die Anfänge der Pharmakotherapie auf primitiver Stufe und im klassische Altertum," *Forschung und Technik der National Zeitung,* no. 104, March 4, 1965.

Castiglioni, A. *A History of Medicine.* New York, Knopf, 1941.

*Cowen, D. L., and Segelman, A. B., eds. *Antibiotics in Historical Perspective.* Rahway, N.J., Merck, 1981.

Davaras, C. *Minoan Art in the Herakleion Museum.* Athens, Editions Hannibal, n.d.

Dressendörfer, W. "Französische Apothekendarstellung aus dem 13. Jahrhundert," *Beiträge zur Geschichte der Pharmazie,* 31[8], 1979, pp. 57–61.

Fejos, P. "Man, Magic and Medicine," in Galdston, I., ed., *Medicine and Anthropology.* New York, International Universities Press, 1959, pp. 11–35.

Goldman, L. "The Balm of Gilead," *Archives of Dermatology,* 112, 1976, p. 881.

Harley, G. W. *Native African Medicine with Special Reference to Its Practice in the Mano Tribe of Liberia.* Cambridge, Harvard University Press, 1941.

Harrison, R. H. *Healing Herbs of the Bible.* Leiden, Brill, 1966.

*Hein, W.-H. "Die Bedeutung der Entzifferung des Linear B für die Arzneimittelgeschichte," *Pharmazeutische Zeitung,* 38, 1961, pp. 1145–48.

Hou, J. P. "The Development of Chinese Herbal Medicine and the Pent-s'ao," *Comparative Medicine East and West,* 5^2, 1977, pp. 117–22.

Huard, P., and Wong, M. *Chinese Medicine.* Trans. from the French by F. Fielding. London, Weidenfeld & Nicolson, 1968.

Jayne, W. A. *The Healing Code of Ancient Civilizations.* New Hyde Park, N.Y., University Books, 1962.

Jonckheere, F. "Le 'Préparateur des remédes' dans l'organisation de la pharmacie Egyptienne," in Firchow, E., ed., *Veröffentlichung Nr. 29, Deutsche Akademie für Wissenschaften zu Berlin: Institut für Orientforschung.* Berlin, Akademie-Verlag, 1955, pp. 149–61.

Kerner, D. "Medizin und Magie in Babylonischen Talmud," *Münchener Medizinische Wochenschrift,* 105, 1963, pp. 464–69.

Kolta, K. S. "swnw' Artz und Hersteller von Heilmitteln im alten Ägypten," *Beiträge zur Geschichte der Pharmazie,* 31^2, 1979, pp. 9–12.

Kramer, S. A. *History Begins at Sumer.* Philadelphia, University of Pennsylvania Press, 1981.

Leake, C. *The Old Egyptian Medical Papyri.* Lawrence, University of Kansas Press, 1952.

Levey, M. "Alberuni and Indian Alchemy," *Chymia,* 7, 1961, pp. 36–39.

———. "A Sumerian Medical Text from Nippur of the 3rd Millennium B.C.," *Actes du VIIIᵉ Congrès International d'Histoire des Sciences, Florence, Sept. 2–9, 1956.* Florence, Gruppe Italiano di Storia della Scienza, 1958, pp. 843–55.

Lu, G.-D. "China's Greatest Naturalist: A Brief Biography of Li Shih-Chen," *Physis* 8, 1966, pp. 383–92.

Majno, C. *The Healing Hand: Man and Wound in the Ancient World.* Cambridge, Harvard University Press, 1975.

*Miller, J. I. *The Spice Trade of the Roman Empire, 29 B.C. to A.D. 64.* Oxford, Clarendon Press, 1969.

Needham, J., and Gwei-Djen, L. "Chinese Medicine," in Poynter, F. N. L., ed., *Medicine and Culture.* London, Wellcome Institute, 1969, pp. 255–84.

*Nutton, V. "The Drug Trade in Antiquity," *Journal of the Royal Society of Medicine,* 78, 1985, pp. 138–45.

*Okazaki, K. *The Pharmaceutical History of Japan.* Tokyo, Naito, 1979.

Oppenheim, A. L. *Ancient Mesopotamia.* Rev. ed. by E. Reiner. Chicago, University of Chicago Press, 1977.

Patel, B., and Schneider, W. "Über Entwicklungsperioden des indischen Arzneischatzes," *Deutsche Apotheker-Zeitung,* 102, 1962, pp. 1292–95.

Pollak, K., and Underwood, E. A. *The Healers: The Doctor, Then and Now.* London, Nelson, 1968.

[Poynter, F. N. L., ed.] *Chinese Medicine: An Exhibition Illustrating the Traditional System of Medicine of the Chinese People.* London, Wellcome Institute, 1966.

Read, B. E. *Chinese Materia Medica: Animal Drugs.* Taipei, Southern Materials Center, 1976.

Rosner, F. *Medicine in the Bible and Talmud.* New York, Ktav Press, 1977.

Saggs, H. W. F. *The Greatness That Was Babylon.* New York, Praeger, 1962.

Said, H. M. *Medicine in China.* Karachi, Hamdard Academy, 1981.

*Scarborough, J. "Theoretical Assumptions in Hippocratic Pharmacology," in Lasserre, F., and Mudry, P., eds., *Formes de pensée dans la Collection Hippocratique,* Actes du IVᵉ Colloque International Hippocratique, Lausanne, Sept. 21–26, 1981. Geneva, Université de Lausanne, Publications de la Faculté des Lettres XXVI, 1983, pp. 307–25.

Sigerist, H. E. *A History of Medicine.* New York, Oxford University Press, 1951.

Solecki, R. S. *Shanidar: The First Flower People.* New York, Knopf, 1971.

*Stannard, J. "Hippocratic Pharmacology," *Bulletin of the History of Medicine,* 38, 1961, pp. 497–518.

Stuart, G. A. *Chinese Materia Medica: Vegetable Kingdom.* Taipei, Southern Materials Center, 1976.

*Temkin, O. "Greek Medicine as a Science and Craft," *Isis,* 44, 1953, pp. 213–25.

————. "Historical Aspects of Drug Therapy," in Talalay, P., ed., *Drugs in Our Society.* Baltimore, Johns Hopkins University Press, 1964, pp. 3–16.

Temkin, O., and Temkin, C. L., eds. *Ancient Medicine: Selected Papers of Ludwig Edelstein.* Baltimore, Johns Hopkins University Press, 1967.

Unschuld, P. U. "The Development of Medical-Pharmaceutical Thought in China," *Comparative Medicine East and West,* 5[2], 1977, pp. 109–15.

————. *Die Praxis des traditionellen chinesischen Heilsystems.* Wiesbaden, Steiner, 1973.

Vaisrub, S. "Medicine," in *Encyclopedia Judaica.* Jerusalem, Encyclopedia Judaica, 1971, vol. 11, cols. 1170–1211.

Veith, I. *Huang Ti Nei Ching Su Wên: The Yellow Emperor's Classic of Internal Medicine.* Baltimore, Williams and Wilkins, 1949.

Wertheimer, A. I. "Pharmacy in China," *American Druggist,* 195[6], 1987, pp. 53–55.

CHAPTER II. THE CLASSICAL WORLD

Berman, A. "The Persistence of Theriac in France," *Pharmacy in History,* 12, 1970, pp. 5–12.

*Cowen, D. L. "Expunctum est Mithridatium," *Pharmaceutical Historian,* 15[3], 1985, pp. 2–3.

Huxley, H. H. "Greek Doctor and Roman Patient," *Greece and Rome,* ser. 2, vol. 4, 1957, pp. 132–38.

Kudien, F. "Celsus," *Dictionary of Scientific Biography.* New York, Scribner's, 1970 etc., vol. 3, pp. 174–75.

Mez-Mangold, L. *A History of Drugs.* Basel, Hoffman-LaRoche, 1971.

Riddle, J. M. "Amber in Ancient Pharmacy," *Pharmacy in History,* 15, 1973, pp. 3–17.

*————. "Dioscorides," *Dictionary of Scientific Biography.* New York, Scribner's, 1970 etc., vol. 5, pp. 119–23.

————. *Dioscorides on Pharmacy and Medicine.* Austin, University of Texas Press, 1986.

Salmon, W. *Pharmacopoeia Londinensis, or, the New London Dispensatory.* London, Dawks, 1679.

*Scarborough, J. "The Drug Lore of Asclepiades of Bythnia," *Pharmacy in History,* 17, 1975, pp. 43–57.

————. "Gnosticism, Drugs and Alchemy in Late Roman Egypt," *Pharmacy in History,* 13, 1971, pp. 151–57.

Stannard, J. "Materia Medica and Philosophic Theory in Aretaeus," *Sudhoffs Archiv,* 48, 1964, pp. 27–53.

Thorndike, L. "Three Texts on Degrees of Medicines," *Bulletin of the History of Medicine,* 38, 1964, pp. 533–37.

*Watson, G. *Theriac and Mithridatium: A Study in Therapeutics.* London, Wellcome Institute, 1966.

CHAPTER III. THE MIDDLE AGES

Anawati, G. C. "Hunayn ibn Isḥāq," *Dictionary of Scientific Biography.* New York, Scribner's, 1970 etc., vol. 15, pp. 230–34.

————. "Ibn Sīnā," *Dictionary of Scientific Biography.* New York, Scribner's, 1970 etc., vol. 15, pp. 494–98.

Arano, L. C. *The Medieval Health Handbook: Tacuinum Sanitatis,* trans. by O. Ratti and A. Westbrook. New York, Braziller, 1976.

Colapinto, L. *Il Nobile Collegio Chimico Farmaceutico Romano: Cenni Storici.* Rome, Stomygen, 1979.

Dillemann, G. "La Pharmacopée au Moyen Age," *Revue d'Histoire de la Pharmacie,* 19, 1968–69, pp. 163–70, 235–43.

Goltz, D. "Mittelalterliche Pharmazie und Medizin: Dargestellt an Geschichte und Inhalt des 'Antidotarium Nicolai'," *Veröffentlichungen der Internationalen Gesellschaft für Geschichte der Pharmazie,* n.f. 44, 1976.

Hamarneh, S. "The Climax of Medieval Arabic Professional Pharmacy," *Bulletin of the History of Medicine,* 42, 1968, pp. 450–61.

————. "Drawings and Pharmacy in Al-Zahrāwī's 10th-Century Surgical Treatise," *United States National Museum Bulletin,* 228, 1961.

————. "The Pharmacy and Materia Medica of al-Bīrūnī and al-Ghāfiqī: A Comparison," *Pharmacy in History,* 18, 1976, pp. 3–12.

————. "The Rise of Professional Pharmacy in Islam," *Medical History,* 6, 1952, pp. 59–66.

————. "Sābūr's Abridged Formulary, the First of Its Kind in Islam," *Sudhoffs Archiv,* 45, 1961, pp. 247–60.

Hamarneh, S., and Sonnendecker, G. *A Pharmaceutical View of Albucasis al-Zahrāwī in Moorish Spain.* Leiden, Brill, 1963.

Hein, W.-H. "Einige Bemerkungen zu den frühen Apothekerstatuten im Königreich Sizilien und im Arelat," *Pharmazeutische Zeitung,* 116, 1971, pp. 1901–1905.

Hein, W.-H., and Sappert, K. "Die Medizinalordnung Friedrich II," *Veröffentlichungen der Internationalen Gesellschaft für Geschichte der Pharmazie,* n.f. 12, 1957.

Iskander, A. Z. "Ibn Sīnā," *Dictionary of Scientific Biography.* New York, Scribner's, 1970 etc., vol. 15, pp. 498–501.

Kallinich, G., and Schnabel, R. "Die Verbindung zwischen Religion und Heilkunde und die sich daraus ergebenden Ursachen für das Entstehen der wissenschaftlichen und praktischen Pharmazie in den abendländischen Klostergründungen," *Deutsche Apotheker-Zeitung,* 103, 1963, pp. 1324–29.

Kennedy, E. S. "Al-Bīrunī," *Dictionary of Scientific Biography.* New York, Scribner's, 1970 etc., vol. 2, pp. 147–58.

Kudlien, F. "Schaustellerie und Heilmittelvertrieb in der Antike," *Gesnerus,* 40, 1983, pp. 9, 91–98.

Levey, M. "The Italian Pharmacopeia and the Influence of Medieval Arabic Pharmacy," *Pharmacy in History,* 12, 1970, pp. 13–15.

————. "Some Facets of Medieval Arabic Pharmacology," *Transactions and Studies of the College of Physicians of Philadelphia,* ser. 3, vol. 30, 1963, pp. 157–62.

————. "Substitute Drugs in Early Arabic Medicine," *Veröffentlichungen der Internationalen Gesellschaft für Geschichte der Pharmazie,* n.f. 37, 1971.

Lloyd, G. E. R. *Magic, Reason and Experience.* Cambridge, Cambridge University Press, 1979.

Lutz, A. "Aus der Geschichte der mittelalterlichen Antidotarien," in Hügel, H., and Hein, W.-H., eds., *Die Schelenz Stiftung II, Veröffentlichungen der Internationalen Gesellschaft für Geschichte der Pharmazie,* n.f. 40, 1973, pp. 115–21.
————. "Die verschollene frühsalernitanische Antidotarius magnus in einer Basler Handschrift aus dem 12. Jahrhundert und das Antidotarium Nicolai," *Veröffentlichungen der Internationalen Gesellschaft für Geschichte der Pharmazie,* n.f. 16, 1960, pp. 97–133.

Matthews, L. G. *The Pepperers, Spicers and Apothecaries of London During the Thirteenth and Fourteenth Centuries.* London, Society of Apothecaries, 1980.

McVaugh, M. "Theriac at Montpellier 1285–1325," *Sudhoffs Archiv,* 56, 1972, pp. 113–44.

Meyerhof, M. "Arabian Pharmacology in North Africa, Sicily and the Iberian Peninsula," *Ciba Symposium,* 6, nos. 5–6, 1944, pp. 1868–72.

*————. "The Background and Origins of Arabian Pharmacology," *Ciba Symposium,* nos. 5–6, 1944, pp. 1847–68.

Müller, I. *Die pflanzlichen Heilmittel bei Hildegard von Bingen.* Salzburg, Müller-Verlag, 1982.

Pagel, W. "Hildegard of Bingen," *Dictionary of Scientific Biography.* New York, Scribner's, 1970 etc., vol. 6, pp. 396–98.

Pines, S. "Maimonides," *Dictionary of Scientific Biography.* New York, Scribner's, 1970 etc., vol. 9, pp. 27–32.

―――. "Al-Rāzī," *Dictionary of Scientific Biography.* New York, Scribner's, 1970 etc., vol. 11, pp. 323–26.

Riddle, J. M. "The Introduction and Use of Eastern Drugs in the Early Middle Ages," *Sudhoffs Archiv,* 49, 1965, pp. 185–98.

―――. "Lithotherapy in the Middle Ages," *Pharmacy in History,* 12, 1970, pp. 39–50.

Schmitz, R. "Die hochmittelalterische Rezeption antiken und arabischen naturkundlichen Wissens in ihrer Bedeutung für die Entwicklung der Pharmazie," *Deutsche Apotheker-Zeitung,* 102, 1962, pp. 923–26.

―――. "Zur Entwicklungsgeschichte und Soziologie des deutschen Apothekerstandes im Hoch- und Spätmittelalter," *Veröffentlichungen der Internationalen Gesellschaft für Geschichte der Pharmazie,* n.f. 13, 1958, pp. 157–65.

Schmitz, R., and Merkelbach, C. "Zur Rechtsgeschichte des älteren Apothekerwesens: 2. über die Datierung des Basler Apothekereides," *Pharmazeutische Zeitung,* 106, 1961, pp. 1138–40.

Schneider, W. "Die geschichtlichen Beziehungen der Mettalurgie zu Alchemie und Pharmazie," *Archiv für das Eisenhüttenwesen,* 37, 1966, pp. 533–38.

Stannard, J. "Marcellus of Bordeaux and the Beginnings of Medieval Materia Medica," *Pharmacy in History,* 15, 1973, pp. 47–53.

―――. "The Theoretical Basis of Medieval Herbalism," *Medical Heritage,* 1^3, 1985, pp. 186–98.

Wankmüller, A. *Die Landshuter Apothekerordnungen der Spätmittelalters.* Tübingen, Tübingen Apothekengeschichtliche Abhandlungen, Heft 10, 1964.

CHAPTER IV. THE RENAISSANCE

Anderson, F. J. *An Illustrated History of the Herbals.* New York, Columbia University Press, 1977.

Arber, A. *Herbals: Their Origin and Evolution.* Cambridge, Cambridge University Press, 1938.

Baudet, J., et al. *Livre d'Or des apothicaireries de France.* Saint-Mande, Éditions Thériaque, 1962.

Blunt, W., and Raphael, S. *The Illustrated Herbal.* New York, Metropolitan Museum of Art, 1979.

Charles, R. H. *The Apocrypha and Pseudepigraphics of the Old Testament,* vol. 1. Oxford, Clarendon Press, 1913.

*Copeman, W. S. C. *The Worshipful Society of Apothecaries of London: A History, 1617–1967.* Oxford, Pergamon Press, 1967.

Correia Da Silva, A. C. *Contributions des Portugais à la connaissance des plantes médicinales des Pays d'Outre-Mer.* Porto, Imprensa Portuguesa, 1961.

*Cowen, D.L. "The Boston Editions of Nicholas Culpeper," *Journal of the History of Medicine and Allied Sciences,* 11, 1956, pp.156–65.

―――. "The British North American Colonies as a Source of Drugs," *Veröffentlichungen der Internationalen Gesellschaft für Geschichte der Pharmazie,* n.f. 28, 1966, pp. 47–59.

―――. "Squill in the 17th and 18th Centuries," *Bulletin of the New York Academy of Medicine,* ser. 2, 50, 1974, pp. 714–22.

―――. "A Store Mixt, Various, Universal," *Journal of the Rutgers University Library,* 25, 1961, pp. 1–9.

Crellin, J. K. *Apothecary Jars: Selections from the Mogull Apothecary Jar and General Pharmacy Collection.* Storrs, School of Pharmacy, University of Connecticut, c. 1981.

Dann, G. E. "Leben und Leistung des Valerius Cordus aus neuerer Sicht," *Pharmazeutische Zeitung,* 113, 1968, pp. 1062–72.

Debus, A. G. "The Chemical Philosophers: Chemical Medicine from Paracelsus to van Helmont," *History of Science,* 12, 1974, pp. 235–39.

―――. *The English Paracelsians.* London, Oldbourne, 1985.

―――. "History With a Purpose: The Fate of Paracelsus," *Pharmacy in History,* 26, 1984, pp. 83–96.

―――. "The Paracelsians in Eighteenth-Century France: A Renaissance Tradition in the Age of Enlightenment," *Ambix,* 28, 1981, pp. 35–54.

————. "The Pharmaceutical Revolution of the Renaissance," *Clio Medica,* 11, 1976, pp. 307–17.

Deutsches Apotheken-Museum im Heidelberger Schloss, Heidelberg. *Führer durch das Deutsches Apotheken-Museum im Heidelberger Schloss.* Frankfurt, Govi, 1976.

Drey, R. E. A. *Apothecary Jars: Pharmaceutical Pottery and Porcelain in Europe and the East, 1150–1850.* London, Faber, 1978.

*Dulieu, L. *La Pharmacie à Montpellier.* Avignon, Les Presses Universelles, 1973.

Duncan, A. *The Edinburgh New Dispensatory.* 3rd ed. Edinburgh, Creech, 1791.

[Fehlmann, H. R.] *Pharmazeutischer Reiseführer Schweiz.* Darmstadt, E. Merck, 1976.

Fleming, A. *Alcohol, the Delightful Poison.* New York, Delacorte, 1975

*Folch Jou, G. *Historia de la farmacia.* 3d ed. Madrid, Catedratico de Historia de la Farmacia de la Universidad de Madrid, 1972.

————. *Museo de la Farmacia Hispaña.* Madrid, Facultad de Farmacia de la Universidad Complutense de Madrid, n.d.

Frothingham, A. W. "Apothecaries' Shops in Spain," *Notes Hispanic,* 1941, pp. 101–24.

Ganzinger, K. "Die heilige Kosmas und Damian als Patrone der Wiener medizinischen Fakultät," *Veröffentlichungen der Schweizerischen Gesellschaft für Geschichte der Pharmazie,* 5, 1985, pp. 33–42.

Giovanni, M. *The Role of Religious in Pharmacy, Upper Canada's "Ancien Régime."* Toronto, 1962.

Griffenhagen, G. B. *Tools of the Apothecary.* Washington, D.C., American Pharmaceutical Association, 1957.

Guerra, F. "Nicholas Bautista Monardes," *Dictionary of Scientific Biography.* New York, Scribner's, 1970 etc., vol. 9, p. 466.

*Hall, M. B. "Apothecaries and Chemists in the 17th Century," *Pharmaceutical Journal,* 199, 1967, pp. 433–36.

Hein, W.-H. *Apotheker Kalender 1961.* Stuttgart, Deutscher Apotheker Verlag, 1960.

————. *Apotheker Kalender 1987.* Stuttgart, Deutscher Apotheker Verlag, 1986.

————. *Christus als Apotheker.* Exhib. cat., Focke-Museum, Bremen, 1975. Frankfurt, Govi, 1975.

*————. *Emailmalereigläser aus deutschen Apotheken.* Frankfurt, Govi, 1972.

————. "Über einige Arzneitaxen des späten Mittelalters," *Veröffentlichungen der Internationalen Gesellschaft für Geschichte der Pharmazie,* n.f. 8, 1956, pp. 99–110.

Hein, W.-H., and Wittop Konig, D. A. *Deutsche Apotheken-Fayencen.* Frankfurt, Govi, 1977.

Hickel, E., and Schneider, W. "Quellen zur Geschichte der pharmazeutischen Chemie in 16. Jahrhundert, 2. Mitteilung: Distillierbücher," *Pharmazeutische Zeitung,* 109, 1964, pp. 51–57.

Ivins, W. M., Jr. *Prints and Visual Communication.* Cambridge, MIT Press, 1985.

Julien, P. "Iconographie et attributs médico-pharmaceutique des Saints Côme et Damien en Piémont," *La Pharmacie Française,* 70³, 1966, pp. 13–20.

————. *Saint Côme et Saint Damien: Patrons des médecins, chirurgiens et pharmaciens.* Paris, Pariente, 1980.

————. "Sur le Célèbre 'Dentiste' ou 'pharmacien' de Pietro Longhi," *Pharmaceutisch, Weekblad* 116, 1981, pp. 1389–92.

Julien, P., and Ledermann, F., eds. "Saint Côme et Saint Damien: Culte et iconographie, "*Veröffentlichungen der Schweizerischen Gesellschaft für Geschichte der Pharmazie,* 5, 1985.

Kuznicka, B. "The Earliest Printed Herbals and Evolution of Pharmacy," *Organon,* 16/17, 1980/81, pp. 255–56.

Laissus, Y. "Le Jardin du roi," in Taton, R., ed., *Enseignement et diffusion des sciences en France au XVIIIᵉ siècle.* Paris, Hermann, 1964, pp. 287–341.

Lloyd, J. U. *Origin and History of the Pharmacopoeial Vegetable Drugs.* Cincinnati, Caxton, 1929.

Lutz, A. "Der zweitälteste Wiener Arzneitaxe in einer Basler Handschrift von 1452," *Österreichische Apotheker Zeitung,* 17, 1963, pp. 333–37.

Matthews, L. G. "Herbals and Formularies," in Poynter, F. N. L., ed., *The Evolution of Pharmacy in Britain*. London, Pitman, 1965, pp. 187–213.

———. *The Royal Apothecaries*. London, Wellcome Institute, 1967.

———. "SS. Cosmas and Damian, Patron Saints of Medicine and Pharmacy: Their Cult in England," *Medical History,* 12, 1968, pp. 281–88.

Minarik, F. "Die Schutzpatrone der Ärzte, Apotheker und Kranken: Kosmas und Damianus in Slowenien," *Veröffentlichungen der Internationalen Gesellschaft für Geschichte der Pharmazie,* n.f. 32, 1969, pp. 117–33.

Nékám, L. *Old Hungarian Pharmacies*. Budapest, Corvina, 1968.

Ornstein, M. *The Role of Scientific Societies in the Seventeenth Century*. Chicago, University of Chicago Press, 1938.

Palmer, R. "Medical Botany in Northern Italy in the Renaissance," *Journal of the Royal Society of Medicine,* 78, 1983, pp. 149–57.

Pelner, L. "Garcia Da Orta," *Journal of the American Medical Association,* 197, 1966, pp. 996–98.

Risley, M. *The House of Healing: The Story of the Hospital*. London, Hale, 1962.

Risse, G. B. "Transcending Culture Barriers: the European Reception of Medicinal Plants from America," *Veröffentlichungen der Internationalen Gesellschaft für Geschichte der Pharmazie,* n.f. 53, 1984, pp. 31–42.

Schmitz, R. "Der Anteil des Renaissance-Humanismus und der Entwicklung von Arzneibüchern und Pharmacopöen," in Krafft, L., and Wuttke, D., eds., *Das Verhältnis der Humanisten zum Buch.* Boppard, Boldt, 1977 (Deutsche Forschungsgemeinschaft, Kommission für Humanismusforschung, Mitteilung IV), pp. 227–43.

[Schmitz, R.] *Pharmazeutischer Reiseführer Norddeutschland*. Darmstadt, E. Merck, 1972.

[Schmitz, R., and Jantz, V.] *Pharmazeutischer Reiseführer Suddeutschland*. Darmstadt, E. Merck, 1972.

Schneider, W. "Arzneirecepte von Paracelsus," *Medizinhistorisches Journal,* 16, 1981, pp. 151–66.

Schullian, D. M. "The Pharmacy of S. Giovanni Evangelista," *Journal of the History of Medicine and Allied Sciences,* 11, 1956, p. 227.

Skrobucha, H. *The Patrons of the Doctors*. Recklinghausen, Bongers, 1965.

Stannard, J. "The Herbal as a Medical Document," *Bulletin of the History of Medicine,* 43, 1969, pp. 212–20.

———. "P. A. Mattioli and Some Renaissance Editions of Dioscorides," *Books and Libraries at the University of Kansas,* 4:1, Oct. 1966, pp. 1–5.

———. "P. A. Mattioli: Sixteenth-Century Commentator on Dioscorides," *Bibliographical Contributions, University of Kansas Libraries,* 1, 1969, pp. 59–81.

[Suñe, J. M.] *Pharmazeutischer Reiseführer Spanien*. Darmstadt, E. Merck, 1967.

[Tergolina, U.] *Pharmazeutischer Reiseführer Rom*. Darmstadt, E. Merck, n.d.

Urdang, G. *Pharmacopoeia Londinensis of 1618, Reproduced in Facsimile with a Historical Introduction by George Urdang*. Hollister Pharmaceutical Library, 2. Madison, State Historical Society of Wisconsin, 1944.

Valverde, J.-L. "The Aztec Herbal of 1552: Martin de la Cruz' 'Libellus de Medicinalibus Indorum Herbis': Context of the Sources on Nahualt Materia Medica," *Veröffentlichungen der Internationalen Gesellschaft für Geschichte der Pharmazie,* n.f. 53, 1984, pp. 9–30.

Vandewiele, L. J. "Introduction," *Den Herbarius in Dyetsche*. Facsimile. Ghent, DeBacker, 1974

Van Tassel, R. *Bezoars and the Collection of Henri van Heurck (1839–1909)*. Antwerp, Koninklijke Maatschappij voor Dierkunde van Antwerpen, c. 1970.

White, C. *Rembrandt and His World*. London, Thames and Hudson, 1964.

Wittop Koning, D. A. *Bronzemörser*. Frankfurt, Govi, 1975.

———. *Die oude Apotheek*. Bussum, Dishoeck, 1966.

CHAPTER V. THE EARLY MODERN AGE: THE NEW SCIENCE

Blake, J. B. *A Short Title Catalogue of Eighteenth-Century Printed Books in the National Library of Medicine.* Bethesda, National Library of Medicine, 1979.

Burnby, J. G. I. *A Study of the English Apothecary from 1660 to 1760.* London, Wellcome Institute, 1983.

Cowen, D. L. *America's Pre-Pharmacopoeial Literature.* Madison, Wis., American Institute of the History of Pharmacy, 1961.

*————. *The Colonial and Revolutionary Heritage of Pharmacy in America.* Trenton, New Jersey Pharmaceutical Association, 1976.

————. "Colonial Laws Pertaining to Pharmacy," *Journal of the American Pharmaceutical Association,* 32, 1934, pp. 1236–42.

————. "The Edinburgh Dispensatories," *Papers of the Bibliographical Society of America,* 45, 1951, pp. 85–96.

————. "The Edinburgh Pharmacopoeia," *Medical History,* 1, 1957, pp. 123–37, 340–51.

*————. "Pharmacy and Freedom," *Pharmacy in History,* 26, 1984, pp. 70–82.

————. "The Spread and Influence of British Pharmacopoeial and Related Literature." *Veröffentlichungen der Internationalen Gesellschaft für Geschichte der Pharmazie,* n.f. 41, 1974.

Crellin, J. K. "Anton Störck (1731–1803) and British Therapeutics," *Clio Medica,* 9, 1974, pp. 103–108.

*————. *Medical Ceramics.* London, Wellcome Institute, 1969.

Debus, A. G. "Quantification and Medical Motivation: Factors in the Interpretation of Early Modern Chemistry," *Pharmacy in History,* 31, 1989, pp. 3–11.

De Francesco, G. *The Power of the Charlatan.* New Haven, Yale University Press, 1939.

Donovan, M. "On the Injurious Effects of the Pharmaceutical Treatment of *Digitalis purpurea,* in Forming Its Tincture, with a Proposal for a More Efficacious Formula," *American Journal of Pharmacy,* 11 (n.s. 5), 1840, pp. 204–15.

Earles, M. P. "Early Scientific Studies of Drugs and Poisons," *Pharmaceutical Journal,* 188, 1962, pp. 47–51.

Estes, J. W. *Hall Jackson and the Purple Foxglove.* Hanover, N. H., University Press of New England, 1979.

Fabre, R., and Dillemann, G. *Histoire de la pharmacie.* Paris, Presses Universitaires de France, 1963.

[Ganzinger, K.] *Neues Quarinisches Dispensatorium Innsbruck 1790.* Facsimile with an intro. by K. Ganzinger. Vienna, Österr. Apotheker-Verlag, 1977.

————. "Die Österreichische Provinzial-Pharmacopöe (1774–1794) und ihrer Bearbeiter," *Zur Geschichte der Pharmazie,* 14³, 1962, pp. 17–24.

————. "Vor 200 Jahren: die Apotheke als ein Beispiel 'klösterlicher und weltliche Mißbräuche'," *Österreichische Apotheker-Zeitung,* 39, 1985, pp. 85–89.

Griffenhagen, G. "Bartholomew Browne, Pharmaceutical Chemist of Salem, Massachusetts, 1698–1704," *Essex Institute Historical Collections,* Jan. 1961, pp. 19–30.

Hein, W.-H. *Die Pharmazie in der Karikatur.* Frankfurt, Govi, 1964.

*Hein, W.-H., and Schwarz, H.-D. *Deutsche Apotheker Biographie,* 2 vols. *Veröffentlichungen der Internationalen Gesellschaft für Geschichte der Pharmazie,* n.s., 43 (A–L) and 46 (M–Z), 1975, 1978.

Helfand, W.H. "The Apothecary General," *Journal of the American Pharmaceutical Association,* n.s. 4, 1964, pp. 124–25.

————. "Medicine and Pharmacy in British Political Prints—The Example of Lord Sidmouth," *Medical History,* 29, 1985, pp. 375–85.

*————. "Medicine and Pharmacy in French Political Prints," *Transactions and Studies of the College of Physicians of Philadelphia,* ser. 4, 42, 1974, pp. 14–33.

[Helfand, W. H., Julien, P., and Cotinat, L.] *La Pharmacie par l'image*. Exposition organisée à l'occasion du Congrès International d'Histoire de la Pharmacie, Paris, Sept. 24–29, 1973. Paris, 1973.

Helfand, W. H., and Rocchietta, S. *Medicina e farmacia nelle caricature politiche italiane 1848–1914*. Milano, Edizioni Scientifiche Internazionali, 1982.

*King, L. S. *The Medical World of the Eighteenth Century*. Chicago, University of Chicago Press, 1958.

Lanning, J. T. *The Royal Protomedicato: The Regulation of the Medical Profession in the Spanish Empire*. Ed. by J. J. TePaske. Durham, Duke University Press, 1985.

Lehmann, H. *Das Collegium Medico-Chirurgicum in Berlin als Lehrstätte der Botanik und der Pharmazie*. Berlin, Triltsch und Hurther, 1936.

Leicester, H. M. *The Historical Background of Chemistry*. New York, Wiley, 1956.

Lesky, E. "Klinische Arzneimittelforschung im 18. Jahrhundert," *Beiträge zur Geschichte der Pharmazie*, 29, 1977, pp. 17–20.

Lewis, W. *The New Dispensatory*. London, Nourse, 1753. 2d ed. London, Nourse, 1765.

Matthews, L. G. *Antiques of the Pharmacy*. London, Bell, 1971.

*McNamara, B. *Step Right Up*. Garden City, N.Y., Doubleday, 1976.

Morton, A. G. *History of Botanical Science*. London, Academic Press, 1981.

Röhrich, H. "Über den akademischen Unterricht in der Materia medica bis zur Einführung eines obligatorischen Studiums für Apotheker," *Veröffentlichungen der Internationalen Gesellschaft für Geschichte der Pharmazie*, n.f. 32, 1969, pp. 147–58.

Urdang, G. *The Apothecary Chemist Carl Wilhelm Scheele*. 2d ed. Madison, Wis., American Institute of the History of Pharmacy, 1958.

————. "Pharmacopoeias as Witnesses of World History," *Journal of the History of Medicine and Allied Sciences*, 1, 1946, pp. 46–70.

Vandewiele, L. J. "Introduction," *Pharmacopoeia Leodiensis 1741*. Facsimile. Ghent, De Backer, 1975.

Van Hoorn, M. "L'Enseigne du protocologue de Musée Gruuthuse de Bruges," *Clio Medica*, 6, 1971, pp. 225–35.

*Wall, C., Cameron, H. C., and Underwood, E. A. *A History of the Worshipful Society of Apothecaries of London*, vol. 1, 1617–1815. London, Wellcome Institute, 1963.

Wankmüller, A. "Die oberbayerischen Klosterapotheken am Ende des 18. Jahrhunderts," *Deutsche Apotheker-Zeitung*, 97, 1957, pp. 919–21.

[Webster, C., and Irving, R.] *The Edinburgh New Dispensatory*. Edinburgh, Elliott, 1786.

Winkler, A. *Carl Spitzweg*. Munich, Südwest, 1968.

Wittop Koning, D. A. "Nederländische Drucke Deutscher Pharmakopoean," *Veröffentlichungen der Internationalen Gesellschaft für Geschichte der Pharmazie*, n.f.10, 1957, pp. 200–208.

Wood, G. B., and Bache, F. *The Dispensatory of the United States of America*. 5th ed. Philadelphia, Grigg and Elliott, 1843.

Woudt, K. *Over de Gaper als Uithangteken*. Chibret, n.p., 1980.

*Zekert, O. *Berühmte Apotheker*. Stuttgart, Deutsche Apotheker Verlag, 1955.

CHAPTER VI. THE NINETEENTH CENTURY: SCIENCE AND PHARMACY

Berman, A. "The Botanic Practitioners of 19th-Century America," *American Professional Pharmacist*, 23, 1957, pp. 868–70, 911–12.

————. "Joseph Bienaimé Caventou," *Dictionary of Scientific Biography*. New York, Scribner's, 1970 etc., vol. 3, pp. 159–60.

————. "Conflict and Anomaly in the Scientific Orientation of French Pharmacy 1800–1873," *Bulletin of the History of Medicine*, 37, 1963, pp. 440–62.

————. "Antoine-Augustin Parmentier," *Dictionary of Scientific Biography*. New York, Scribner's, 1970 etc., vol. 10. pp. 325–26.

————. "Pierre-Joseph Pelletier," *Dictionary of Scientific Biography*. New York, Scribner's, 1970 etc., vol. 10, pp. 497–99.

————. "The Problem of Science in 19th-Century French Pharmaceutical Historiography," *Proceedings of the 10th International Congress of the History of Science, Ithaca, 1962*. Paris, Hermann, 1964, vol. 1, pp. 891–94.

*————. "The Scientific Tradition in French Hospital Pharmacy," *American Journal of Hospital Pharmacy*, 18, 1961, pp. 110–19.

————. "A Striving for Scientific Respectability: Some American Botanics and the Nineteenth-Century Plant Materia Medica," *Bulletin of the History of Medicine*, 30, 1956, pp. 7–31.

————. *The Thomsonian Movement and Its Relation to American Pharmacy*. Madison, Wis., American Institute of the History of Pharmacy, 1952.

Bynum, W. F. "Chemical Structure and Pharmacological Action: A Chapter in the History of 19th-Century Molecular Pharmacology," *Bulletin of the History of Medicine*, 44, 1970, pp. 518–38.

Coulter, H. L. *Homeopathic Influences in Nineteenth-Century Allopathic Therapeutics*. Washington, D.C., American Institute of Homeopathy, 1973.

*Cowen, D. L. "Ehrlich, the Man, the Scientist," *American Journal of Pharmaceutical Education*, 26, 1962, pp. 4–11.

*————. "Materia Medica and Pharmacology in American Medical Schools," in Numbers, R., ed., *The Education of American Physicians*. Berkeley, University of California Press, 1979, pp. 95–121.

*————. "The Role of the Industry," in Blake, J. B., ed., *Safeguarding the Public*. Baltimore, Johns Hopkins University Press, 1970, pp. 72–82.

"End of American Homeopathy: Closing Pharmaceutical Era," *SKF Hospital Pharmacy News*, July, 1965.

Helfand, W. H. "Mariani et le vin de coca," *Revue de l'Histoire de la Pharmacie*, 27, no. 198, pp. 227–34.

————. "Vin Mariani," *Pharmacy in History*, 22, 1980, pp. 12–19.

The Homeopathic Pharmacopoeia of the United States, Philadelphia, Boericke & Tafel, 1964.

Irissou, L. "Au Sujet de la création de l'École gratuite de Pharmacie de Paris," *Revue de l'Histoire de la Pharmacie*, 6, no. 120, 1948, pp. 279–80.

Kaufman, M. *Homeopathy in America*. Baltimore, Johns Hopkins University Press, 1971.

King, M. M. "Dr. John S. Pemberton: Originator of Coca-Cola," *Pharmacy in History*, 29, 1987, pp. 85–89.

*Liebenau, J. M. *Medical Science and Medical Industry*. Baltimore, Johns Hopkins University Press, 1987.

Mahaffey, F. T., et al., eds. *Survey of Pharmacy Law, 1986–87*. Park Ridge, Ill., National Association of Boards of Pharmacy, 1987.

*McCollum, E. V. *A History of Nutrition*. Boston, Houghton Mifflin, c. 1957.

*Parascandola, J. "Reflections on the History of Pharmacology," *Pharmacy in History*, 22, 1980, pp. 131–40.

Parascandola, J., and Swann, J. "Development of Pharmacology in American Schools of Pharmacy," *Pharmacy in History*, 25, 1983, pp. 95–115.

Paterson, G. R., and Locock, M. J. "The History of Cardiac Glycosides," *Applied Therapeutics*, 9, 1967, pp. 60–65.

*Schmitz, R. "Friedrich Wilhelm Sertürner and the Discovery of Morphine," *Pharmacy in History*, 17, 1985, pp. 61–74.

*Schneider, W. "Aus der Geschichte der deutschen pharmazeutischen Industrie im 19. Jahrhundert," *23. Kongreßder Pharmazeutischen Wissenschaften, Münster/Westfalen, 1963*. Frankfurt, Govi, 1964.

Sedgwick, W. T., and Tyler, H. W. *A Short History of Science*. New York, Macmillan, 1927.

Selwyn-Brown, A. *The Physician Throughout the Ages*. New York, Capehart-Brown, 1928.

Singer, C. *A Short History of Science*. Oxford, Clarendon Press, 1941.

Sonnedecker, G. "Contribution of the Pharmaceutical Profession Toward Controlling the Quality of Drugs in the Nineteenth Century," in Blake, J. B., ed., *Safeguarding the Public*. Baltimore, Johns Hopkins University Press, 1970, pp. 97–111.

Urdang, G. "Materials and Outline for a Short History of Pharmacognosy," *American Journal of Pharmaceutical Education,* 9, 1945, pp. 199–206.

Wankmüller, A. "Deutschsprachige Lehrbücher der Pharmakognosie im 19. Jahrhundert," *Deutsche Apotheker-Zeitung,* 126, 1986, pp. 1786–88.

CHAPTER VII. THE NINETEENTH CENTURY: THE PHARMACEUTICAL ESTABLISHMENT

Bell, J., and Redwood, T. *Historical Sketch of Pharmacy in Great Britain.* London, Pharmaceutical Society of Great Britain, 1880.

Bonnemain, H. "L'Académie de Pharmacie," *Bulletin Ordre des Pharmaciens,* no. 200, May 1977.

Bourquelot, E. "Les Origines de la Société de Pharmacie de Paris," *Journal de Pharmacie et Chimie,* ser. 6, 18, 1903, pp. 443–89.

Bouvet, M. "Comment on limitait autrefois le nombre des officines," *Revue d'Histoire de la Pharmacie,* 23, no. 89, 1935, pp. 54–56.

Büsch, G. "Approbationsordnung für Apotheker erschienen," *Pharmazeutische Zeitung,* 116, 1971, pp. 1229–30.

Cowen, D. L. "America's First Pharmacy Laws," *Journal of the American Pharmaceutical Association, Practical Pharmacy Ed.,* 3, 1942, pp. 162–69, 214–21.

———. "Pharmacy in the Curriculum of American Medical Schools," *Pharmacy in History,* 20, 1978, pp. 17–21.

———. "George Bacon Wood," in Kaufman, M., et al., eds., *Dictionary of Medical Biography,* Westport, Conn., Greenwood Press, 1984, vol. 2, pp. 819–20.

Dale, J. R., and Appelbe, G. E. *Pharmacy Law and Ethics.* 2d ed., London, Pharmaceutical Press, 1979.

De Mari, J. *La Société Libre des Pharmaciens de Paris (1796–1803).* Strasbourg thesis, Grenoble, Prud-homme & Cie, 1944.

Earles, M. P. "The Pharmacy Schools of the Nineteenth Century," in Poynter, F. N. L., ed., *The Evolution of Pharmacy in Britain.* London, Pitman, 1965, pp. 79–95.

England, J. W. *The First Century of the Philadelphia College of Pharmacy, 1821–1921.* Philadelphia, Philadelphia College of Pharmacy and Science, 1922.

*Gathercoal, E. N. *The Prescription Ingredient Survey.* Washington, D.C., American Pharmaceutical Association, 1933.

Hickel, E. "Der Einfluß von Botanik und Pharmakognosie auf die Arzneimittelkontrolle in den Pharmakopöen des 19. Jahrhunderts," *Medizin Historisches Journal,* 7, 1972, pp. 279–300.

Huard, P., and Grmek, M.D. *Sciences, médicine, pharmacie de la Révolution à l'Empire (1780–1815).* Paris, Dacosta, c. 1970.

Linstead, H. N. *Poisons Law.* London, Pharmaceutical Press, 1936.

London Cigarette Card Company. *The Catalogue of International Cigarette Cards.* Exeter, England, Webb & Bower, 1982.

Mondor, H. *Doctors and Medicine in the Works of Daumier.* Trans. by C. de Chabanne. Boston, Boston Book and Art Shop, 1960.

Phillippe, A. *Geschichte der Apotheker,* trans. by H. Ludwig. 2d ed. Wiesbaden, Sändig, 1966.

Schmitz, R. *Die deutschen pharmazeutisch-chemischen Hochschulinstitute und ihre Entstehung und Entwicklung in Vergangenheit und Gegenwart.* Ingelheim, Boehringer, 1969.

"The Schools of Pharmacy," *Pharmaceutical Journal,* 237, 1986, pp. 446–48.

Wallis, T. E. *History of the School of Pharmacy, University of London.* London, Pharmaceutical Press, 1964.

Wankmüller, A. "Pharmazeutische Privatinstitute und Universitäten zu Beginn des 19. Jahrhunderts," *Tübingen Apothekengeschichtliche Abhandlungen,* Heft 23, 1973.

———. "Die Stellung der Pharmazie an den süddeutschen Hochschulen um 1840," *Veröffentlichungen der Internationalen Gesellschaft für Geschichte der Pharmazie,* n.f. 36, 1970, pp. 159–67.

Wittop Koning, D. A., *Het Etiket in de Apotheek.* Amsterdam(?), Coöperatieve Apothekers Vereeniging, 1984.

CHAPTER VIII. PHARMACY AND THE INDUSTRIAL REVOLUTION

Bender, G. A. *Great Moments in Pharmacy.* Detroit, Northwood, 1966.

Chapman, S. *Jesse Boot of Boots the Chemists: A Study in Business History.* London, Hodder & Stoughton, 1974.

Ciba. *The Story of Chemical Industry in Basel.* Olten and Lausanne, Urs Graf, 1959.

Cowen, D. L. "The Foundations of Pharmacy in the United States," *Journal of the American Medical Association,* 236, 1976, pp. 83–87.

———. *The New Jersey Pharmaceutical Association, 1870–1970.* Trenton, New Jersey Pharmaceutical Association, 1970.

Cowen, D. L., and Helfand, W. H. "The Progressive Movement and Its Impact on Pharmacy," *Pharmaceutica Acta Helvetiae,* 50, 1979, pp. 317–22.

Engel, L. *Medicine Makers of Kalamazoo.* New York, McGraw-Hill, 1961.

Ernst, E. *Das "Industrielle" Geheimmittel und seine Werbung.* Dissertation, Marburg, 1969.

Francis, A. *A Guinea a Box.* London, Hale, 1963.

Griffenhagen, G. B., and Young, J. H. "Old English Patent Medicines in America," *United States National Museum Bulletin,* 218, 1959, pp. 153–83.

Gunn, C. "A History of Some Pharmaceutical Presentations," in Poynter, F. N. L., ed., *The Evolution of Pharmacy in Britain.* London, Pitman, 1965, pp. 131–49.

Helfand, W. H. "Ephemera of the American Medicine Show," *Pharmacy in History,* 27, 1985, pp. 185–91.

———. "James Morison and His Pills: A Study of the Nineteenth-Century Pharmaceutical Market," *Transactions of the British Society for the History of Pharmacy,* 1^3, 1974, pp. 101–35.

Helfand, W. H., and Cowen, D. L. "American Pharmaceutical Posters," *Veröffentlichungen der Internationalen Gesellschaft für Geschichte der Pharmazie,* n.f. 50, 1981, pp. 207–19.

*———. "Evolution of Pharmaceutical Oral Dosage Forms," *Pharmacy in History,* 25, 1983, pp. 3–18.

Hickel, E. "Die Auseinandersetzung deutscher Apotheker mit den Problemen der Industrialisierung im 19. Jahrhundert," *Pharmazeutische Zeitung,* 118, 1973, pp. 1635–44; 119, 1974, pp. 12–19.

"How Warner-Lambert Got Its Name," *Resident and Staff Physician,* November 15, 1969, pp. 52–59.

Kahn, E. J., Jr. *All in a Century: The First 100 Years of Eli Lilly and Company.* n.p., 1976.

Kogan, H. *The Long White Line.* New York, Random House, 1963.

Krantz, J. C., Jr. *Historical Medical Classics Involving New Drugs.* Baltimore, Williams & Wilkins, 1974.

Mahoney, T. *The Merchants of Life.* New York, Harper, 1959.

Marion, J. F. *The Fine Old House.* Philadelphia, SmithKline Corporation, 1980.

Mayer, A. C. *Earlier Years of the Drug and Allied Trades in the Mississippi Valley.* St. Louis, 1948.

E. Merck AG. *From Merck's "Angel Pharmacy" to the World-Wide Merck Group.* Darmstadt, E. Merck, c. 1968.

Mohr, F., Redwood, T., and Proctor, W., Jr. *Practical Pharmacy.* Philadelphia, Lea & Blanchard, 1849.

Moore, J. T. "The Early Days of Pharmacy in the West," *Journal of the American Pharmaceutical Association,* 25, 1936, pp. 705–15.

*Nelson, G. L. *Pharmaceutical Company Histories*. Bismarck, N.Dak., Woodbine, 1983.

Oliver, J. W. *History of American Technology*. New York, Ronald, 1956.

Parascandola, J. "Patent Medicines in Nineteenth-Century America," *Caduceus*, 1, Spring 1985, pp. 1–41.

Parke, Davis & Co. *Scientific Contributions from the Laboratories, 1866–1966, Parke, Davis & Co.* n.p., Parke, Davis & Co., 1966.

Partington, J. R. *A History of Chemistry*, vols. 3, 4. London, Macmillan, 1962, 1964.

Pollay, R. W. "Pills, Potions and Palliatives: Some of the Social History of Drug Usage," *History of Medicine*, 6, 1975, pp. 58–63.

Remington, J. P., and Cook, E. F. *The Practice of Pharmacy*. 6th ed. Philadelphia, Lippincott, 1917.

"The Revolutions of a Pill," *Chemist and Druggist*, 59, 1901, pp. 154–56.

Rusek, V. "The Development of the Injection Form of Drugs. 2. The Development of the Technology of Injections," *Ceskoslav. Farm.*, 12, 1963, English summary, p. 57.

Sandoz. *Fiftieth Anniversary Sandoz USA*. N.p., Sandoz, c. 1969.

———. *Sandoz 1886–1961*. Basel, Gasser, n.d.

Schäfer, R. *Alt Hoechst*. Königstein, Langewiesche, 1966.

Sonnedecker, G. "The Rise of Drug Manufacture in America," *Emory University Quarterly*, 21, 1965, pp. 73–87.

Sonnedecker, G., and Griffenhagen, G. "A History of Sugar Coated Pills and Tablets," *Journal of the American Pharmaceutical Association, Practical Pharmacy Ed.*, 18, 1957, pp. 486–88, 553–55.

Urdang, G. "The Invention of Gelatin Capsules," *Pharmaceutical Archives*, 14, 1943, pp. 58–59.

Young, J. H. "From Hooper to Hohensee," *Journal of the American Medical Association*, 204, 1968, pp. 100–104.

*———. *The Medical Messiahs*. Princeton, Princeton University Press, 1967.

———. "Patent Medicines: An Early Example of Competitive Marketing," *Journal of Economic History*, 30, 1960, pp. 648–56.

———. "Patent Medicines in the Early Nineteenth Century," *The South Atlantic Quarterly*, 48, 1949, pp. 557–65.

———. *The Toadstool Millionaires*. Princeton, Princeton University Press, 1961.

CHAPTER IX. SCIENCE, TECHNOLOGY, AND PHARMACY

Applezweig, N. *Steroid Drugs*. New York, McGraw-Hill, 1962.

Autio, D. E. "Development of Radiotherapy in America: A Brief Survey," *Pharmacy in History*, 18, 1976, pp. 13–16.

*Bandelin, F. J. *Our Modern Medicines*. Hankinson, N.Dak., Woodbine, 1986.

Bickel, L. *Rise Up to Life*. New York, Scribner's, 1972.

Biomedical Information Corporation. *The Compendium of Drug Theory*. New York, Biomedical Information Corporation, 1986.

Blane, G. F. "Review of European Clinical Experience with Fenofibrate," *Cardiology*, 76, supp. 1, 1989, pp. 1–9.

Boston Women's Health Book Collective. *The New Our Bodies, Ourselves: A Book by and for Women*. New York, Simon & Schuster, 1984.

Brown, M.S., and Goldstein, J. L. "Drugs Used in the Treatment of Hyperlipoproteinemias," in Goodman, L. S. and Gilman, A. G., eds., *The Pharmacological Basis of Therapeutics,* 7th ed, New York, Macmillan, 1985.

Bullough, V. "James Lind," *Dictionary of Scientific Biography*. New York, Scribner's, 1970 etc., vol. 8, pp. 361–63.

Caldwell, A. E. "History of Psychopharmacology," in Clark, W. G., and Del Giudice, J., eds., *Principles of Psychopharmacology*, 2d ed., New York, Academic Press, 1978, pp. 9–40.

———. *Origins of Psychopharmacology from CPZ to LSD*. Springfield, Ill., Thomas, 1970.

Cowen, D. L. "Nutrition and Vitamins," in *Dictionary of American History*. New York, Scribner's, c. 1976, vol. 5, pp. 127–29.

———. "Pharmaceutical Scientists and Pharmacokinetics," *Veröffentlichungen der Internationalen Gesellschaft für Geschichte der Pharmazie*, n.f., 57, 1989, pp. 53–68.

De Haen, P. "Compilation of New Drugs 1940 thru 1975," *Pharmacy Times*, 42[3], March 1976, pp. 40–74.

*———. *Drug Product Index: International*, vol. 1, 1987–1988. Englewood, Colo., De Haen, 1988.

De Haen's Drugs in Research: Annotated Cumulative Bibliography 1969–1972. New York, De Haen, 1973.

Deniker, P. "Discovery of the Clinical Use of Neuroleptics," in Parnham, M. J., and Bruinvels, J., eds., *Discoveries in Pharmacology*, vol. I: *Psycho- and Neuro-pharmacology*. Amsterdam, Elsevier, 1983, pp. 163–80.

Diamond, M. C., and Korenbrot, C. C. *Hormonal Contraceptives, Estrogens, and Human Welfare*. New York, Academic Press, 1978.

Dowling, H. F. *Fighting Infection: Conquests of the Twentieth Century*. Cambridge, Harvard University Press, 1977.

*———. *Medicines for Man: The Development, Regulation and Use of Prescription Drugs*. New York, Knopf, 1970.

Eder, H. A. "Drugs Used in the Prevention and Treatment of Atherosclerosis," in Goodman, L. S., and Gilman, A., eds., *The Pharmacological Basis of Therapeutics*. 5th ed. New York, Macmillan, 1975, pp. 744–52.

*"EEC Soon to Accede to European Pharmacopoeia," *Scrip: World Pharmaceutical News*, 1427, July 7, 1989.

Haber, L. F. *The Chemical Industry During the Nineteenth Century*. Oxford, Clarendon Press, 1958.

Harvey, S. C. "The Barbiturates," in Goodman, L. S., and Gilman, A., eds., *The Pharmacological Basis of Therapeutics*. 5th ed. New York, Macmillan, 1975, pp. 102–23.

Helfand, W. H., Woodruff, H. B., Coleman, K. M. H., and Cowen, D. L. "Wartime Industrial Development of Penicillin in the United States," in Parascandola, J., ed., *The History of Antibiotics*. Madison, Wis., American Institute of the History of Pharmacy, 1980, pp. 31–56.

Hermann, W., Baulieu, E.-E., et al. "Effet d'un stéroide anti-progestérone chez la femme: Interruption du cycle menstruel et de la grossesse au début," *Comptes Rendus*, 294, 1982, pp. 933–38.

*Hoffman-LaRoche. *50 Years of Progress, 1928–1978*. Nutley, N.J., Hoffman-LaRoche, 1978.

Illingworth, D. R. "Lipid-Lowering Drugs," *Drugs*, 33, 1987, pp. 259–79.

Jarvik, M. E. "Drugs Used in the Treatment of Psychiatric Disorders," in Goodman, L. S., and Gilman, A., eds., *The Pharmacological Basis of Therapeutics*. 4th ed. New York, Macmillan, 1970, pp. 151–203.

*Kondrates, R. A. "Biologics Control Act of 1902," in Young, J. H., ed., *The Early Years of Federal Food and Drug Control*. Madison, Wis., American Institute of the History of Pharmacy, 1982, pp. 8–27.

Krugman, S. "The Newly-Licensed Hepatitis B Vaccine," *Journal of the American Medical Association*, 247, 1982, pp. 2012–15.

LaRosa, J. "Review of Clinical Studies of Bile Acid Sequestrants for Lowering Plasma Lipid Levels," *Cardiology*, 76, supp. 1, 1989, pp. 55–61.

Lehmann, H. E., and Kline, N. S. "Clinical Discoveries with Antidepressant Drugs," in Parnham, M. J., and Bruinvels, J., eds., *Discoveries in Pharmacology*, vol. 1: *Psycho- and Neuro-pharmacology*. Amsterdam, Elsevier, 1983, pp. 209–21.

Levy, G., and Nelson, E. "Pharmaceutical Formulation and Therapeutic Efficacy," *Journal of the American Medical Association*, 177, 1961, pp. 689–94.

Liebenau, J. M. "Industrial R & D in Pharmaceutical Firms in the Early Twentieth Century," *Business History*, 26, 1984, pp. 329–46.

Merck & Co. *Hydrocortisone and Cortisone*. Rahway, N.J., Merck, 1956.

————. *The Merck Manual*. 14th ed. Rahway, N.J., Merck, 1982.

Mitchell, A. G. "Pharmaceutical Factors Affecting Drug Availability," *Australasian Journal of Pharmacy*, 47, 1966, pp. 558–61.

Mitsuya, H., et al. "3′-Azido-3′-Deoxythyamidine (BW A509U): An Antiviral Agent that Inhibits the Infectivity and Cytopathic Effect of Human T-lymphotropic Virus Type III/lymphadenopathy-associated Virus in Vitro," *Proceedings of the National Academy of Science (USA)*, 82, 1985, pp. 7096–7100.

Mitsuya, H., et al. Letter re AZT, *New York Times*, Sept. 28, 1989.

Moe, G. K., and Abildskov, J. A. "Antiarrhythmic Drugs," in Goodman, L. S., and Gilman, A., eds., *The Pharmacological Basis of Therapeutics*. 5th ed. New York, Macmillan, 1975, pp. 683–704.

Moore, T. J. "The Cholesterol Myth," *The Atlantic*, 264, no. 3, Sept. 1989, pp. 37–40, 42–44, 46–52, 54, 56–57, 60.

*Nichols, O., ed. *By Their Fruits*. Rahway, N.J., Merck, c. 1962.

Nickerson, M. "Vasodilator Drugs," in Goodman, L. S., and Gilman, A., eds., *The Pharmacological Basis of Therapeutics*, 5th ed., New York, Macmillan, 1975, pp. 727–43.

Nickerson, M., and Ruedy, J. "Antihypertensive Agents and the Drug Therapy of Hypertension," in Goodman, L. S., and Gilman, A., eds., *The Pharmacological Basis of Therapeutics*. 5th ed. New York, Macmillan, 1975, pp. 705–26.

Parascandola, J. "The Controversy Over Structure-Activity Relationships in the Early Twentieth Century," *Pharmacy in History*, 16, 1974, pp. 54–63.

*————. "Industrial Research Comes of Age," *Pharmacy in History*, 27, 1985, pp. 12–21.

"Production of Hepatitis B Vaccines in Yeast," *WHO Chronicle*, 38, 1984, pp. 260–61.

Richman, D. D. "The Treatment of HIV Infection: Azidothymidine (AZT) and Other New Antiviral Drugs," *Infectious Disease Clinics of North America*, 2^2, 1988, pp. 397–407.

Rosenberg, H. R. *Chemistry and Physiology of the Vitamins*. New York, Interscience, 1942.

Sandström, E. G., and Kaplan, J. C. "Antiviral Therapy in AIDS: Clinical Pharmacological Properties and Therapeutic Experience to Date," *Drugs*, 34, 1987, pp. 372–90.

Schwartzman, D. *Innovation in the Pharmaceutical Industry*. Baltimore, Johns Hopkins University Press, 1976.

Seaman, B., and Seaman, G. *Women in Crisis*. New York, Rawson Associates, 1977.

Sheehan, J. C. *The Enchanted Ring: The Untold Story of Penicillin*. Cambridge, MIT Press, 1984.

Sonnedecker, G. "The Concept of Chemotherapy," *American Journal of Pharmaceutical Education*, 26, 1962, pp. 1–3.

Swann, J. P. "Insulin: A Case Study in the Emergence of Collaborative Pharmacomedical Research," *Pharmacy in History*, 28, 1986, pp. 3–13, 65–74.

Swintosky, J. V. "Personal Experiences in the Early Days of Biopharmacy and Pharmacokinetics," in Benet, L. Z., Levy, G., and Ferraiolo, B. L., eds., *Pharmacokinetics: A Modern View*. New York, Plenum, 1982, pp. 37–54.

Szent-Györgyi, A. "Observations on the Function of Peroxidase Systems and the Chemistry of the Adrenal Cortex," *Biochemical Journal*, 22, 1928, pp. 1386–1409.

Wagner, J. G. "The History of Pharmacokinetics," *Drug Intelligence and Clinical Pharmacy*, 11, 1977, pp. 747–48.

Westoff, L. A., and Westoff, C. F. *From Now to Zero: Fertility, Contraception and Abortion in America*. Boston, Little, Brown, 1971.

Woodward, T. E., and Wisseman, C. L., eds. *Chloromycetin*. New York, Medical Encyclopedia, 1958.

Yarchoan, R., et al. "Administration of 3′-Azido-3′-Deoxythymidine, an Inhibitor of HTLV-III/LAV Replication, to Patients with AIDS or AIDS-Related Complex," *Lancet*, 1, 1986, pp. 575–80.

CHAPTER X. THE ROLE OF THE INDUSTRY

Bobst, E. H. *Bobst: The Autobiography of a Pharmaceutical Pioneer*. New York, McKay, 1973.

*Cowen, D. L. "The On-going Pharmaceutical Revolution: The Role of the Industry," in *Farmacia y Industrialización: Libro Homenaje al Doctor Guilermo Folch Jou*. Madrid, Sociedad Española de Historia de la Farmacia, 1985, pp. 95–104.

————. "The Swiss-American Pharmaceutical Houses of New Jersey," in Schramm, G., ed., *Neue Beiträge zur Geschichte der Pharmazie: Festschrift für Herrn Dr. phil. Hans-Rudolf Fehlmann*. Zurich, 1979.

*Faust, R. E. "Envisioning the Future of R & D," *Pharmaceutical Executive*, vol. 4 nos. 9 and 10 (1984).

Furman, B. *United States Public Health Service, 1798–1948*. Bethesda, U.S.D.H.E.W., 1973.

Harden, V. A. *Inventing the NIH: Federal Biomedical Research Policy 1887–1937*. Baltimore, Johns Hopkins University Press, 1986.

Letsch, S. W., Levit, K. R., and Waldo, D. P. "Health Care Financing Trends," *Health Care Financing*, 10^2, Winter 1988, pp. 109–22.

Liebenau, J. "Scientific Ambitions: The Pharmaceutical Industry, 1900–1920," *Pharmacy in History*, 27, 1985, pp. 3–11.

McLean, J. "The Discovery of Heparin," *Circulation*, 19, 1959, pp. 75–78.

*Pharmaceutical Manufacturers Association. *Facts at a Glance*. Washington, D.C. Pharmaceutical Manufacturers Association, 1983.

————. *PMA Fact Book 1980: Prescription Drug Industry*. Washington, D.C. Pharmaceutical Manufacturers Association, 1980.

————. *PMA Statistical Fact Book, January 1986*. Washington, D.C. Pharmaceutical Manufacturers Association, 1986.

————. *PMA Statistical Fact Book, August 1988*. Washington, D.C. Pharmaceutical Manufacturers Association, 1988.

Tomita, D. K., et al. *Drug Utilization in the U.S. 1987: Ninth Annual Review*. Washington, United States Department of Health and Human Services, 1988.

CHAPTER XI. THE TWENTIETH-CENTURY PHARMACIST

The American Council on Pharmaceutical Education: Accredited Professional Programs of Colleges and Schools of Pharmacy, Annual Directory. July 1986.

Appraisal of Subscriber Attitudes [to American Pharmacy] Made by the T. A. Miller Co., Inc., at the Request of the Amerian Pharmaceutical Association and Media for Medicine. c. 1987.

Bardell, E. B. "America's Only School of Pharmacy for Women," *Pharmacy in History*, 26, 1984, pp. 127–33.

Blauch, L. E., and Webster, G. L. *The Pharmaceutical Curriculum*. Washington, American Council on Education, 1952.

The British Health Care System. London, Economic Models, Ltd., 1976.

Brodie, D. C., and Benson, R. A. "The Evolution of the Clinical Pharmacy Concept," *Drug Intelligence and Clinical Pharmacy*, 10, 1976, pp. 506–10.

Cohen, J. L. "Health Insurance," *Encyclopaedia Britannica*. 13th ed. London and New York, Encyclopaedia Britannica Co., 1926, vol. 30, pp. 491–93.

"Common Market: The Pharmacy Directives," *Pharmaceutical Journal*, 235, 1985, pp. 781–83.

Conacher, J. B. *Waterloo to the Common Market*. New York, Knopf, 1975.

Courtwright, D. T. *Dark Paradise: Opiate Addiction in America Before 1940*. Cambridge, Harvard University Press, 1982.

Cowen, D. L. "A Century of American Pharmacy," in *A History of the Activities of the Pennsylvania Pharmaceutical Association, 1878–1978,* Harrisburg, Pennsylvania Pharmaceutical Association, 1978, pp. 3–13.

————. "Pharmacy," in *Encyclopedia of Bioethics*. New York, Free Press, 1978, vol. 3, pp. 1211–15.

Cowen, D. L., King, L. D., and Lordi, N. G. "Nineteenth Century Drug Therapy," *Journal of the Medical Society of New Jersey,* 78, 1981, pp. 758–61.

Crellin, J. K. "Apothecaries, Dispensers, Students and Nineteenth-Century Pharmacy at St. George's Hospital, London," *Medical History,* 9, 1962, pp. 131–45.

Demichel, A. *Le Droit pharmaceutique*. Paris, Papyrus, c. 1986.

Duffy, J. *The Rudolph Matas History of Medicine in Louisiana,* vol. 1. Baton Rouge, Louisiana State University Press, 1958.

Encyclopedia of Associations: International Associations, 1989. Detroit, Gale, 1989.

Francke, D. E., and Whitney, H. A. K., Jr. "Patterns of Clinical Pharmacy Education and Practice in the United States," *Drug Intelligence and Clinical Pharmacy,* 10, 1976, pp. 511–21.

The French Health Care System. London, Economic Models, Ltd., 1976.

Ganzinger, K. "Zür Geschichte der Wiener Krankenhausapotheken," *Österreichische Apotheker-Zeitung,* 18, 1964, pp. 34–38.

Gelfand, T. "Medicine in New France," in Numbers, R. C., ed., *Medicine in the New World*. Knoxville, University of Tennessee Press, 1987.

Hoffmann, F. "The International Pharmaceutical Conferences," *American Journal of Pharmacy,* 73, 1901, pp. 315–25, 373–83, 431–46.

Jackson, C. O. *Food and Drug Legislation in the New Deal*. Princeton, Princeton University Press, 1970.

Kaplan, A., and Becker, R. "An Examination of the ANDA/Patent Restoration Law," *Pharmaceutical Executive,* 60, Dec. 1984, pp. 62–63.

Kushner, D., and Feierman, R. "The Class of '88," *American Druggist,* 198[2], Aug. 1988, pp. 36–42.

Macarthur, D. *The EEC Environment for Medicines: Progress Toward Harmonization*. Richmond, England, PJB Publications [Scrip], 1987.

Marino-Bettolo, G. B. Preface to *European Pharmacopoeia,* vol. 1. Sainte-Ruffino, Maisonneuve, 1969, pp. 9–19.

Matthews, L. G. "The Apothecaries of the Royal Hospital," in *Atti del Congresso Internazionale di Storia della Farmacia, Aosta, 1969*.

Mrtek, R. G. "Pharmaceutical Education in These United States: An Interpretive Historical Essay of the Twentieth Century," *American Journal of Pharmaceutical Education,* 40, 1976, pp. 339–65.

Nielsen, J. R. *Handbook of Federal Drug Law*. Philadelphia, Lea & Febiger, 1986.

"NJPhA Proposes Third Class of Drugs," *New Jersey Journal of Pharmacy,* 57[1], 1984, p. 14.

Orzack, L. H. "Competing Professions and the Public Interest in the European Economic Community: Drugs and Their Quality Control," in Blume, S.S., ed., *Perspectives in the Sociology of Science*. London, Wiley, 1977, pp. 95–129.

Penna, R. P., and Sherman, M. S. "Degrees Conferred by Schools and Colleges of Pharmacy, 1987–1988," *American Journal of Pharmaceutical Education,* 53, 1989, pp. 266–83.

"Pharmacien: Une profession qui attire les femmes," *Flash,* Winter, 1986–87, p. 46.

Pharmacists for the Future: Report of the Study Commission on Pharmacy ["The Millis Report"]. Ann Arbor, Mich., Health Administration Press, 1975.

Pharmacopoeia Internationalis. Geneva, W.H.O., 1951, Preface.

Pharmacy News Briefs. New Jersey Pharmaceutical Association, Trenton N.J. June 1986.

A Profession in Transition: The Changing Face of Pharmacy, Schering Report X. Kennilworth, N. J., Schering Laboratories, 1988.

Pubis-Braunstein, M. "The First Polish Women Pharmacists," *Pharmacy in History,* 31, 1989, pp. 12–15.

Ried, L. D., and McGhan, W. F. "Pharm.D. or B.S.: Does the Degree Really Make a Difference in Pharmacists' Job Satisfaction?" *American Journal of Pharmaceutical Education,* 50, 1986, pp. 1–5.

Risse, G. B. *Hospital Life in Enlightenment Scotland: Care and Teaching at the Royal Infirmary of Edinburgh.* Cambridge, Cambridge University Press, 1986.

Rodowskas, C. A., Jr. "The Impact of Clinical Pharmacy on the Curriculum," *Drug Intelligence and Clinical Pharmacy,* 10, 1976, pp. 522–27.

Roeske, W. *Women of Polish Pharmacy.* Warsaw, Polish Medical Publishers, 1976.

Sappert, K. "Vergleich des Niederlassungsrechtes der Apotheker in 56 Staaten der Erde," *Pharmazeutische Zeitung,* 90, 1954, pp. 923–28.

Schramm, G. "Krankenhaushygiene, eine Aufgabe des Apothekers," *Krankenhauspharmazie,* 2, 1981, pp. 92–95.

Sonnedecker, G. "American Pharmacy: A Retrospective Future," *Journal of the American Pharmaceutical Association,* n.s. 13[3], 1976, pp. 128–31.

———. *Emergence of the Concept of Opiate Addiction.* Madison, Wis., American Institute of the History of Pharmacy, c. 1963.

———. "Women as Pharmacy Students in 19th-Century America," *Veröffentlichungen der Internationalen Gesellschaft für Geschichte der Pharmazie,* n.f. 50, 1973, pp. 135–41.

Stieb, E. W., Coulas, G. C., et al. "Women in Ontario Pharmacy, 1867–1927," *Pharmacy in History,* 28, 1986, pp. 125–34.

"Uniformity of Potent Medicaments," *Pharmaceutical Journal,* ser. 4, 24, Jan. 26, 1907, p. 76.

Urdang, G., and Murphy, J. *Position of Pharmacy in Sickness Insurance.* Madison, Wis., American Institute of the History of Pharmacy, 1942.

Vogelenzang, E. H. "The European Pharmacopoeia," *Journal of the American Pharmaceutical Association,* n.s. 15, 1975, pp. 705–6.

White, J. P. "Breakthroughs for Pharmacists: Prescribing Privileges," *Drug Topics,* 129[14], 1985, pp. 26–30.

Zalai, K. "Pharmaceutical Education in Central Europe: A Historical View," *Pharmacy in History,* 28, 1986, pp. 138–45.

PHOTOGRAPH CREDITS

The authors and the publisher thank the museums, libraries, and private collectors who permitted the reproductions of works in their possession and supplied the necessary photographs.

Numbers refer to pages.

AP/Wide World: 130 top; W. Bertsch/H. Armstrong Roberts: 13; Caisse Nationale, Paris: 32; ©Camerique/H. Armstrong Roberts, Inc.: 240 top; Ludovico Canali: 45 top, 98 bottom; Jean-Loup Charmet: 46 top, 82, 91 top; Junebug Clark, Photo Researchers, Inc.: 216 left center; ©Comstock: 212 top; Cooperman-Bridgeman, London: 125 bottom right; ©Tim Davis 1986 Photo Researchers, Inc.: 224 top; Denver Public Library: 237; Fotoabteilung Stadtspital Waid, Zurich: 238; Fotofast, Bologna: 37 top; Michael Freeman: 93 top, 176; Klaus Grieshaber: 37 bottom left; Hirmer Fotoarchiv, Munich: 30; Courtesy of Hoffmann-LaRoche: 84 bottom right, 133 top; Kansas State Historical Society, Topeka: 189; ©Susan Leavines 1986 Photo Researchers, Inc.: 224 bottom; ©Will & Demi McIntyre Photo Researchers, Inc.: 212 bottom, 213, 216 bottom left, 216–217; Courtesy of Merck: 204; National Library of Medicine, Bethesda: 132 top; John Parnell: 161 bottom; Philadelphia Museum of Art, Given by William Helfand: 228 top; Philadelphia Museum of Art, William S. Pilling Collection: 74; Philadephia Museum of Art, SmithKline Beckman Corporation Fund: 232; ©Photo Researchers, Inc.: 201 top, 202, 216 top, 227; Copy photos by Philip Pocock: 8 upper left, 9 upper left, 9 center left, center, and right, 9 bottom left and right, 27, 48 bottom, 76 top and bottom right, 84 top, 93 bottom, 96 bottom, 98 top, 102, 103, 114 bottom left and right, 119 bottom, 132 bottom, 150 top, 156, 169 bottom, 172 top, 173 bottom, 178–179, 193, 201 bottom, 228 bottom; H. Armstrong Roberts: 240 bottom; ©Kjell B. Sandved: 133 bottom; Ronald Sheridan/Ancient Art and Architecture Collection: 31 left, 33 top, 51 bottom; The Smithsonian Institution: 209 bottom; Dr. Ralph Solecki: 17 bottom; Courtesy of Squibb: 210 bottom; Photo by Leonard Von Matt: 33 bottom; Photo from *Die Wesser Renaissance*: 75.